Modern Equine Dentistry for Horse Owners

Understand what you need to know...

to get the best dental care for your horse's comfort and safety

Modern Equine Dentistry for Horse Owners

Understand what you need to know...

to get the best dental care for your horse's comfort and safety

By

Elizabeth A. Thompson
BA (HONS.), DVM, MANZCVS, GRADDIPTEACH
&
Lizzi Tremayne

Blue Mist
Publishing

COPYRIGHT

Modern Equine Dentistry for Horse Owners is a work of nonfiction. The details in this book are accurate to the best of the author's ability, although some names and details have been changed to protect the privacy of others.

DISCLAIMERS: These disclaimers are designed to help educate my readers about the risks involved in equine dentistry and emphasize the importance of safety and professional supervision. See the entire *chapter* entitled DISCLAIMER for the full disclaimer.

Blue Mist Publishing (A Division of Blue Mist Holdings Ltd.)

Franklin Road, RD 2, Waihi, New Zealand 3682

EquineVetToday@gmail.com | https://equistillstocks.com

Amazon Case Hardcover V6 26 June 2024

ISBN 978-1-99-115960-1 (eBook)

ISBN 978-1-99-115961-8 (paperback Amazon)

ISBN 978-1-99-115965-6 (hardcover Amazon)

Book 1 of the Equine Vet Today series

Library of Congress Control Number: 2023920681

Formatting, cover design, interior design, photos, images, and artwork by Blue Mist Holdings Ltd. [Elizabeth Thompson, BA (Hons) DVM MANZCVS (EqDent) GradDipTeach (SecSci)] DBA Blue Mist Publishing, Waihi, NZ, unless credited on the Image and Graphics Credits page.

Interior graphics created in Canva, interior layout and design created in Scrivener, Vellum, and Affinity Publisher by Blue Mist Holdings Ltd., DBA Blue Mist Publishing, Blue Mist Equine Veterinary Centre, and Equi-Still Portable Equine Stocks and Dental Instrumentation, Waihi, NZ.

Cover photo credit to Joan E. Gilchrist.

Author photos credit to James Hewitt and Kajai@gmail.com.

Images and graphics by Blue Mist Holdings Ltd., (Elizabeth Thompson), unless otherwise credited. Full credits details on Image and Graphics Credits page.

TABLE OF CONTENTS

APPENDICES

DEDICATION

To my NZ human family, who make life worth living. I love you all:

Matthew
Stuie, Tamiee and Odin
Elliot and Amelia

&

To my equine and canine family, who have given me so much:

Lady, Milly, Sunshine, Princess, Uri, Sasha, Sky High, Jules, Micky, Rugger, Minty, Living Word and her two colts Montoya and Shemaya, Tango, Drive, Jasmine, and my precious little Lena...

all of whom are over the rainbow bridge,

either grazing away or tirelessly chasing bunnies.

ACKNOWLEDGEMENTS

ONE DOESN'T WRITE A BOOK LIKE THIS alone. I am indebted to:

Dr Colin Dunlop for his unique and lifesaving advice regarding sedation in the older, anxious, or compromised patient.

Professor Gary J Wilson for his many years of putting up with my inane and not so inane questions as my mentor, and always encouraging me to do more.

Those who started me off and sustained me on my equestrian and dental journeys: Kirsten and Gary, Muriel and Jesper, Leslie, Jerry, Veronica, Eric, Elliot, Stuart & Matthew.

My forever dental colleague friends: Dr Glenn Beeman, Dr Marieke van den Enden, and Dr Katie Kindleysides, and all the new online "colleague friends" I've made while writing this book!

My Beta Readers, Editors, and Foreword Writers: As an Indie Author (self-publishing), I owe a great debt of gratitude to my beta readers for keeping me on track. They make my writing life worth living! My heartfelt appreciation to my veterinary and horse-owning beta readers and foreword writers: Dr Ingrid Bill, Michelle Bolger, Dr Eric Davis, Professor Padraic Dixon, Cathie Heald Greenwell, Patrick Hearty, Dr Lucy Holdaway, Dr Kirsten Jackson, Dr Olivia James, Dr Ray Lenaghan, Hannah Lowry, Dr Scott Marx, Matthew Mole, Dr Rob Pascoe, Dr Elke Pollaris, Laura Roy, Dr Ruth V. Sobek, Dr Manfred Stoll, Lenora Till, Dr Tracy Tinsley, Dr Marieke van den Enden, Professor Dr Denis Verwilghen, Dr Jenny Weston, and Professor Gary Wilson.

My Image Providers: The generous provision of so many images for this book has made all the difference in its quality. Without these amazing contributors, this would be one boring book with only my images. Their full credits are on the Image and Graphics Credit page. My forever thanks to: Dr Amy Ardern, Dr Glenn Beeman, Professor Padraic Dixon, Dr Nicole du Toit, Dr Jack Easley, Equine Veterinary Education (Journal), Joan E. Gilchrist, Cathie Heald Greenwell, Dr Maxwell Hall, Dr Barbara Hunter, Dr Kirsten Jackson, Dr Olivia James, Dr Oliver Liyou, Matthew Mole, New Zealand Equine Veterinary Journal (NZVA), Dr Laurinda Oliver, Dr Chris Pearce, Dr Elke Pollaris, Katrina Price, Dr Manfred Stoll, Elliot Thompson, Dr Tracy Tinsley, Dr Marieke van den Enden, and Professor Dr Denis Verwilghen.

My Advance Readers: An Indie Author needs to know how their book is going to be received. My *Modern Equine Dentistry Advanced Reader Copy (MEDARC) Team* gave me the final input and honest reviews I needed. I hope you loved the book! Thank you so much to: Dr Abu Sufyan, Amanda, Amy Gough, Dr Andrew Cribb, Dr Anne Lowe, Anni Kurze, Bex Tasker, Dr Brendon Bell, Dr Caroline Bagshaw, Catherine, Dr Celia Grant, Charlotte Ellis, Dr David Evertson, Deb Lawton (nee Tarr), Emily, Dr Georgia Beasley, Gina, Graham Gillard, Hannah Lowry, Ishbel Black, Dr James Alcorn, Dr James Chatterton, Professor Jenny Weston, Dr Jocelyn Woodd (and thanks for making me go to NZ in the first place in 1991), Kathleen Sutton, Kate, Katie Hill, Katrina & Garth, Kylie, Laura Roy, Dr Laurinda, Leanne Fecser, Lenora, Lisa Coulson, Lisa Lydon, Dr Lydia Uddstrom, Dr Mark Braunschmidt, Marsha, Matthew Mole,

Michelle Bolger, Dr Michelle Logan, Molly Mills, Dr Muhammad Tayyab, Rebekah, Rena, Richard L Vetter, DVM, Rochelle Thomson, Rya, Sally, Dr Tia Nelson, Tyla Remkes, Wendy Felton, and Yohann.

R.L. Parker - Fantasy Author for his tech support with a program he only *uses*. He posted some great Affinity Publisher videos and unfortunately for him, they caught my eye. He subsequently has spent several hours of his time helping me understand how APub works. Without his help, the print version of the book would be nothing like what it has become. Thank you Rick!

Avril Sabine - Author for her eleventh-hour salvage operation export of the PDF ... my profound appreciation!

But most of all, my humblest appreciation to all the pioneers in equine dentistry: Only a small sampling of the publications of these leaders are listed in the Bibliography and Further Reading. Their writings have been the source of all of the information I have gleaned throughout my study of equine dentistry and attempted to translate into the language of the horse owner. I can claim only the mistakes, which are mine alone. I am indebted to each and every one of these authors and researchers, leaders in this field.

And they are still pioneering.

My most grateful thanks to you all.

Dr Elizabeth Thompson
Waihi, NZ 30 May 2024

Forewords

"IN MY FORTY-SEVEN YEARS AS A veterinarian, I have been fortunate to see a great number of innovations benefitting the health and welfare of horses. From modern imaging techniques such as MRI to unlocking the metabolic cause of laminitis, the whole practice of equine medicine has moved light years ahead in past decades. However, as a technologic advancement that affects the everyday life of our horses, mules, and donkeys perhaps the most cosmic change has been in the field of dentistry. New science, technology, and techniques have brought the treatment of the equine tooth from the days of a box of rusting "floats", into a universe of possibilities that will make horses live longer, better lives. There are plenty of textbooks, scientific publications, and continuing education courses for the veterinary professional interested in dentistry. However, these often leave the person who knows and cares the most about their horse, the owner, in the dark. What is needed today is a good text that lays out the anatomy, physiology, and clinical techniques for the horse owning public, in an understandable and readable style. I have often advocated for a well-illustrated book, written by a knowledgeable professional, whose only motivation is to educate. Today's owner wants to know the details so that they can talk to their veterinarian, and understand not only treatment options, but disease prevention. This is especially true in a time when uncurated information, produced by those with something to sell, is flooding the internet and social media. Fortunately, a wonderful young veterinarian, Dr. Elizabeth Anne Thompson, who has all the credentials and writing skills, has come to the rescue and produced this excellent, owner friendly, dentistry text. Besides being a long-time horseperson and veterinarian, Lizzi has made an assiduous study of the field and become a sought-after equine dental practitioner and teacher. She currently serves as the President of the Dentistry Chapter of the ANZCVS and as an NZEVA Dental Subcommittee member. Besides this, she has also engineered and produced a very useful and humane equine dental stocks, which provides both horse and human safety, while minimizing mental trauma to the equine patient. Every horse owner should have a copy of this book. All horses have teeth, and we want them all to be healthy and content. Educating yourself with Dr. Thompson's book will be an important step in achieving this for the horses that you love."

—**Dr Eric W. Davis** DVM, MS, DipACVS, DipACVIM, Davis, CA, USA

"THIS NEW BOOK FOR HORSE OWNERS DESCRIBES in an eminently readable format the complete topic of equine dentistry. It details the different range of personnel who perform equine dentistry and clarifies the training and knowledge of these different groups, from the untrained lay person up to the highest level, i.e. equine veterinary dental specialists who have passed post-graduate professional examinations in this subject. The book describes equine dental anatomy, physiology , the different dental examination techniques and the very wide range of dental diseases that horses suffer from. It also notes that dental diseases may cause greatly different problems, from subtle behavioural changes that owners may not instantly recognise, up to severe infections of teeth and their supporting bones. The different range of treatments for these disorders and who should perform them are set out clearly. This text will be a very useful addition to horse owners."

—**Professor Padraic M. Dixon,** MVB, PhD, FRCVS, Diploma EVDC (Equine), RCVS Specialist in Equine Surgery (Soft Tissue), European Specialist in Equine Dentistry. Edinburgh, Scotland, UK

"THOUGH LACKING IN ANY FORMAL VETERINARY TRAINING, I am a life-long owner and breeder of American Quarter Horses. I marvel and appreciate the world of information Dr Thompson has laid out in Modern Equine Dentistry in a clear format, understandable to the average horse owner. I have known Liz for a number of years and can attest to the thoroughness of her research and attention to detail. Both we and our equine friends are greatly benefited."

—**Patrick Hearty**, National Pony Express Association. Utah, USA

"IN "MODERN EQUINE DENTISTRY FOR HORSE OWNERS," Dr. Liz Thompson delivers a valuable guide for anyone devoted to the health and care of horses. Equine dentistry has undergone a worldwide revolution in the last two decades, with an explosion of research, new knowledge and innovative diagnostic techniques and treatments. This progress has empowered veterinarians with a deep-seated passion for equine dentistry - affectionately known as 'equine dental nerds' - to enhance our expertise and be better equipped to care for our patients. After all, the love of the horse is why many of us choose our profession.

Dr. Thompson's clear, engaging explanations make complex topics accessible and easily understood, without oversimplifying the science. You almost feel that you are both sitting by a cosy fire, glass of wine in hand, while you are taken on a captivated adventure of the horse's mouth. Dr Thompson's prowess as a highly successful published author is evident in her penmanship of this book, with the high degree of 'readability' enabling anyone who can read to educate themselves! Her book fills a crucial gap in contemporary literature, providing insights into the proper diagnosis, treatment, and maintenance of equine dental health for horse owners, veterinary students, and veterinarians.

Congratulations Dr. Thompson for crafting such an informative and accessible resource for all horse lovers and professionals alike. To the readers of this book – enjoy the enlightening journey through equine dentistry!"

—**Dr Olivia James**, BVSc(Hons) MANZCVS(Eq Dentistry), CMAVA, DipICEVO, DAVDC(Equine), Board Certified Veterinary Dentist™, Diplomate of the American Veterinary Dental College Equine Speciality

"EQUINE DENTISTRY HAS UNDERGONE SOMETHING OF A revolution in veterinary care in the past twenty years. Horses owners are more aware than ever that their animals need regular dental care. However, with a large number of providers offering these services, it can be almost impossible to ascertain the standard of work being performed in an area of anatomy that is hard to visualise. Added to this mix are a large number of theories on equine dentistry which hold little truth when subjected to scientific rigour, leaving owners confused about where to turn and what to expect when their four-legged friend needs their teeth looked at.

Modern Equine Dentistry for Horse Owners sets out all the key information they need to know about the dental care their horse needs. Dr Thompson, one of many veterinary surgeons who have pushed equine dentistry to the forefront across the globe in recent years, has set out a comprehensive text which informs and educates horse owners on the standards to expect in modern dental care, as well as some of the problems we can encounter in the mouths of horses. The text not only serves this purpose, it can also be considered a useful resource for all veterinary surgeons undertaking equine dentistry - a reminder of what modern equine dentistry really entails!"

—**Dr Rob Pascoe** BVSc F/NCED DipAVDC-Eq MRCVS, Fellow Nordic College of Equine Dentistry, RCVS/ American Specialist in Equine Veterinary Dentistry. Kent, UK

"EVERYTHING STARTS WITH EDUCATION. As a horse owner, it is important to know what to do and what to have done to keep your horse in optimal health. That's why these type of books are so important!

In equine dentistry, common misconception exists about horses 'needing to have their teeth done' (read: need to have their teeth floated) once a year. However, this type of mindset belongs to the past when only limited knowledge was available. Current extensively available scientific literature shows the great value of a yearly dental check in every horse. And that's what its about in equine dentistry! I would say dig in, read, educate yourself and you will soon understand what I mean! I hope you enjoy reading it as much as I did! Kudos Dr. Thompson!"

—**Dr Elke Pollaris**, MSc, PhD, Diplomate EVDC (Equine). Asse, Belgium

"EXCELLENT INFORMATION TO GET A DETAILED OVERVIEW of the different aspects of equine dentistry! I am convinced that this comprehensive client education book will bring the dental care and well-being of horses up to date with current research and understanding today. Through the described details and hints herein, the knowledge gained by horse owners will progressively improve the understanding of the chewing system in equidae, and also increase the expectations of veterinarians for the practice of evidence-based dentistry."

—**Dr Manfred Stoll**, Fellow of the Nordic College of Equine Dentistry, Diplomate of the European Veterinary Dental College, Specialist Veterinarian in Equine Dentistry LTK Hessen (Germany), Teaching Faculty Equine Dentistry LTK Hessen. Breithardt, Germany

"HORSES' TEETH HAVEN'T EVOLVED IN OUR LIFETIME, but how amazing is it to see such a wide development in the diagnosis and treatment options available. In my short lifetime I have seen this area booming. Once a black box, now a well lit space. The horse's mouth keeps fascinating me and many others, and it was time someone took up the task to write an understandable, informative text to share all the current knowledge available on the topic. Great work Dr Thompson. To the reader, I hope you will be as fascinated as I am about equine dentistry and agree with me at the end. Your horse's teeth are his capital of life, its pension, its superannuation. Don't attack (read rasp) it without proper indication. Have a great read."

—**Professor Dr. Denis Verwilghen**, DVM, MSc, PhD, DES, Diplomate of the European Veterinary Dental College Diplomate EVDC (Equine), MRCVS. Victoria, Australia

"LIZ THOMPSON HAS DONE A WONDERFUL JOB with this masterpiece bringing the immense amount of information available down to a very readable edition suitable for the advanced to the beginner in the realm of equine dentistry. Her explanations allow the reader to follow the information without being overwhelmed. This book has filled an obvious void in the available literature and is a welcome addition to any library for all those involved with horses."

—**Professor Gary Wilson**, Registered Specialist in Equine Dentistry: BVSc, MVSc, MACVSc (Veterinary Dentistry), Diplomate ICEVO, FAVA, Cert Teach, Founding Diplomate of the American Veterinary Dental College Equine Speciality. Queensland, Australia

AUTHOR PREFACE

Hello and welcome! This preface is designed to give you the keys to best understand this book. Please read it!

FOR MY FIRST FOURTEEN YEARS OF EQUINE veterinary practice, I prided myself on my dental abilities—while in truth, I was only providing a "Fourth Level dental exam and treatment" (you will soon know what that means.). I "floated" teeth without mirrors, lights, or a full mouth speculum, and often without sedation. I possessed a clunky old museum piece of a speculum—which quite frankly I was terrified to use, especially without sedation—so I only used a unilateral (one-sided) wedge speculum and hand floats. Thanks to my friend and colleague Dr Glenn Beeman, a Canadian New Zealand vet, I saw the light (literally), when he came up from the South Island and placed a proper speculum and light into my horse's mouth. He showed me what modern dentistry was all about. I was appalled at the pathology I knew I must have missed in my patients' mouths all those years. It seems I left the USA twelve years before that, those early years when the rapid advancement of modern equine dentistry had truly begun. During this time, I'd been immersed in my new country's joys of farming and motherhood, plus a few spinal fractures, and somehow missed the revolution.

The once-accepted idea that "floating", or removing the sharp enamel points, is all a horse needs for dentistry is long gone. Times have changed and many of us are trying to get the word out to owners who haven't heard. We now diagnose and treat most of the same conditions your human dentist does. It simply isn't good enough to perform equine dentistry without carefully examining the mouth, diagnosing dental disease, and treating it before your horse shows outward signs of disease. It's high time owners were given the opportunity to learn what's really inside that dark cavern called "their horse's mouth".

Equine dentistry is not a regulated modality in most areas of the world. As such, it is imperative that owners of equids understand what comprises modern equine dentistry. Understanding the principles and limitations of the techniques used to maintain good dentition (teeth) and treat suboptimal dentition allows you, as the owner, to safeguard your horse. By understanding the horse's oral anatomy, growth, wear patterns, tooth eruption, and diseases, you will be in an excellent position to safeguard your animal's health. Modern equine dentistry can offer your horse the best life has to offer.

A few points about this book:

1- When I say horse, I include all equids, including horses, ponies, donkeys, mules, zebras and the like.

2- You will find I use many medically correct terms but remain calm: I will briefly define some of them in the text, or you will find them in the glossary. Learning more of these words will enable you to understand dental disease more clearly and to more precisely explain your horses' dental issues to those trying to help you. Words in ***bold italic*** or ***links*** (in ebook) are defined in the ***Glossary***

3- A survey of my equine practice clients and other horse-keen readers on social media regarding their preference for regular book or question & answer (Q & A) format revealed an interest in both, so for those readers who prefer it, I have included Part Two (Q & A). The items in Part Two refer to relevant chapters in Part One (The Book) for more detail and images. Because those choosing Part Two format will be entering Part One at various points, I have referred to the glossary items the first time they are used in *every* chapter, rather than once per book, as is the usual. Glossary words will be in ***italic bold links*** (in the ebook), or in ***italic bold*** (in the print version). So remember, words in ***bold italic*** or ***links*** are defined in the ***Glossary***.

4- I use the term ***vet*** as an abbreviation for a veterinarian who has completed a full course in veterinary medicine at an accredited veterinary school and is licensed to practice in the country (state in the USA, province in CA and other countries) in which he or she is practicing medicine and dentistry. In many places, dentistry is legally limited to veterinarians registered in that state, province, or country.

5- In many countries, a wide variety of people perform equine dental procedures. Some may be veterinarians, some may be well trained and appropriately qualified as an Equine Dental Technician (EDT, see below). Other may be inexperienced people with no or some training (but with no appropriate externally-monitored qualification), who still perform advanced dental procedures. Some of these last unqualified people create injuries, some of them serious or life-threatening, to equid teeth, jaws, and throats.

I reserve the term ***Equine Dental Technician (EDT)*** in this book for those who have qualified with a BAEDT (UK) or IGFP (Germany), or an equivalent, though I don't believe there are others currently operational. The other non-veterinary operators are, for the purposes of this book, termed ***lay dental operators*** (lay indicates non-veterinary).

Depending upon where you live, there are different rules for who may perform dentistry. In the UK, for example, non-veterinarians who are not BAEDT-qualified are only allowed to float or rasp small dental overgrowths. Many places (country, state, or province) define equine dentistry as the practice of veterinary medicine. In these places, there may be no regulation or required education of EDTs or lay dental operators. In areas where this is the case, no one other than a veterinarian in that state, province or country is meant to be doing dentistry, unless under veterinary supervision. Several USA states and CA provinces require lay dental operators and EDTs to be registered, but there may be little to no enforcement. In New Zealand, there is currently no non-veterinary regulatory board for equine dentistry, no examination procedure, no continuing education, nor is proof of fitness required of anyone to perform tooth floating or dentistry. This is similar to many places in the USA and many other countries. Because of the lack of uniform rules and regulations regarding who can perform equine dentistry around the world, horse owners should check with their local, state, province, or country regulatory boards to determine the qualifications and legitimacy of individuals offering equine dental services.

6- Technical stuff for the digital edition: With most eReading devices, clicking or double tapping and then spreading fingers apart on an image or graphic enlarges it for ease of viewing. The graphics and images use full-colored images, labels, filled parts, and arrows. If you want to get the most out of the book, it is recommended to use either a full-colored eReader OR download a free Kindle or other colored eReading app onto your iPhone or android phone, tablet, or computer, which will provide you with full color images and graphics.

In the eBook, sub-subheadings appear like this: ". *Diastemata and periodontal disease*", with three spaces and a dot before the italicized sub-subsection. This is not an error, but to make the Table of Contents work. :) This will not be the case in the paper versions!

7- Disclaimers: Reading past this Author Preface is taken as evidence that you understand and acknowledge all concepts in the following subclasses (7a, 7b, and 7c) and fully accept the responsibilities outlined here, in the Disclaimer shown on the Copyright page , and also on the DISCLAIMER page just after the Glossary.

7a- Disclaimer 1: This book has been written with the intent of informing and educating you about the possible dental and other pathologies which may occur in your equids. It is *not* intended to diagnose disease or pathology, or substitute for the proper diagnosis, treatment, and recommendations of your equine dental veterinarian. It is not a substitute for the consultation or recommendations of your equine dental veterinarian. Call your veterinarian for examination and treatment of your equids.

7b- Disclaimer 2: Regarding you personally attempting to view, touch, or smell any of the anatomical landmarks, teeth, gingiva, skin, and/or any other part of an equid discussed in this book, you are doing this of your own free will. Horses, zebras, donkeys, mules, and any other equids are inherently dangerous creatures. They have teeth to bite with and hooves to kick with. They outweigh us by about ten times. If you get near an equid, you are responsible for your own life and your own safety. No person associated with this book, publishing, images, or information in any way takes any responsibility for any injury to you or anyone else you know if you try to check out anything mentioned in this book. Any injury, loss of income, or loss in any way you sustain is entirely your choice and none of us are responsible nor liable.

7c- Disclaimer 3: This book is not a manual to teach you or anyone else how to perform equine dentistry. The book has been created with **solely three intents:** 1- to offer you the information which will enable you to understand more about equine dentistry, 2- to enable you to determine and choose the level of dentistry you desire for your horse— for your horse's and your own benefit, and 3- to enable you to judge, to a greater degree than you might be able to right now, the competency of the person you schedule to perform dental work on your horse. This book is a summation, in layman's language, of the current information (as of 01 March 2024) available in equine veterinary medicine from the literature. Reading this book will not turn you into a dental practitioner in any way.

Any use of this information for other than the **three intents**, above, is wilful ignorance. No one associated with this book in any way will be liable for any losses— physical, mental, monetary, or any other loss you can dream up. Just learn the information and use it for the betterment of you and your horse in your dealings with your chosen dental practitioner.

TRIGGER WARNING: there are images of portions of deceased horses, blood, etc., and detailed descriptions used to illustrate disease conditions. If any of these both you, ***do not read this book***.

FOR FULL DISCLAIMER NOTICE, SEE COPYRIGHT PAGE and the DISCLAIMER page (listed in the Table of Contents).

8- My upcoming online courses for horse owners are nearly complete: one for Equine Emergency Care and another for Modern Equine Dentistry. I wanted this book published first!

If you are interested in these topics, please join my Equine Vet Today VIP list by clicking on the link or on the QR Code. This will invite you to my Equine Vet Today VIP List!

9- I am creating more books in parallel to this one. One of them is an adaptation for younger horse enthusiasts, their parents, or owners who want a less technical explanation in a shorter, handbook version.

If you have specific items you think your young friends would like to read about, or if you would be interested in a copy, please let me know by leaving a message at **https://equistillstocks.com/equine-vet-today-contact-us/**

I also write historical and veterinary fiction (relatively horsey, of course) as Lizzi Tremayne.

You can join my:

1) Equine Vet Today VIP List by going to: **https://bit.ly/EqVetToday** *or* **use the QR code!**

2) Lizzi Tremayne Author VIP list by going to**: https://bit.ly/44oYeOR** *or* **use the QR code!**

Enjoy!

Dr Elizabeth (Lizzi) Thompson
Blue Mist Holdings Ltd, DBA Blue Mist Equine Veterinary Centre

Part One: The Book

CHAPTER ONE

HOW DO I KNOW MY HORSE HAS DENTAL DISEASE?

"Saying floating is all a horse needs is like saying if you brush your teeth, you won't get cavities, periodontal disease, or cracked teeth."
–Jack Easley, DVM, MS, DBVP (EqPract), AVDC (Equine)

Hello and welcome! If you have not yet read the Author Preface (just before this chapter) please go back and read it! The preface is designed to give you the keys to best understand this book.

SOMETIMES HORSES SHOW you clearly that their mouth is bothering them, or show you "signs" of dental pain. And sometimes they don't, or at least not in ways we can always understand. Despite this, there are many clinical signs, or "what the vet sees", which may indicate dental disease or "dental ***pathology***". We use "signs" rather than "symptoms", because "symptoms" are the signs of the disease noticed by the patient, and since the patient is a horse, herein lies the problem with using "symptoms" for a non-human.

The definition of pathology as it pertains to dental disease is defined by the Cambridge Dictionary as "medical characteristics of a disease" and "a disease or medical condition". Merriam-Webster further defines pathology as "the structural and functional deviations from the normal that constitute disease or characterize a particular disease". It isn't only the teeth themselves which may be affected by dental pathology; other problems may occur as a direct or indirect result, such as choke, colic, poor performance, recurrent fertility problems, and aggression.

By paying close attention, you may recognize subtle signs of painful dental disease. If you've ever had a serious toothache, you may remember how debilitating the pain can be. It probably affected your performance at work, school, or sport. Unsurprisingly, if your horse has dental pain, it may strongly influence *their* comfort level, and their performance, as well.

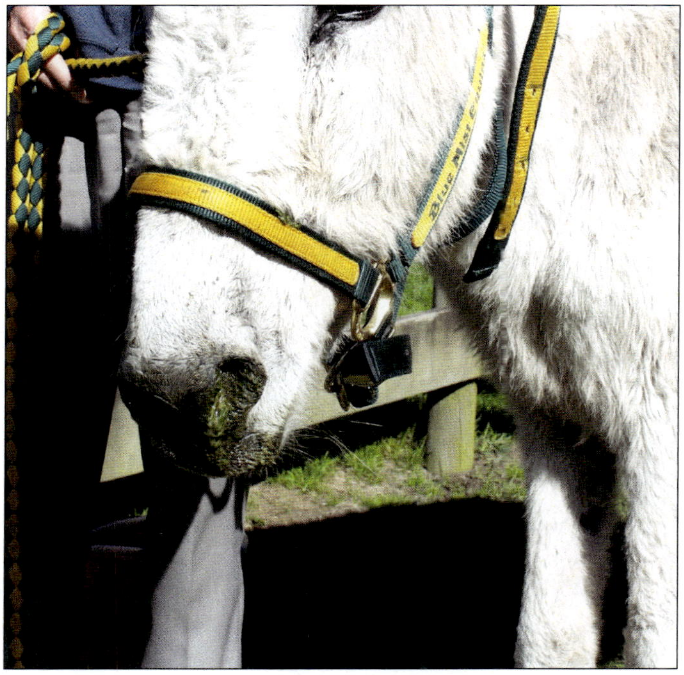

Donkey discharging chewed-up feed from nostrils in a case of "choke" likely secondary to poor dentition. Image credit Author.

Clinical Signs of Dental Pain

Signs during work

- pulling or "lugging" on one or both reins
- resisting turns or other evasion
- head tossing or head shaking
- unexplained subtle lameness
- mouthing or chewing the bit
- head tilt or playing with the tongue
- sticking the tongue out of the mouth, or over the bit

- resisting bridling
- refusing to maintain a frame or vertical head carriage
- sensitivity of cheeks to touch
- irritability or aggression when asked to perform certain movements

These behavioral or training issues may be a sign that something is amiss in your horse's mouth, although they may be attributable to other causes like lack of effective training or problems in musculoskeletal, neurological, or skeletal areas other than the mouth. It is relatively straightforward for someone well-trained in veterinary dentistry to evaluate your horse for oral conditions which could cause these problems.

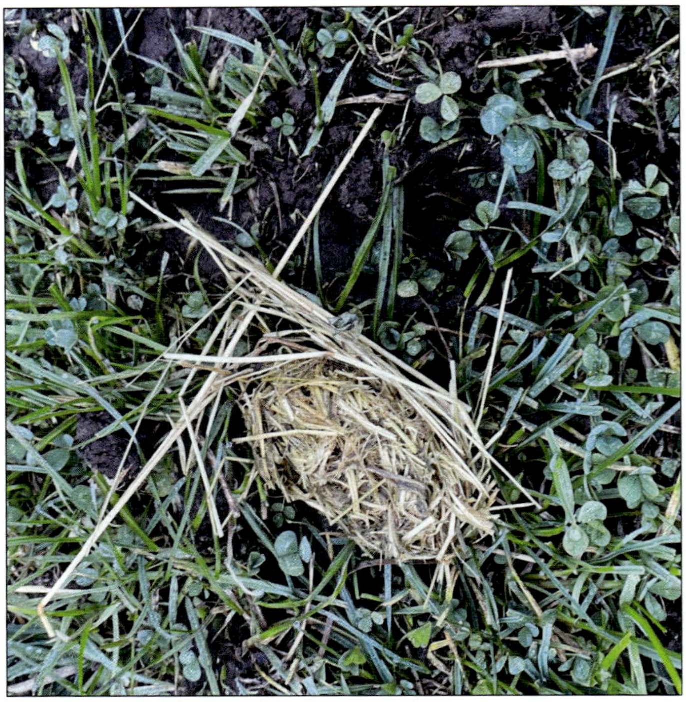

This 30+-year-old pony has significant dental disease but does well on grass and soaked pelleted feeds. Sometimes she manages to sneak hay from the other horses and chews it 'round and 'round, but she cannot chew it well enough to swallow the "quid" of twisted hay that forms in her mouth . She then has to drop these "quids" on the ground. Image credit Dr Laurinda Oliver.

Signs at rest in the stable or field

- dropping grain/***hard feed***, hay, or grass
- ***quidding*** – dropping "quids", or twisted wads of hay or grass
- excessive salivation/ drooling
- foul odor from mouth
- head tilt while eating
- grain/hard feed in water bucket
- playing with the tongue
- whole grains in manure
- > 3.5 mm hay particles in manure: increased fecal fiber length
- refusal to eat, or slow to eat
- weight loss usually only occurs when dental disease is severe
- swellings along the jaw or on the side of the face
- ***purulent*** discharge from face or beneath the jaw

The most common sign of all?

The most common sign is... ***NO OBVIOUS SIGN AT ALL, or none that we notice**, **anyway!*** Surprised? Many people are. Horses tend to be stoic and usually hide even severe dental pain. A regular, thorough, six-monthly or yearly clinical examination can identify early signs of disease, allowing your horse's dental care to be based on examination and diagnosis, or prophylactic (preventative) dental care, as with your own dentist. Your dental vet can offer early intervention based on examination and advanced diagnostics, rather than having to resort to being the ambulance at the bottom of the cliff, attempting catch-up treatment of disease which has advanced to a severe stage where your horse may show signs of advanced clinical disease — which will be difficult, time-consuming, and expensive to treat.

But why don't they seem to show pain?

Why Don't Horses Display Obvious Pain? Or do they?

HOW CAN THE most common sign of dental disease be "no obvious sign at all?"

There are many potential reasons, but it's partly because horses are a "prey" species, which means in their evolutionary history, they were "preyed upon" (eaten) by meat-eating predators. While they are sentient beings, there is no advantage in displaying that they are weak or in pain, as it would encourage these predators. Your horse may not be surrounded by hungry wolves anymore, but a few hundred years of keeping the wolves away hasn't changed the defense mechanisms evolved in his species over millions of years. However, this is only part of the reason. I see the primary problem here is our failure to notice the subtle signs horses show us every day.

Pain and the Horse Grimace Scale

Sometimes it's hard to tell they're in pain, but fortunately they do actually show signs of pain from dental disease—it's up to us to learn what these look like! Several new studies have been published which look at "pain faces", or a pain coding system called the Horse Grimace Scale (HGS). Many of us have known of these signs intuitively long ago, the tight muzzles and the wrinkles around their eyes, to name just a few, but finally vet researchers have looked at this and quantified the signs. Many vets and techs in veterinary hospitals are using pain scoring to recognize and quantify (to determine the amount of) signs of pain in hospitalized animals. Many of the signs evaluated in the HGS may have been attributed to anger or grumpiness in the past, but people are finally recognizing them for what they are... signs of pain.

Facial expression changes have been used in human medicine for some time now. They have been adapted to equine medicine as the HGS, which has proven to be an easily learned, sensitive tool with a high reliability between different observers. HGS has been used to evaluate pain levels in different areas of the body by evaluating six characteristics of equine facial expression:

- ears held stiffly backwards
- tension above eye area
- tightening around the eye
- prominent and strained chewing muscles
- mouth strained with pronounced chin
- strained nostrils with flattening of the profile

Some of the newest papers are specific to HGS observations of horses with dental pain and are showing that dental disorders result in different levels of pain or discomfort for horses, which hadn't been clearly demonstrated before. They found these levels of pain or discomfort could be reliably evaluated and quantified using the HGS, whether the observer was standing beside the horse or looking at photographs of the horse.

This makes the HGS extremely useful, as it can be clinically significant in the routine evaluation of horses by general practitioners and realistically, it could be utilized by owners as well! Check out the papers on it in the Bibliography and Further Reading.

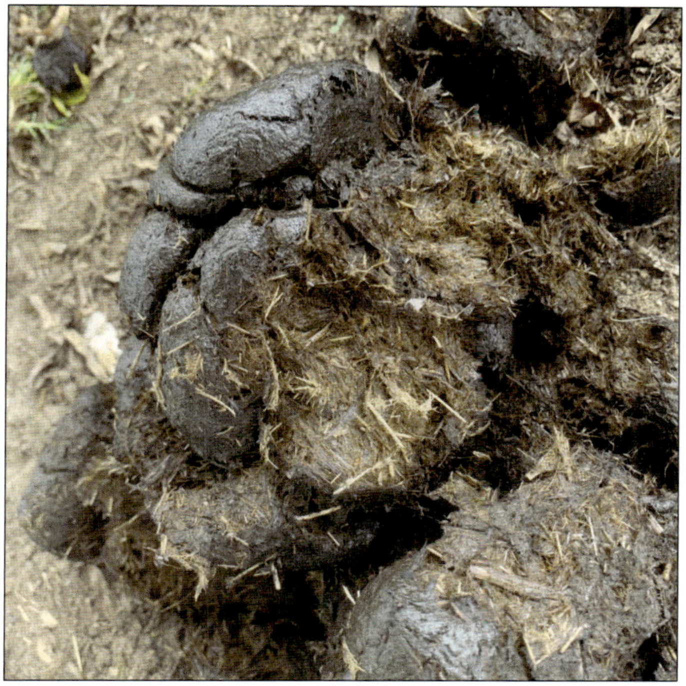

Manure with hay stems longer than 3.5 mm in a horse with significant oral pain. Image credit Author.

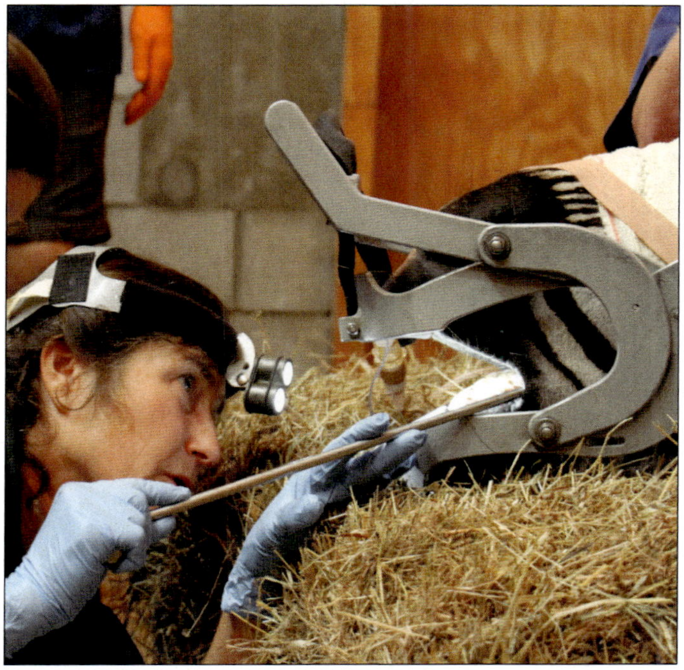

While signs of dental pain in captive, unhandled zoo zebras may only be evident by recognition of increased fecal fiber length and observation of facial expressions, they need dental care, too! This is Itika, a Plains Zebra at the Auckland Zoo in New Zealand with Dr Elizabeth Thompson. Itika is having a planned ***odontoplasty*** *(dental examination and tooth floating) under general anesthesia. Image credit Vanessa Marsh, used with permission of Auckland Zoo.*

Believe me, I'm sure a fractured tooth will cause him constant pain every time he chews or moves. Now, due to these studies, many other people will understand just how painful dental conditions can be! The pain caused by dental pathology is often underestimated. When your horse is asked to work, it is likely worse. Can you imagine the effect this may have upon your horse's performance?

Think back to when you were last in serious pain from a tooth and how it affected you every moment of every day. And then realize many of us have treated horses with serious dental conditions, including fractured teeth, who were in *full work* up until the time they were examined. The relief they showed after extractions makes it clear how much pain they were in before the treatment. The effect of this pain cannot be underestimated.

So how do we diagnose these painful conditions? Read on!

THERE ARE EIGHT LEVELS OF EQUINE DENTISTRY?

"Many people don't understand that when you have an emergent, objectively established truth by the methods and tools of science, you do not have the luxury of standing in denial of it because it is true, whether or not you believe in it,"
—Neil deGrasse Tyson

THE WEATHER IS great, you have more time off, and it's time to get that horse fit! Unfortunately, he's doing funny things with his mouth and not taking rein contact. Is he just out of condition, or is something in his mouth bothering him?

Just as there are different ways to treat most health conditions, there are different levels of dentistry. Multiple levels of dentistry have been described, which are defined by how the examination is performed, the equipment and pharmaceuticals utilized, and the treatment itself. More information about the condition of the horse's mouth is available at each subsequent level.

The level you select is your choice, as the owner, but it is vital you understand what those levels mean before you make your choice. Consider, as you read through this chapter and the rest of the book, what is involved at these different levels, what may be missed, and what degree of thoroughness you desire for your horse. We will come back to this question later, in Chapter 13.

What Are These Levels?

The First Level

The First Level involves only the use of a hand ***float*** (a dental file) or a motorized power float. Information obtainable at this level is severely limited. Removal of ***sharp enamel points*** is possible in cooperative horses who will let one work without continually closing their mouth on the float. Large ***distal hooks*** and subtle problems will be missed or ignored due to the difficulty in treating them. It is difficult to remove distal hooks on the far edge of the teeth furthest back in the mouth ('11s, which you will learn about in Chapter 3) because there is often pain in the soft ***tissues*** near these hooks and horses tend to be less than cooperative when you are hurting them.

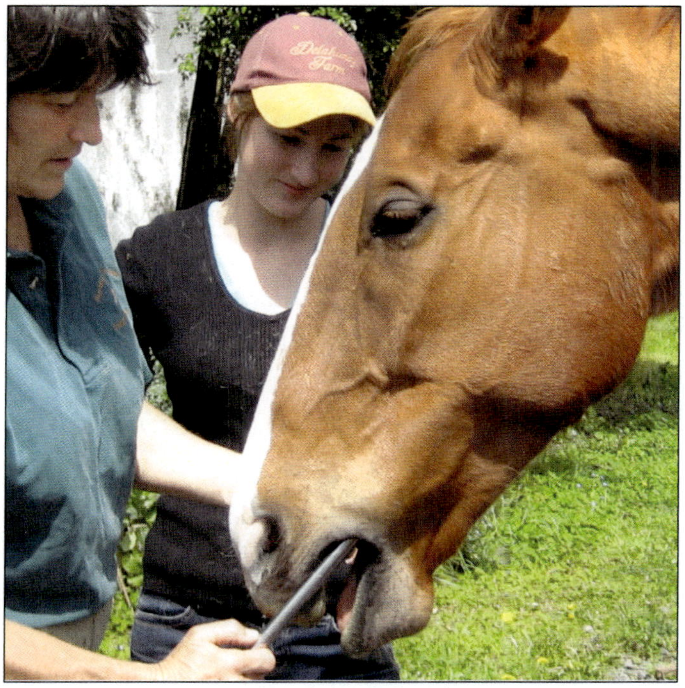

Image of Dr Elizabeth Thompson and Hannah Lowry performing a hand float at the First Level of Equine Dentistry, for illustrative purpose only. Image credit Elliot Thompson.

There is no visibility into the mouth as it's dark and the mouth is full of food. One may see the ***incisors, canines, wolf teeth*** and the more ***mesial*** portions of the first ***cheek tooth***. It is difficult and unsafe to check the ***buccal*** (toward the cheek) and ***lingual*** (toward the tongue) edges of the more distal ***cheek teeth***. These usually need the most attention but are unfortunately the most neglected. Obviously, one cannot see any detail on most of the teeth, and thus most of the ***pathology*** giving your horse problems will be missed.

At this level, one is merely waving a rasp at an unknown quantity of pathology.

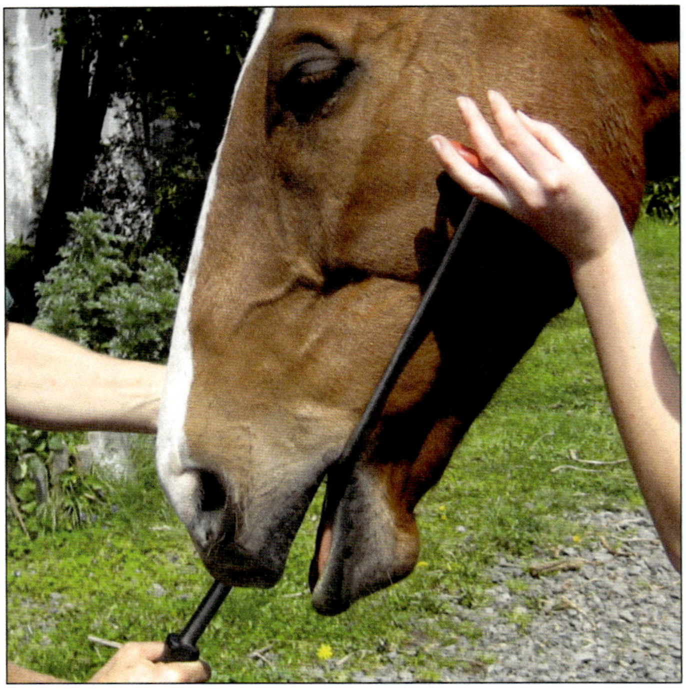

Image of Dr Elizabeth Thompson and Hannah Lowry using a unilateral (one-sided) gag and hand float at the Second Level of Equine Dentistry, for illustrative purpose only. Image credit Elliot Thompson.

The Second Level

In the Second Level, a one-sided gag is added. These go by the name of Bayer, Schouppe, spool, coil, Landmeisser, wedge, and the like. They have a bite piece which fits between the cheek teeth made of either:

- cylindrical spring steel or a solid metal cylinder (the "spool" types), or
- a wedge of metal, plastic, or rubber (the wedge types).

The only benefit from using either of these types of gag is slightly easier floating of the teeth because one side of the mouth is held open to some degree. However, these gags ***are not recommended*** because at best, they do not significantly assist in examination or floating, and at worst, they frequently cause serious damage. The reasons for this are as follows:

- A horse ***masticates*** (chews) a lot with a unilateral (one-sided) gag in place. This makes it difficult to examine the teeth (the primary purpose of a dental examination), which should be performed before the teeth are filed.
- As the gag occupies mouth space on the side where it is placed, the tongue is pushed toward the other side where examination or floating is being attempted. This decreases visibility inside the mouth, already minimal at this level, and makes floating more difficult.
- The ***temporomandibular*** or jaw joint, commonly known as the TMJ, may be damaged when a horse bites down hard on only one side at a time
- If the gag slips from *between* the teeth to the inside of the teeth, the palatine artery may be ruptured. It bleeds. A lot. For a long time.
- Most seriously, however, the danger of fracturing cheek teeth is very real. The cylindrical shape of the "spool" types causes the entire force of both sides of the strong masseter (chewing) muscles to be focused on a narrow line across two opposing teeth, which may lead to a fractured cheek tooth or teeth, with severe consequences. A fractured tooth

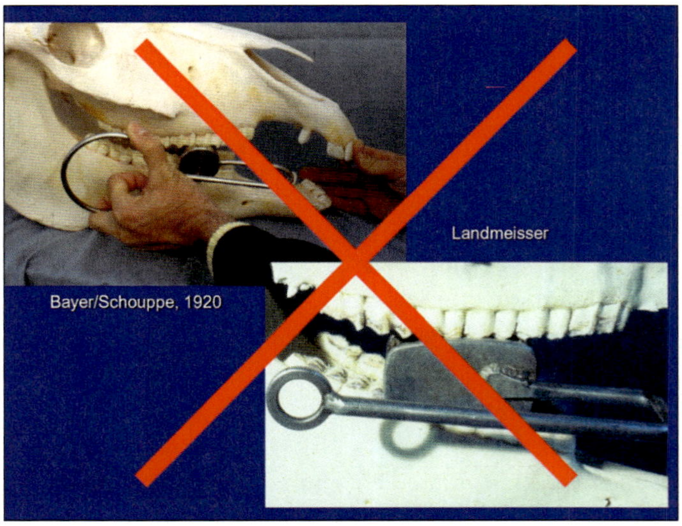

The image shows two of the many NON-recommended gags which are sometimes used at The Second Level: Shown are the Bayer/Schouppe (1920) and the Landmeisser. These can seriously damage teeth and other tissues, including causing fracture of cheek teeth. Unmarked image credit Dr Jack Easley, graphic credit Author.

needs to be extracted. A fractured tooth will cause your horse a lot of pain until the tooth is actually *discovered* and extracted. Make no mistake, this is major surgery, especially because that recently-healthy tooth will be firmly stuck in place. And the worst thing? The fracture *never had to happen* in the first place.

Back to the levels, if there is any pathology at Level Two in your horse's mouth, it will most likely be missed as well. One is still merely waving a rasp around in the darkness.

The Third Level

Addition of a full mouth speculum assists, but pathology will be missed as the mouth is still dark and full of feed. The image on the right shows what the inside of the mouth would look like with a light, but no light is used at this level. You wouldn't even see this green mess, which hasn't been flushed out at this level.

In the middle right image, you see a speculum being utilized, but a speculum on the head of an unsedated horse, especially if the horse is not in ***stocks***, can be dangerous for the handler, operator and the horse itself. Imagine what could happen if the horse swings its heavy head around while wearing a heavy speculum and you or a young owner is standing in the way.

Unfortunately, the Third Level is still rasp-waving.

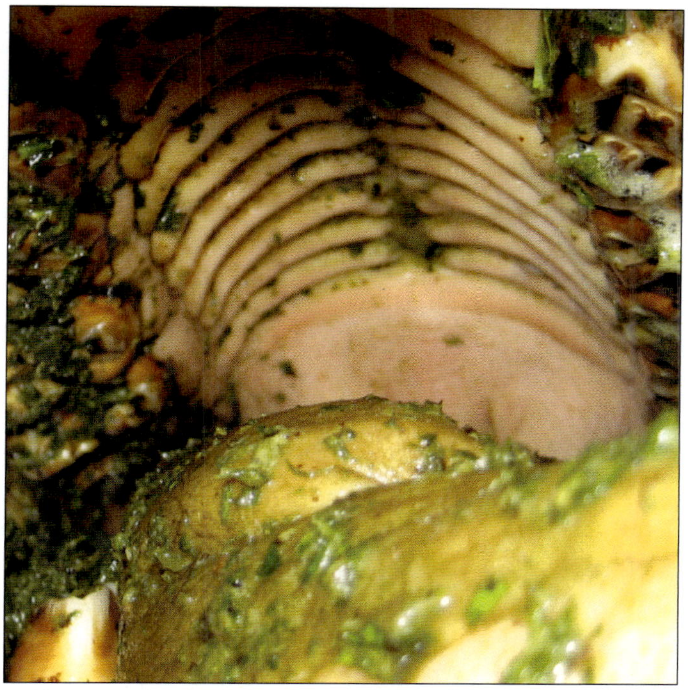

This is not The Third Level, but to show you what the mouth would look like even if you had a light at The Third Level, which you do not.

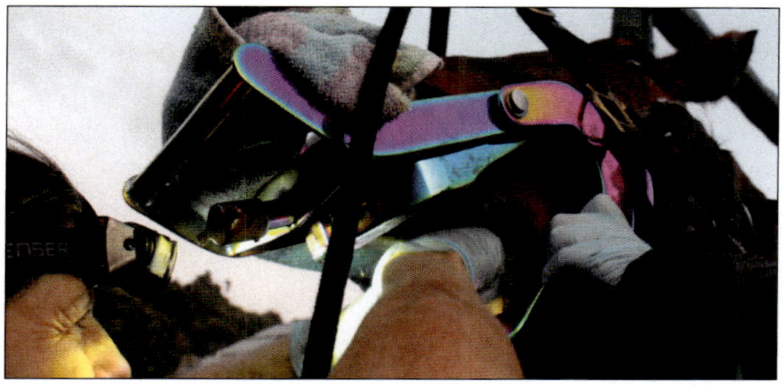

Speculums are heavy. Using one of these on an unsedated horse with an already heavy head is a recipe for disaster in this day and age. Image Credit Matthew Mole.

The Fourth Level

Addition of flushing of the mouth reveals some pathology, but one can only see that pathology if it's in the very front of the mouth, as it's still dark in there. Yes, this is still rasp-waving as well.

The Fifth Level

Addition of intraoral light, sedation, and headstand or dental halter significantly enhances the practitioner's ability to diagnose problems in the mouth. Thorough oral exams are important because horses often do not display what we would consider obvious signs of pain, even when oral pathology is well-advanced. Even while the patient is sedated, a well-trained dental practitioner will find painful areas during a thorough dental examination. At this level without mirrors, the operator can unfortunately only see the teeth and gums in the very front of the mouth. Without mirrors, many malocclusions, periodontal disease, tumors, foreign bodies, wriggling bot larvae, or other abnormalities will be missed. The ***occlusal***, or chewing, surface of the teeth in the very front of the mouth may be evaluated for pulp horn defects or ***pulp exposure***, but one cannot see the occlusal surfaces of the more distal teeth without a

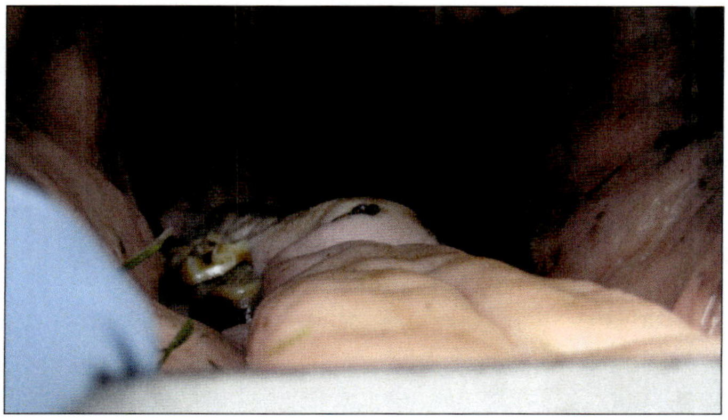

Trying to see into the mouth at the Fourth Level of Equine Dentistry. Image credit Author.

mirror or oroscope. Pulp horn defects (black areas or holes on the occlusal surfaces) may indicate dead or dying teeth, which need further evaluation by modalities included in the eighth level.

At this point, it is are still rasp-waving. Although things are improving, until you have properly examined every surface of every tooth in the mouth, you're not fully informed and the floating you're doing cannot yet be called odontoplasty.

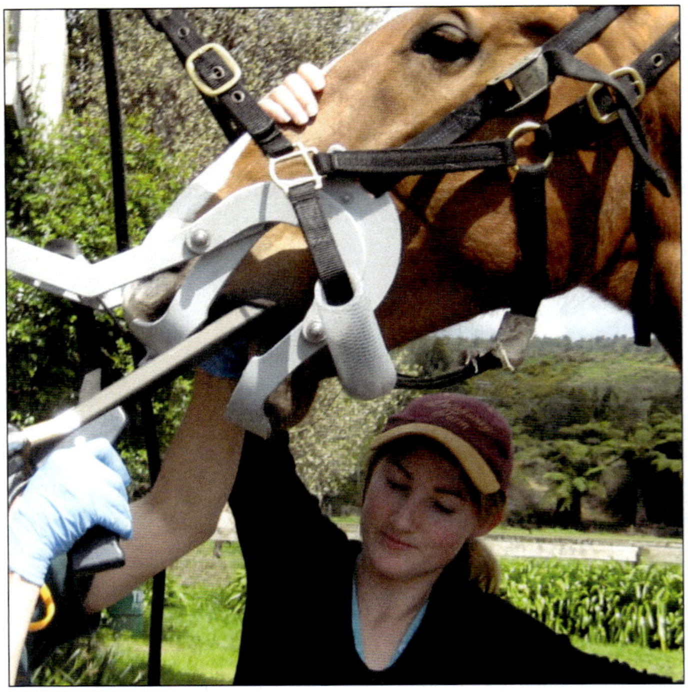

Dr Elizabeth Thompson and Hannah Lowry utilizing a full-mouth speculum, head lamp, dental halter, and sedation at the Fifth Level of Equine Dentistry. For illustrative purposes. Image credit Elliot Thompson.

The Sixth Level

Addition of mirror and probes or picks allows a thorough visual examination of all surfaces of the teeth and correct diagnosis of problems, as well as documentation of oral pathology. These instruments are required to offer prophylactic dentistry (rather than bottom-of-the-cliff dentistry). This additional instrumentation allows early intervention in the treatment of disease, saving your horse pain, and you, dental dollars. Now that the mouth has been properly examined, the dental treatment provided may, if the float is informed by the examination and specific to the pathology discovered within the entire mouth, be called *odontoplasty*, or "the informed redefining, contouring, or ***rasping*** of the teeth". To achieve the "informed" portion of this definition requires a thorough oral examination be performed prior to rasping teeth, otherwise it is simply waving a rasp around in the darkness. Floating, or smoothing down the sharp buccal or lingual enamel points of the cheek teeth of horses with a rasp (hand or power), can be done in the absence of an examination, but in this situation, not only will pathology be missed, but unnecessary reduction of teeth in this situation can shorten a horse's life. While floating has been performed for over hundreds of years, there is little to no scientific-based evidence to support general floating. The enamel ridges, sharp points, and transverse ridges may likely improve your horse's ability to chew forage, but at some point, these "malocclusions" can cause problems such as interference with other teeth or injury to soft tissue. This, then, is what "odontoplasty" is meant to be: the crown reduction which is performed after a thorough examination dictates which teeth should have their crowns shaped and reduced, and exactly how this should be done.

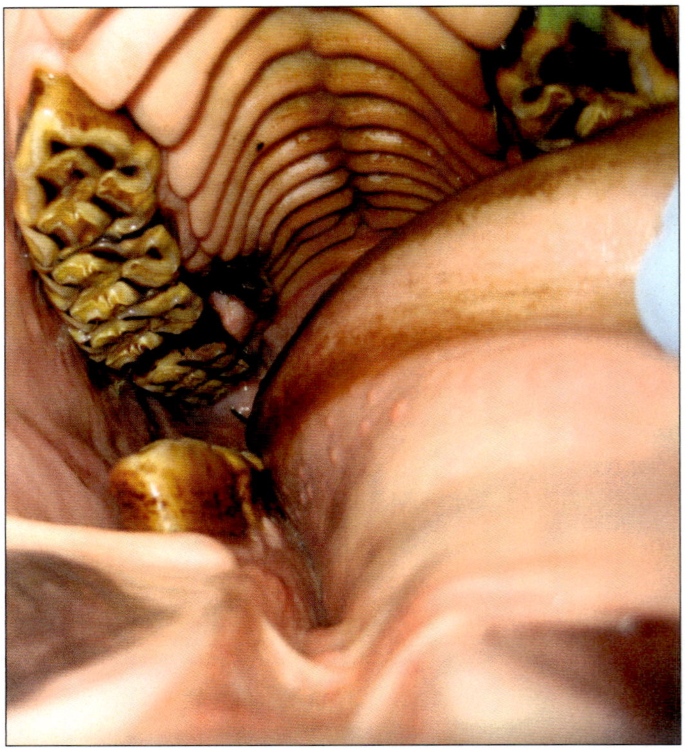

The Fifth Level of Equine Dentistry: What you can see intraorally, (inside the mouth) in a flushed mouth with sedation, bright lights and head support. Image credit Author.

The Seventh Level

Addition of oroscopy, or oral endoscopy, allows the practitioner to see the fine detail of every surface of every tooth and photograph and video all of these. This takes the oral examination truly to "the next level". Oroscopy clearly defines pathology of a much more subtle nature, allowing

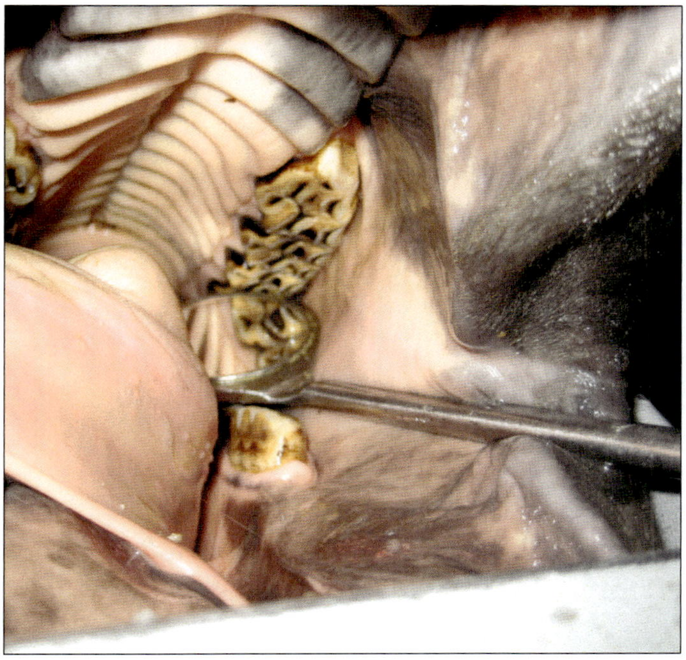

Using an intraoral mirror at the Sixth Level of Equine Dentistry. Image credit Author.

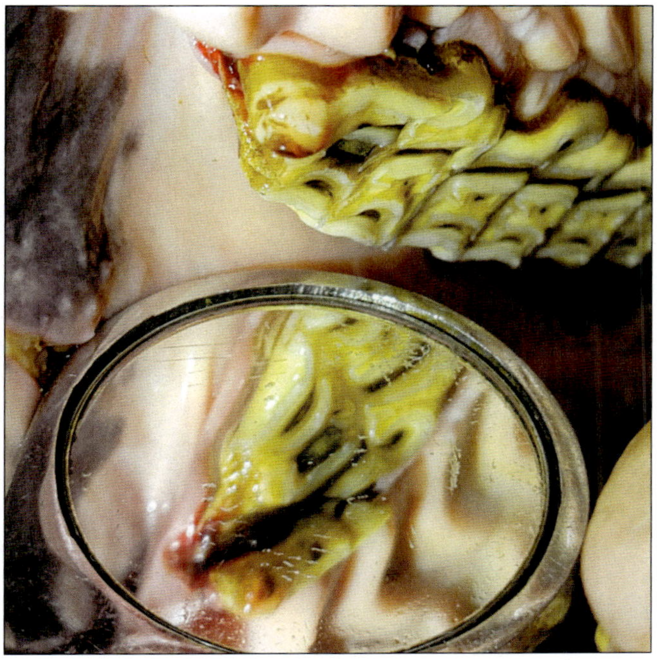

Without a mirror (and the blood), seeing this fracture might be difficult. Image credit Cathie Heald Greenwell.

your ***vet*** to pick up previously undetectable early signs of disease before they become serious. While having a mirror is an advance on *not* having one, the oroscope opens up a whole new world for your horse's comfort and pain relief.

Oroscopy is now the standard of care for a good oral examination, even for general practitioners. This is the best way of showing you, the owner, the true pathology in the mouth of your horse.

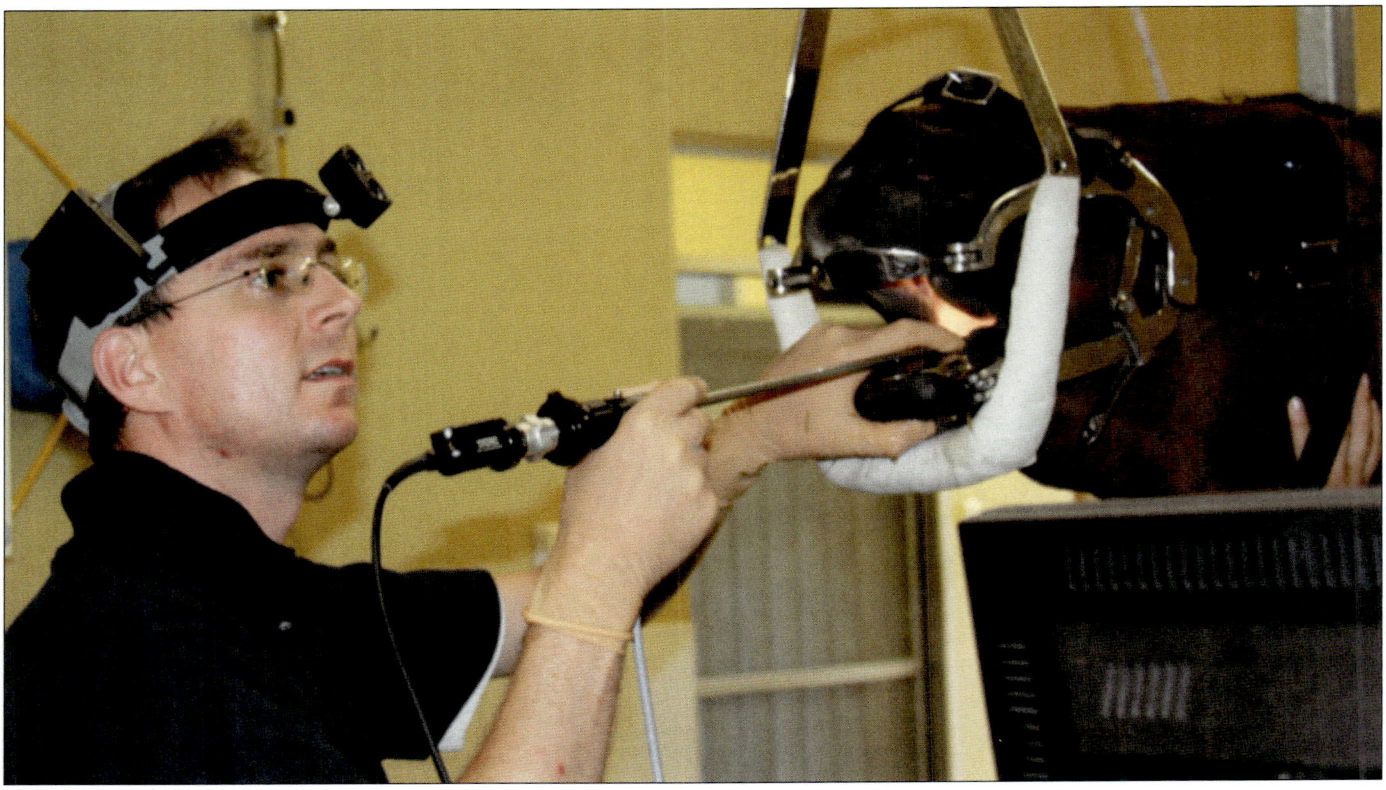

Oroscopy performed at Ugglarps Gard Equine clinic in Sweden. This technique clearly displays the fine and necessary dental details to Dr Denis Verwilghen and his equine patient's owner. He is looking at the screen as he works. Image credit Dr Denis Verwilghen.

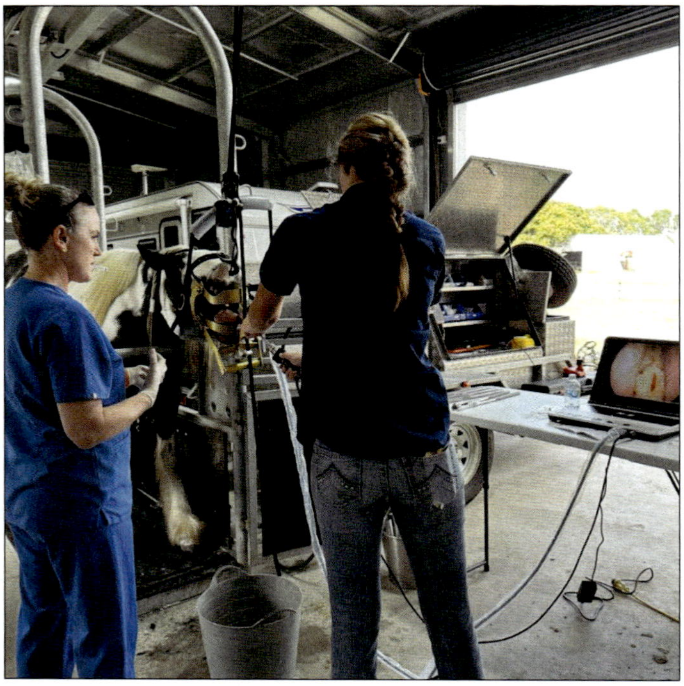

Oroscopy shows you exactly what your veterinarian is seeing in your horse's mouth. It's great for teaching as well, as displayed by Dr Olivia James of Australian Veterinary Equine Dentistry. Image credit Dr Olivia James.

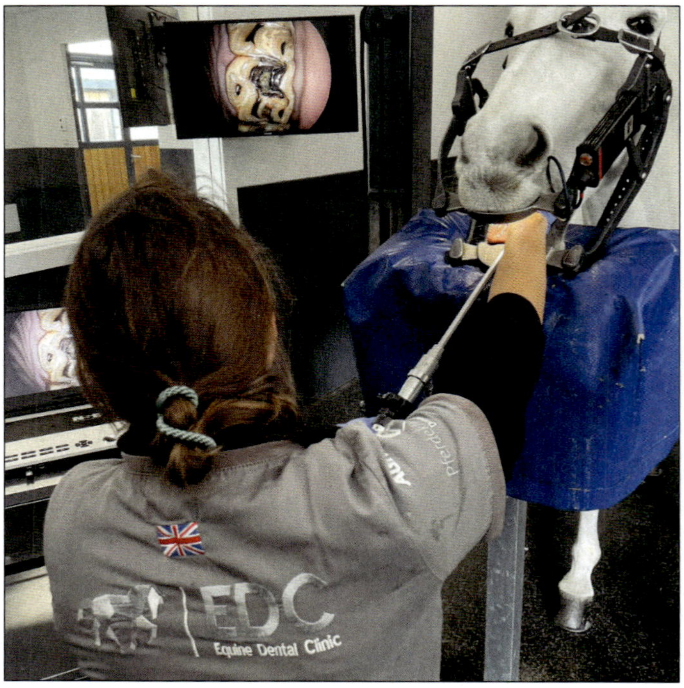

Oroscopy at EDC (Equine Dental Clinic) lets Dr Nicole du Toit grade the **infundibular caries** *in this patient. Image credit Dr Nicole du Toit.*

The Eighth Level

The eighth level includes addition of other diagnostic modalities including digital radiography (X-Rays), ultrasound, scintigraphy, CT, and MRI. Radiographs may be effectively taken in the field, and even cheek tooth extractions are readily managed in the standing patient without general ***anesthesia***, with the aid of portable stocks and the excellent sedation and ***perineural anesthesia*** (nerve blocks) now available.

How are Floating or Odontoplasty Related to the Eight Levels?

YOU PROBABLY NOW realize there are significant differences between a first or second level "float" and a thorough seventh or eighth level "dental examination and odontoplasty". Even a sixth level examination should include recording a detailed history, a whole horse examination (particularly of the head and mouth for disease and abnormal wear), good record keeping, and progress charting. A veterinarian with postgraduate equine dentistry training has the knowledge of disease conditions and whole-body systems essential to undertaking this examination.

International standard of practice in veterinary equine dentistry requires that the small intraoral structures be evaluated, which is difficult in the unsedated horse. Would you want a mirror in your unsedated horse's mouth? Sedation provides safety for the owner or handler as well as for the horse, plus it enables a thorough examination every time, not just when the horse "allows" it. X-rays and laboratory analysis of blood or abnormal tissues may be

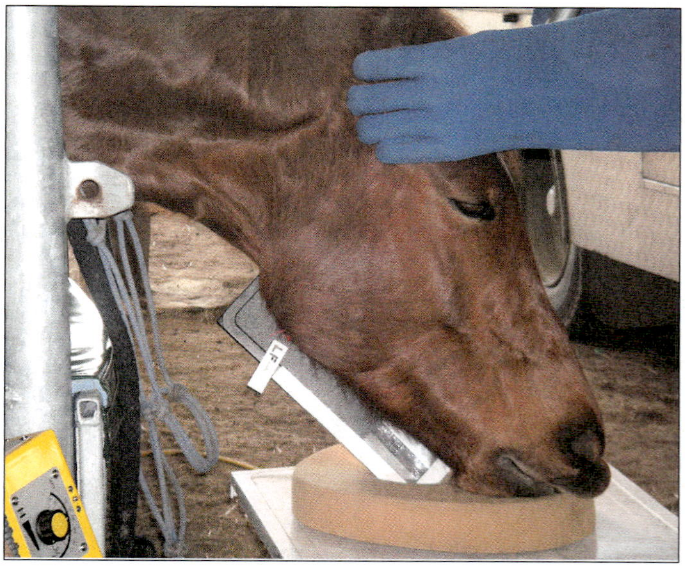

Taking radiographs at the Eighth Level of Equine Dentistry. Image credit Author.

used to diagnose pathologic conditions and monitor response to therapy.

Sedation and anesthesia may only be administered by your veterinarian, along with any (if necessary) antibiotic and anti-inflammatory treatment.

Portable or stationary stocks provide support and stabilization. They appear to make sedated horses more relaxed and require less sedation, as the equid can lean against the walls of the stocks, which may minimize ***ataxia***.Their head can be supported in one position, rather than you having to lift and lower their heavy head multiple times onto your shoulder, which tends to waken them from sedation prematurely (as well as tire you out!).

Geriatrics (older equids) require special consideration: pre-operative bloods are recommended, and special sedative techniques are useful to enhance the safety in these older patients. See more in Chapter 12, Special Equids.

After all this is addressed and proper sixth or seventh level examination completed, appropriate odontoplasty is performed to correct abnormalities (See Chapter 14, Odontoplasty). Horses should awaken promptly from sedation after dentistry and should be keen to eat short grass as soon as they awaken. Unwillingness to eat after dentistry may indicate a serious problem which should be addressed within 24 hours by a veterinarian well-trained in modern equine veterinary dentistry.

The equipment and examination utilized at each level dictates the amount of information available to your dental operator. Here is a summary:

You can look at this in reverse: if your dental operator arrives with only a set of floats and nothing else, know that you'll only be getting a first level exam. If she rocks up with a full mouth speculum, a large dose syringe, and floats, you know you're probably in for a level four.

So, can you think of some pathology which may be missed at each of these levels? Maybe come back and answer that later, after you've read this book!

How is Equine Dentistry Changing?

IN THE PAST, it was accepted practice to merely look for problems when a horse showed us what we thought were the signs of dental pain. Things have changed to a more proactive approach:

- Today, we can perform thorough dental examinations with lights, safe speculums, stocks, and customized instruments. By doing great dental examinations every ear, we can identify early dental issues before they become deeply seated, even more painful, and more expensive to treat. Comprehensive dental examinations are a must.

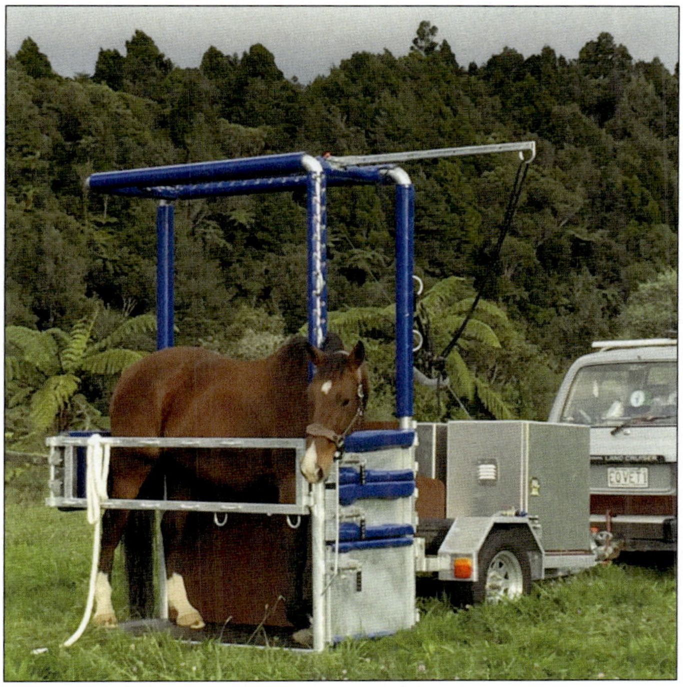

Maya checks out the new 2018 version of the Equi-Still Portable Stocks. He is completely happy in these padded, comfortable stocks. Image credit Author.

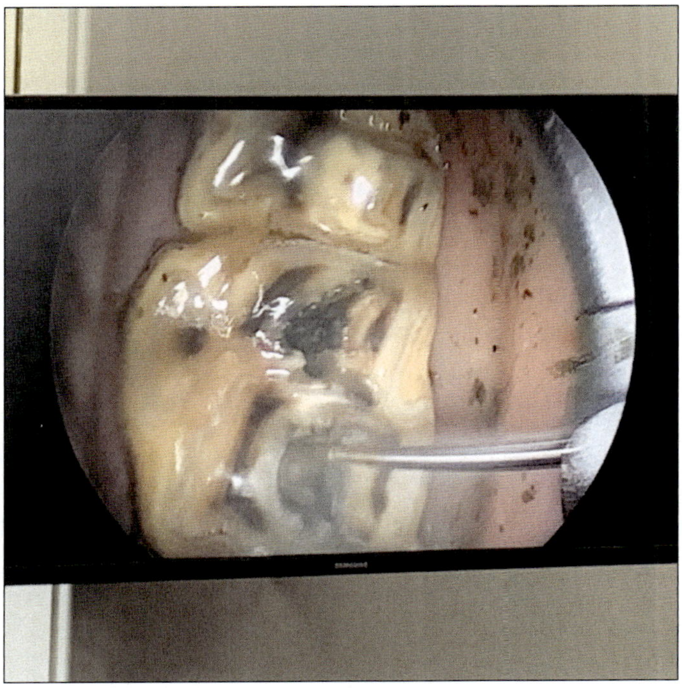

Restorative treatment under endoscopic guidance by Dr Nicole du Toit of Equine Dental Clinic in the UK. Image credit Nicole du Toit.

- Today, your own dentist would never give you a quick brush-up and send you on your way without properly examining your entire mouth as well as radiographing and perhaps scanning your teeth (some dentists use an oroscope, but it's not standard practice yet), both to evaluate problem areas and to screen for as-yet invisible but developing issues. Your veterinarian can provide thorough dental, radiographic, and oroscopic examinations to ensure your horse's mouth is the best it can be. Dental radiography and oroscopy are rapidly becoming standard of practice for the provision of equine dental care. Ask your dental veterinarian about it.
- Today, the advent of improved sedation and anesthetic protocols allows us to perform most dental surgeries standing without the need for general anesthesia. Added to that, the development of better equipment, including portable, water cooled, battery-operated high and low speed drills and odontoplasty equipment, all combine to provide the opportunity for every horse to have the care it deserves.

Levels of Dentistry: Equipment and Inclusions

First	hand or power float only
Second	add a wedge or spool gag
Third	add a full-mouth speculum
Fourth	add effective flushing unit to flush the mouth
Fifth	add light, sedation, headstand/dental halter,vet
Sixth	add mirror, probes, and picks, thorough dental exam
Seventh	add oroscope, precision dental exam
Eighth	add any indicated diagnostics: X-ray, ultrasound, scintigraphy, CT, MRI, laboratory analysis

Table of equipment and examinations utilized at each of the Eight Levels of Equine Dentistry. Image credit Author.

What Can Vets Do That Others Can't?

THERE'S A SAYING: "What vets can do, only vets can do". How's that? I may be biased towards veterinarians for performing dentistry, but it's probably not for the reason you think.

It's not because I'm protectionist of veterinarians. There are many reasons, beginning with the fact that veterinarians have completed a full course in veterinary medicine at an accredited veterinary school and are licensed to practice in the country (and state or province, in CA, the USA and many other places) in which they are practicing medicine and dentistry. Veterinarians have a full working understanding of anatomy, physiology, anesthesiology, cardiology, critical care, endocrinology, microbiology, neurology, radiology and radiography, surgery, dental pathology, infection control, nutrition, health and safety, veterinary ethics, current legislation, etc., all of which enable them to properly care for the entirety of your horse, *including* their mouth. They are also subject to comprehensive regulation as to the quality of their practice, plus they are usually insured. Veterinarians who perform a lot of equine dentistry have likely also taken significant postgraduate or postdoctoral courses in advanced equine veterinary dentistry and dental surgery. I term these *equine dental veterinarians* throughout this book. Veterinarians who have studied advanced equine dentistry and attained board certified equine dental qualifications are *specialist equine dental veterinarians*.

If you have a horse, you know that *things* happen. Your vet can be the best help when those *things* happen. The teeth are live tissue and are not an isolated part of your horse. Teeth are not blocks of wood. The tissues around the teeth, as well as the teeth, have nerves plus an exceptional blood supply. Teeth are attached to ligamentous and other tissues which anchor them to bone. All these tissues need proper veterinary care, as does the rest of your horse. Sedation is not something to be taken lightly. Sedation is vet-only for good reason. In untrained hands, sedation drugs and the results of sedation in an animal that outweighs us by ten times can be lethal—not only for your horse, but for those around him, including you and yours.

As such, I believe veterinarians with postdoctoral or postgraduate equine veterinary dental training are best placed to care for your horse's mouth. The exception is well-trained EDTs who work alongside veterinarians with the above training. Your opinion? Please wait to make a firm decision until you've read this whole book. I'll leave it up to you to decide for yourself at that time!

What Does the Title of a Person Performing Dentistry Really Mean? I'm Confused!

VARIOUS PEOPLE WHO work on equid teeth call themselves by many different titles: veterinarian, lay "dentist", equine dental technician (EDT), dental technician, equine "dentist", horse "dentist", etc. What do these terms really mean? Do they give you any indication of their education, proven competency, or continuing education? Have they passed examinations by an outside consumer or government regulatory board? For most of these, the short answer is no.

Why not use the term Dentist for these, or for non-specialist dental veterinarians?

First, because in most countries, the term "dentist" is a registered title and only registered human dentists are legally entitled to use it. In New Zealand, it falls under the HPCA Act 2003.

Second, because the term "Dentist" denotes a certain level of scholastic and practical achievement, not to mention qualification by rigorous examination. For humans, a significant course in dental science and demonstrated competency is required, along with regulatory licensing and continuing education to keep abreast of current therapy.

Third, veterinarians are not able to use the term Dentist unless they have earned the trademarked term "Veterinary Dentist" or "Specialist in Veterinary Dentistry". These are reserved for those veterinarians who have achieved a postgraduate specialty in veterinary dentistry, which is a post-doctorate diploma or fellowship equivalent to a four-year postgraduate residency and examination with demonstrated competency by examination, along with continuing education to keep abreast of current therapy. This compares to a human Dentist qualification, but a veterinary dental specialty is in total a longer course, when one includes veterinary school years.

Why not use EDT, dental technician, or dentist and instead use the term "lay dental operator" for non-veterinary operators of horse dentistry other than BAEDTs and IGFPs?

The term "technician" usually implies a certain level of education and demonstrated competency. While there *are* equine dental technicians who *do* have this level of education and demonstrated competency, especially the BAEDTs and IGFPs, unfortunately, this is not always the case. In many places, this "certain level of education and demonstrated competency" is not required of many non-veterinary operators of horse dentistry, and they can still use the title of "technician", "equine dental technician", or "EDT" as they desire.

Veterinarians with postgraduate training and certification in veterinary dentistry, but *not* holding a specialist equine dentistry qualification, may be known as equine dental veterinarians. They are *not* Veterinary Dentists. Neither should lay (non-veterinary) dental operators or EDTs be called "dentists", as first of all, "Dentist" is a reserved term for human dentists and veterinary specialist veterinarians, and second, this implies a certain level of education and demonstrated competency as well. Not all non-veterinary dental courses are equal. Even if a layperson (a non-veterinarian) calls themself a "dentist", it doesn't mean they are the best choice, no matter now nice they are to you and your horse. The dental education of non-veterinary lay dental operators varies from "learned from a friend" to a formal program with proper examination and certification by an outside consumer or government board. Unfortunately, many schools of horse dentistry create their own certification and are not answerable to anyone but themselves, other than to the humane and welfare laws of their domicile. Unfortunately, having these certifications gives the appearance of legitimacy, which can be problematic, as it gives credibility to a system which cannot be legitimate. Depending upon the area in which they work and reside, most lay dental operators are not regulated by outside consumer bodies or boards, their workmanship is not usually insured, and they don't usually have a requirement for annual continuing education. Notable exceptions are 1-BAEDT (UK) dental technicians, who often hold insurance through BAEDT, and 2- dental technicians employed by and working directly with veterinarians, who are usually deemed part of the practice of the veterinarian who is supervising and responsible for the work of that technician.

For all the reasons detailed above, in this book I refer to non-veterinary operators of horse dentistry as either EDTs (if they have one of the two qualifications described above) or "lay dental operators". This is not intended to be derogatory, but to ensure everyone is perfectly clear on the possible limitations on education, qualification, and accountability of those working with your horses.

What do you call veterinarians who have postgraduate veterinary dental training but are not specialists?

Dental veterinarians, or *equine dental veterinarians*. They have obtained postgraduate training in equine dentistry after passing a five- to eight-year (depending upon the country) course in pre-veterinary and veterinary medicine including anesthesiology, cardiology, critical care, endocrinology, ethics, neurology, physiology, radiology and radiography, surgery, etc. They are examined and regulated by outside consumer bodies or governmental veterinary boards. Their professional workmanship is usually insured, and they must complete prescribed, regular continuing education to stay up to date on current therapies and procedures. All of this training and practice enables them to properly care for the entirety of your horse, *including* its mouth.

What is the Minimum Instrumentation Needed for a Thorough Examination?

I HOPE IT is clear to you by now that to perform dentistry to a thorough level, your dental practitioner needs at minimum the following equipment:

- safe, full-mouth speculum
- large dose syringe or hose to flush the mouth with water
- strong light source
- intraoral mirror
- dental picks and probes
- dental floats or a power floating unit
- veterinarian to examine and sedate the horse if a veterinarian is not performing the dentistry.

I once thought I did a pretty good job of dentistry without sedation, until I started learning more about it and began looking much deeper.

I recently manned a booth for the NZ Equine Veterinary Association at an equestrian event called Equifest in New Zealand and spoke with hundreds of people during the event. I started by asking nearly every person walking past our booth if they'd like to look inside a horse's mouth. Most of them took up the offer, so I seated them on my rolling stool in front of a clean horse skull which had been set up on a headstand and covered with a towel to mimic the darkness inside of a mouth.

They first peered up into the darkness, frowning slightly, until I gave them a headlamp.

"OOOH!", most said, at the brilliance of the interior of the mouth.

"Do you see all of the teeth now?" I asked each of them.

"Yes!" they all exclaimed, whether they were three years old or 83.

"And can you see every surface of every tooth?"

Most said no, but a few said "Yes".

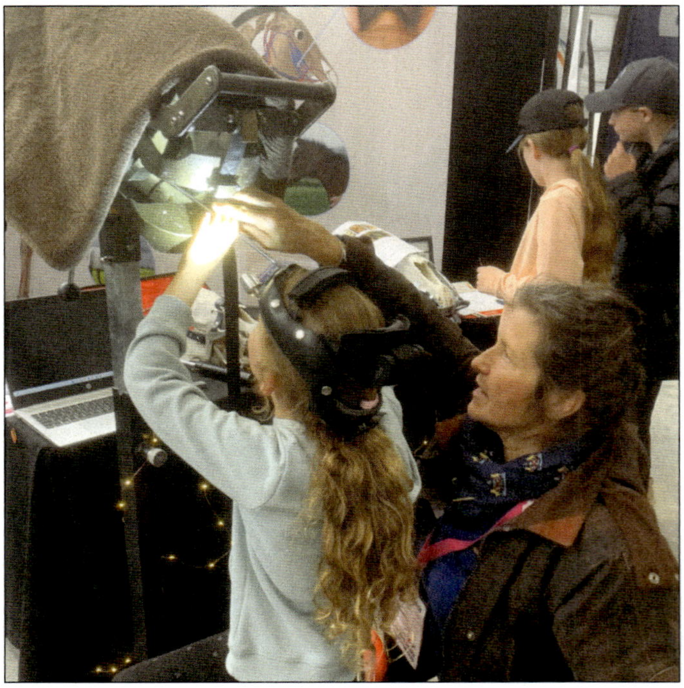

Young attendee at a horse event learning what can be discovered with a dental mirror, speculum, and good light inside a clean horse's mouth. Image credit Dr Holly Blue.

"You're better than I am, then! I can't see every surface, especially when the cheeks and tongue are in there!"

"I guess not," these all agreed.

"How about if I give you a mirror?" I asked, showing them how to hold it and see all the surfaces.

"Now I can see them all!", most of them exclaimed, the light coming on in their eyes.

"So, do you agree you need a mirror to do a thorough dental examination?"

"Yes, absolutely," was the most common response, but all agreed.

"But do you want me to put a mirror in your horse's mouth if it's unsedated and awake? And do you think you could do a really good dental exam with a mirror in an unsedated horse?"

"Definitely not!", or "No!" they said, with a look of horror.

If these keen horse people got nothing else from the show, I would be happy.

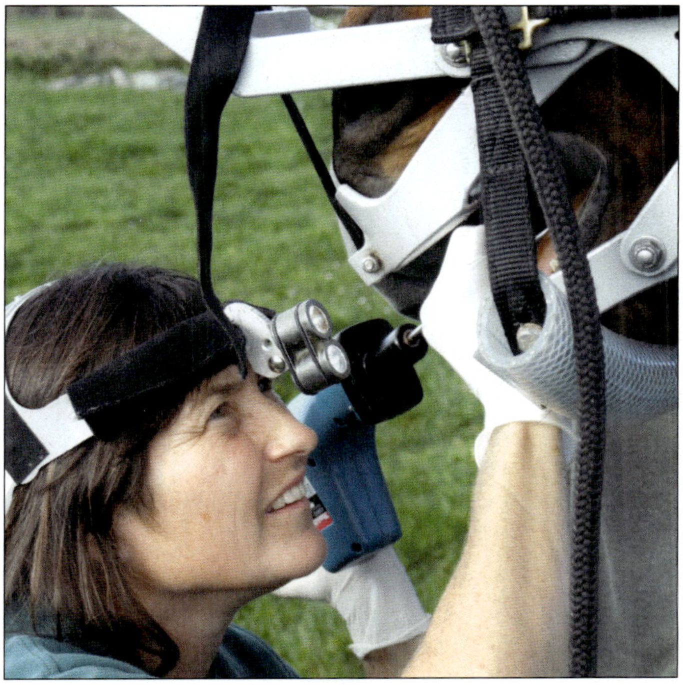

Working in the mouth of a properly supported and sedated horse, with a good headlamp and safe equipment. Image credit James Hewitt.

Sedation allows a thorough examination to be performed on every horse, every time. Not just when the horse prefers. Sedation is excellent for safety while using a mirror in a horse's mouth, but just as importantly, it offers safety for the handler and the horse as well. Visualization of many small intraoral structures is next to impossible in the unsedated horse, and the international standard of practice in veterinary equine dentistry dictates that these structures are evaluated. The use of X-Rays by your veterinary dental practitioner is required for the diagnosis, treatment, and monitoring of many of the more challenging (and unfortunately, common), conditions. Does your dentist take radiographs of your own teeth? Think about it.

Who Can Use Power Filing Instruments? Can't Anyone Buy Them?

While power dental grinding instruments are replacing many hand instruments for the educated equine dental practitioner, they are not for use by the untrained nor insufficiently trained. Power floating instruments require significant training in their proper use. They also require the judicious use of water to cool the teeth and *especially*, a thorough knowledge of dental anatomy and physiology to understand why this is so important to the life of your horse. Proper use of instruments and water cooling minimizes the potential for thermal (heat) damage to the tooth pulps.

Used judiciously in well-trained hands, they are a time- and effort-saving tool which allows the practitioner to work on specific portions of the individual teeth they wish to treat, which is difficult-to-impossible with hand rasps. This allows the operator to leave the mouth of every horse the best they can possibly make it within the constraints of the teeth themselves. The last horse of the day can receive the same quality of care as the first one.

Power dental instruments should never be used by untrained floaters, or even experienced practitioners untrained in their use, as damage can occur rapidly.

Pulps may be exposed by the aggressive hand floats now in use, but with power instruments it can happen much more quickly. Whether using power or hand instruments, your equine dental practitioner must understand and take into account that the ***dentinal tubules*** which contain extensions of the pulp may reside as little as one millimeter (3/64 of an inch) beneath the surface of an overgrown tooth. Removing more than this, whether by grinding or cutting, may expose pulp. If any pulp is exposed, indicated by a pink or red (bleeding!) spot on the surface of the tooth, vital pulpotomy is needed, ideally within 24–36 hours, to try to prevent death of that tooth over the next few years. Even a pulp "near exposure" may put the tooth at risk. A vital pulpotomy will be explained in detail in later chapters, but in short, it is a procedure to cover the exposed live part of the tooth with dental composites to protect it from further trauma and infection. The vital pulpotomy surgery itself is a "painful procedure" and to perform it, one must enter live tissue.

As such, this procedure should only be (and depending upon your location, may legally *only be*) performed by a registered veterinarian trained in the procedure.

Red Flags: Instruments Which can Seriously Damage Your Horse

What are molar cutters or molar shears, and how are they dangerous?

While molar shears or cutters are not power instruments, they are probably even more dangerous for two main reasons:

First, their usage is not incremental, as is odontoplasty, and they do not allow the operator to evaluate the distance to live pulp, which increases the risk of ***pulpar exposure***. When you cut off a piece of tooth with this modified bolt cutter, you cannot see if pulp is in the way of your cut. These have historically been used for long crown ***eruptions***, or ***overgrowths*** on teeth which were not in apposition to another tooth.The position of the pulp in an "unopposed" tooth is extremely close to the occlusal surface and pulps can readily be exposed.

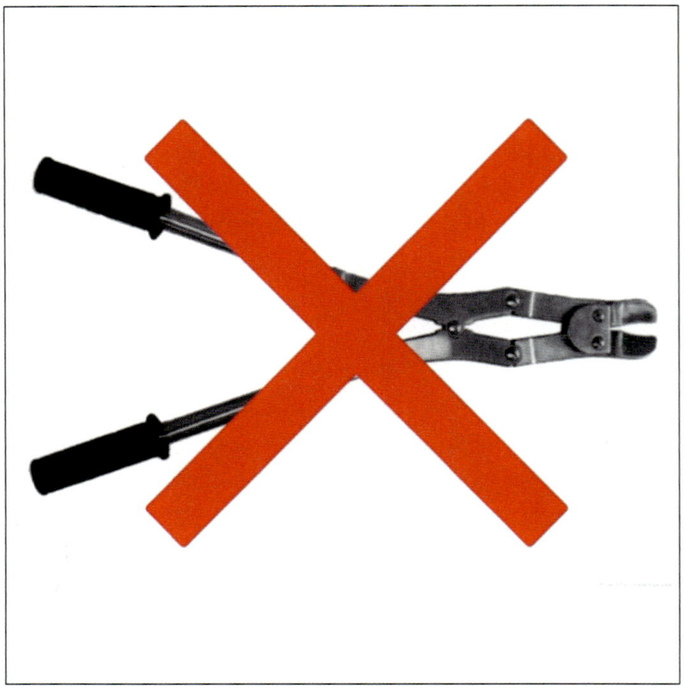

Molar cutters or molar shears are best used as bolt cutters for cutting steel. Not for teeth, which are best left alive. Image credit Author.

Second, teeth cut with molar cutters tend to crack on a longitudinal, or ***apex***-to-occlusal line, which will require extraction of a live tooth (significance: still alive, painful, and stuck tightly in place), which will shortly die, causing excruciating pain to your horse before that happens, but will be difficult to remove in its entirety. Molar cutters are best used as bolt cutters for cutting steel, which is not alive. The only exception to this is during extraction of a tooth, for a veterinarian to section a tooth in a transverse plane (cutting across the tooth) by a sectioning burr. This is only necessary when a cheek tooth is partially extracted but is too long and is blocked from fully exiting the ***alveolus*** due to lack of available height in the mouth. This tends to occur in young horses (relatively long cheek teeth) with a small mouth.

Cut-off wheels? How can they hurt my horse?

The flat surface of a powered cut-off wheel may be safely used in a sedated horse by a veterinarian to carefully reduce tooth overgrowths by grinding with the *flat* of the blade, when coupled with water cooling and careful observation. This

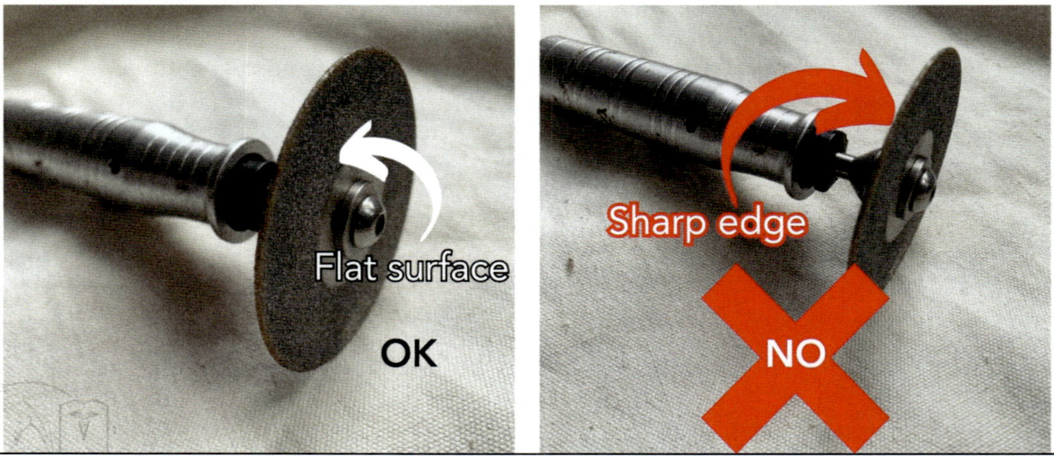

Using the sharp edge of a cut-off wheel to slice across a live tooth is contraindicated, as it is likely to lead to pulp exposure and tooth death. The flat side may be used carefully with intermittent water cooling and observation to watch for disappearance of dentinal staining to prevent pulp exposure, as with other power dental instruments. Image credit Author.

is *not* the same as using the edge of the cut-off wheel. When the sharp edge of a cut-off wheel is used to cut transversely across a tooth, cutting off a slice of ***crown elongation***, the operator may expose living pulp or some of the pulp's tiny extensions, both of which endanger the life of a tooth. Vital pulpotomy by a veterinarian is indicated if a ***pulp exposure*** or near-pulp exposure occurs. See Chapter 3, Anatomy of the Mouth and Chapter 9, Iatrogenic Disease.

How could one-sided or unilateral gags be seriously dangerous?

These go by the name of Bayer, Schouppe, spool, coil, Landmeisser, wedge, and the like. They have a bite piece which fits between the ***cheek teeth*** made of either:

- cylindrical spring steel or a solid metal cylinder (the "spool" types), or
- a wedge of metal, plastic, or rubber (the wedge types).

The only benefit from using either of these types of gag is slightly easier floating of the teeth because one side of the mouth is held open to some degree. However, these gags are not recommended because at best, they don't significantly assist in examining the mouth or floating, and at worst, they frequently cause serious damage. The reasons for this are as follows:

- A horse ***masticates*** (chews) a lot with a unilateral (one-sided) gag in place. This makes it difficult to examine the teeth, which should be done before the teeth are filed.
- As the gag occupies mouth space on the side where it is placed, the tongue is pushed toward the other side where examination or floating is being attempted. This decreases visibility inside the mouth, already minimal at this level, and makes floating more difficult.
- The ***temporomandibular*** or jaw joint, commonly known as the TMJ, may be damaged when a horse bites down hard on only one side at a time
- If the gag slips from between the teeth to the inside of the teeth, the palatine artery may be ruptured. It bleeds. A lot. For a long time.

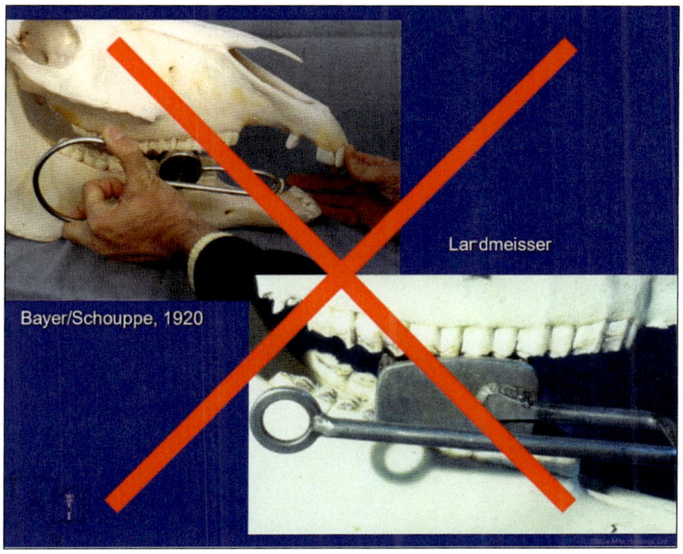

The image shows two of the many NON-recommended gags which are sometimes used at The Second Level: Shown are the Bayer/Schouppe (1920) and the Landmeisser. These can seriously damage teeth and other tissues, including the fracture of cheek teeth. Unmarked image credit Dr Jack Easley. Graphic credit Author.

- *Most seriously, however,* the danger of fracturing cheek teeth is very real. The cylindrical shape of the "spool" types causes the entire force of both sides of the strong masseter (chewing) muscles to be focused on a narrow line across two opposing teeth, which may lead to a fractured cheek tooth or teeth, with severe consequences. A fractured tooth needs to be extracted. A fractured tooth will cause your horse a lot of pain until the tooth is discovered and extracted. Make no mistake, this is a major surgery, especially because that recently-healthy tooth will be firmly stuck in place. And the worst thing? ***The fracture never had to happen in the first place.***

What about a captive bolt percussion tooth cutter, that "chips" off the tooth? They're slick!

These are ***not*** slick. These captive bolt tooth cutters are dangerous to the life of your horse. These tools (I won't give them the credit of calling them instruments...) are placed over the crown elongation of a tooth and with a slam of the attached weight, cut off the elongation in one go, cutting the tooth at whatever level they are placed (or wherever they happen to slip to). I imagine by now you understand what can also happen... Not only will it remove the elongation, but it may also cause an unintended tooth fracture, and will most likely (almost 100% of the

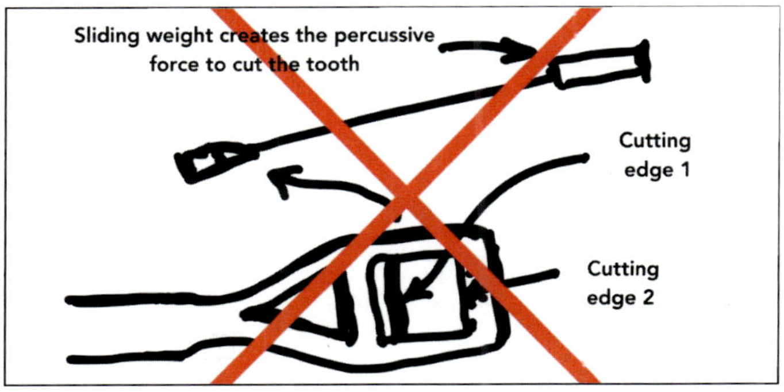

Captive bolt percussion cutting tool. Totally contraindicated. Sorry, but luckily I could not find one to photograph. Image credit Author.

time) expose the pulp, which you also probably now also know will cause a pulpitis, with likely tooth death sometime down the road... The tooth will fracture in any direction it chooses... not ideal, and disastrous for the horse. If a horse has a weakened jaw, perhaps from underlying ***osteomyelitis***, the use of this captive bolt percussion tooth cutter could also fracture the skull. I think it's fair to say these are ***contraindicated*** at all times.

ANATOMY OF THE MOUTH? HOW MUCH COULD THERE BE?

"First, then, let there be no mistake about the age. If the horse has lost his mark [...] not only will the purchaser's hopes be blighted, but he may find himself saddled for ever with a sorry bargain."
—Xenophon, On Horsemanship, Gutenberg translation

WHY DO WE need to understand anatomy? Because without it, we cannot understand what we need to know to help our horses. I will use images of "cleaned" skulls (only the bone, no soft ***tissue*** like skin, muscle, tendon, cartilage, etc.) to illustrate many of the anatomical concepts and parts below, as it is much clearer when there is no hair, tongue, cheeks, or personalities to mask what I'm trying to describe.

Equid teeth are very unlike ours. While humans have ***brachydont*** (short-***crowned***) teeth, horses have ***hypsodont*** (long crowned) teeth, with exposed ***enamel*** ridges throughout the tooth to help grind rough grasses and grains.

You will find more descriptions of the teeth and mouth later in this chapter, and remember, you'll find words in ***bold italics*** in the glossary.

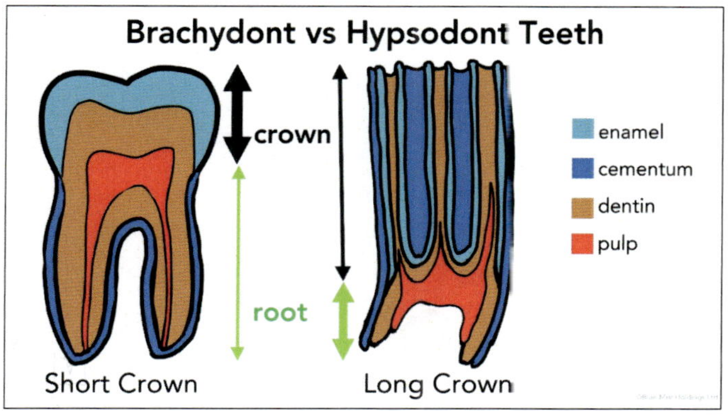

The long-crowned hypsodont tooth has short roots and the short-crowned brachydont tooth has the reverse. Image credit Author.

How did Equid Teeth, or Dentition, Evolve?

AROUND 50 MILLION years ago, the evolutionary predecessors of the horse had evolved to Eohippus, or Hyracotherium, which were medium dog-sized foraging-browsers living in a forest environment and dining on leaves, fruit, vines, and twigs. They had short-crowned, brachydont teeth, similar to ours, and dogs, for example. Over the next 30 million years, as the environment changed, becoming drier, and more grasslands-like, the fossil record shows evolution of the next of our horse's predecessors, some overlapping in the same strata, through the presence of Orohippus, Epihippus, Mesohippus, Parahippus. As the available feeds changed gradually to rougher grass which required more grinding to extract the nutrition needed to survive, many changes occurred in the evolving lines of animals toward becoming hypsodont, such as 1) ***premolars***, starting with the ones furthest back in the mouth and progressing toward the front of the mouth, 2) increasing numbers of paired cusps on the teeth, and 3) gradual increase in length of the teeth. These changes all facilitated the grinding of harder feeds.

This evolution progressed gradually until around 10-15 million years ago, when the pony sized *Merychippus* evolved, with its longer face and longer legs to escape predators. Its teeth had made a major jump to become the first true hypsodont in its lineage, with long crowns and ***cementum*** coating the entire tooth. The fossil record showed further development of Equus, with six molarized ***cheek teeth***, as seen in our modern *Equus caballus*. There are more detailed discussions of equid dentition elsewhere, but for our purposes, this will suffice.

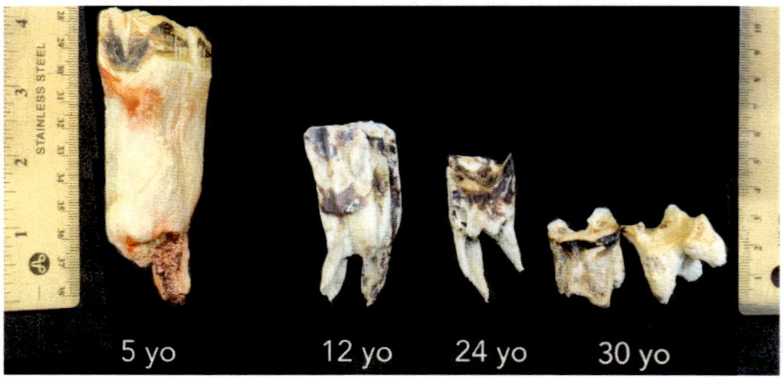

These teeth are lined up by their apices. These are all pathologic teeth from extractions, but this illustrates how long teeth truly are in young horses! Image credit Author.

What are Chewing and Grinding Patterns?

WHILE IT MAY appear that horses pull grass with their ***incisors***, they actually use their strong lips to grasp the feed or grass and pull it between their incisors. Their incisors are used to cut the grass or feed, but the real grinding is done by the cheek teeth. The feed material is moved toward the back, or ***distally*** (***caudally***) through the mouth by the auger-like action of the palate, tongue, and cheek teeth.

Horses have a chewing pattern which enables them to build up huge grinding forces with their cheek teeth. They begin with an opening stroke followed by a closing stroke, then a power stroke, and finishing with a recovery stroke toward a resting position. The force generated by the closing stroke and the power stroke is huge, and studies have shown the force increases as one measures from the '06s toward the '11s. The power stroke can generate an astonishing 1800 Newtons of force on the cheek teeth at the back of the mouth. To give you an idea of what that amount of force equals, imaging dropping a weight of 10 kg from a height of approximately 1600 meters (around 1.6 km), or a mile high. This would generate around 1800 Newtons of force upon impact. Safety Alert: You really don't want your fingers between a horse's teeth, especially the cheek teeth!

Horses without teeth, or with few effective teeth, are still able to eat feed if it is presented in a ground-up or pelleted form due to this auger-action. However, if feed is presented to these horses in a form they cannot grind well, such as hay or long-stemmed grass, they tend to drop spirally-wound, unground boluses of feed ("quids"), or swallow them, which may be the cause of "choke", or esophageal obstruction. Finding these ***quids*** in your horse's paddock or stall indicates your horse is probably having significant problems with its mouth.

What are Some Anatomical and Historical Considerations?

WE HAVE SEEN that horse teeth differ from those of humans in their structure, but they also differ in their timing of ***tooth eruption***. Equids have ***prolonged eruption***. An equid's individual ***permanent*** (adult) teeth continue to erupt for most of their lives, (approximately 20–30 years for cheek teeth), unless the teeth or their supporting structures become diseased. Unlike rats and rabbits, their teeth do not continue to grow after the roots develop (for the cheek teeth, that is about two years after they erupt into the mouth), which accounts for a horse tooth's finite life. See below. The tooth on the far right is nearly "used up" and would soon be ***exfoliated*** (shed, lost, or fallen out).

Tooth wear is the result of three processes: ***abrasion*** (wear produced by interaction between teeth and other materials), ***attrition*** (wear through tooth-to-tooth contact) and ***erosion*** (dissolution of hard tissue by acidic substances).Teeth undergo wear as they grind rough feeds against the teeth of the opposing ***arcade,*** or row of teeth, until the teeth become ***cupped***, and then ***expired*** (the hard enamel has worn away) and only the softer tooth structures called ***dentin*** and cementum remain. After some time, the short stubs of roots are exfoliated.

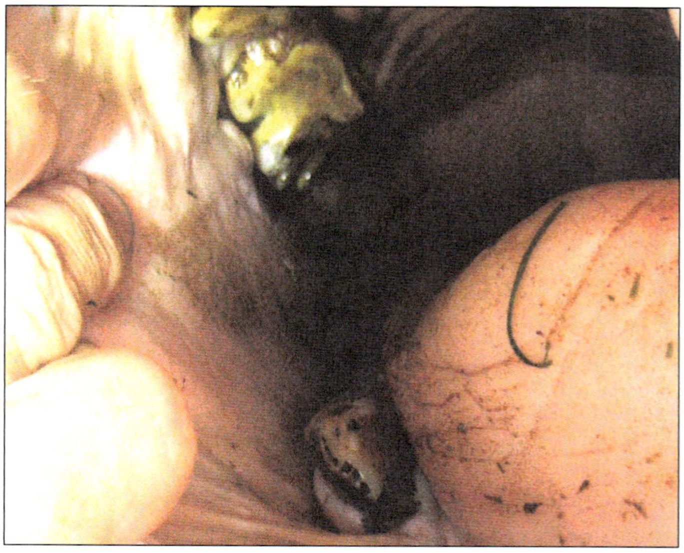

Cheek teeth are cupped in this aged horse. Image credit Author.

So, we need to help them take care of their teeth. Since we don't tend to keep domestic equids in the same environment in which they evolved, the feeds we offer them differ from those they have evolved to eat, so we need to help them. But why?

Let's start with the wild or feral horses. Why do our horses need dental care when wild horses don't? First, we have selectively bred domestic horses for things like speed and jumping ability, rather than for "good teeth". In the wild, a process called "natural selection", or "survival of the fittest" allows only the strongest and fittest to survive. Natural selection keeps horses with suboptimal or "not so perfect" teeth out of the gene pool, as horses who cannot eat well tend to become undernourished. Undernourished horses cannot run as fast nor fight as well as their healthier herd-mates and thus become easy prey for predators—and therefore are less likely to survive to reproduce. Second, our horses don't live under the wild conditions under which horses evolved. Think of the frigid steppe of Mongolia, for example. The natural diet there is devoid of copious amounts of grains and easily fermented sugars, and comprises primarily relatively soft grasses. Most of these grasses cause significantly less wear on teeth than grains, even though horses on the Mongolian steppe graze for twelve to sixteen hours per day. Refined sugars, honey, sugar beet, and low pH feeds in the modern domesticated horse's diet may also contribute to dental disease. Increased bacterial growth encouraged by readily available sugars produces acid, which results in a relative acidity, or a lower pH, inside the mouth. This lower pH may lead to ***periodontal*** disease, infundibular and ***peripheral caries***, and premature tooth loss. All told, our modern feeding may contribute detrimentally to our horses' dental disease, although it allows us to maintain our horse's weight more easily than with feeding grass or hay alone.

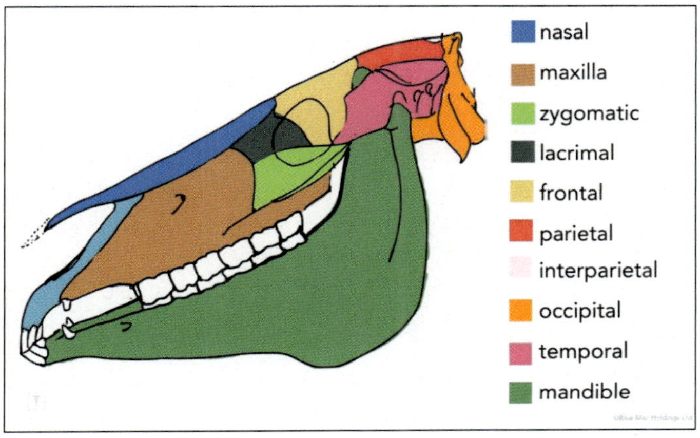

Major bones of the skull are given in the legend to the right. The lines where two bones join are called the "sutures", which will become significant later in Chapter 6 and 10. Image credit Author.

Here's a Skull: Let's Start With the Basics!

A BARE SKULL best illustrates what I'm trying to describe in many of the images below.

Primary bones of the skull

The top portion of the skull is the ***maxilla***. Along with many other structures, it contains the maxillary (upper), teeth. The bottom portion is the ***mandible***, or jawbone. It contains the mandibular (lower) teeth.

When viewing the head from the outside, we use the terms ***rostral*** (toward the nose) and ***caudal*** (toward the tail) to indicate direction. The front twelve teeth that you can see when a horse's lips are open are called the incisors, the back teeth are called cheek teeth, and in between are the ***canines*** and the ***wolf teeth***. These teeth are arranged in well-defined blocks called arcades. The line between the central teeth of the incisor arcades is referred to as the ***midline***, which will be discussed below. Note that where two bones of the skull join is called a ***suture***.

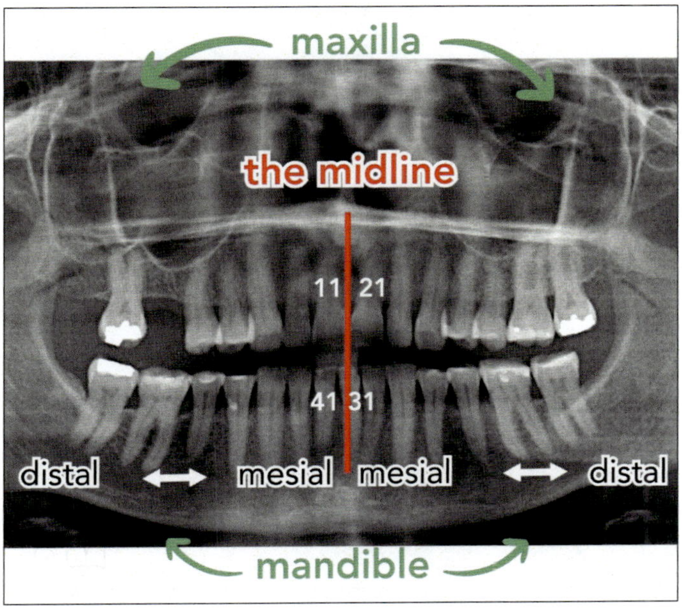

Here is the OPG of a human (see next page). Note the midline (red), the maxilla, the mandible, and how the toward the midline is mesial and away from the midline is distal. Since there are less than ten teeth in each grade, only two digits are used to name teeth, compared to the horse's three digits in the Modified Triadan nomenclature system. The horse's right is to your left.

Once we are inside the mouth, we can see the incisors. The line between the two central incisors on the mandible and maxilla becomes important in naming the the teeth, just like in human dentistry. ***Veterinary*** dentistry is becoming more like human dentistry, so we are using more of their terms like ***mesial*** (toward the midline) and distal (away from the midline) to describe their positions. You may be used to hearing the terms rostral and caudal inside the mouth, but we are getting away from using these terms (which we still use on the outside of the head) like rostral and caudal.

The midline in a horse's mouth (and in yours!) is located between the central incisors, at the red lines in the two images to the right and below. The tooth surfaces closest to the midline (the red line) are called the mesial surfaces. The space between the surfaces of two teeth touching each other are called the ***interproximal spaces.*** To help understand this better, think about a human full-mouth X-ray, called an OPG (see previous page). The middle of a human's dental arcade is usually at the red line marked "midline" in the image. This X-ray is taken around a person's face and then it is turned into a flat picture for the dentist to study.

Now think of a horse. If we were able to take an OPG of your horse and lay it out flat, a schematic of it would look like this, which is also a dental chart for a horse (see above right)!

Everyone's brain works differently, and the diagram below may make more sense to some readers (see right).

Now let's translate that back to a 3-D horse. If you wrap that dental chart around its skull, voila! (See below)

In case you have trouble remembering ***mesial*** vs ***distal***, here is help (see image to right): **"Mes**ial" is towards the **mid**line of the curve of the incisor dental arcade while "**dist**al" is **dist**ant, or further away from the that same midline. **Remember: mesial and distal apply to both tooth surfaces and the entire inside of the mouth. Rostral and caudal should only be used outside the mouth.**

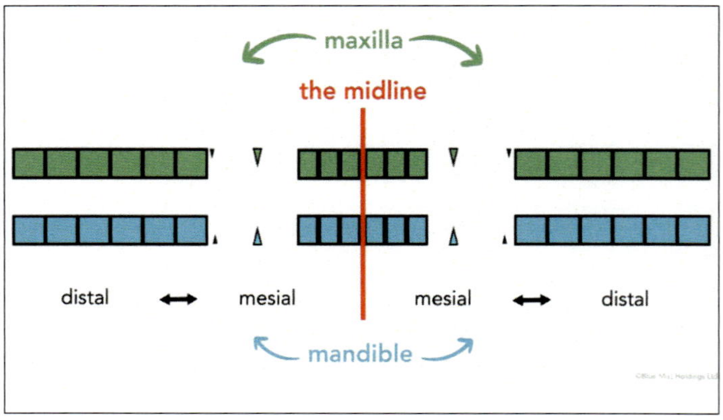

Compare this equine dental chart to the human OPG to see the horse's teeth laid out flat so one can see how the "mesial" direction is toward the midline and "distal" is away from the same midline. The horse's right is to your left. Image credit Author.

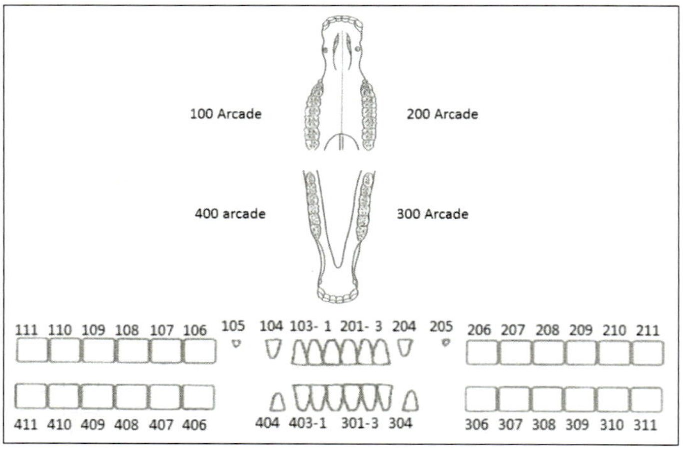

Another image illustrating the Modified Triadan tooth numbering system. Image credit Dr Kirsten Jackson, Dental Vet.

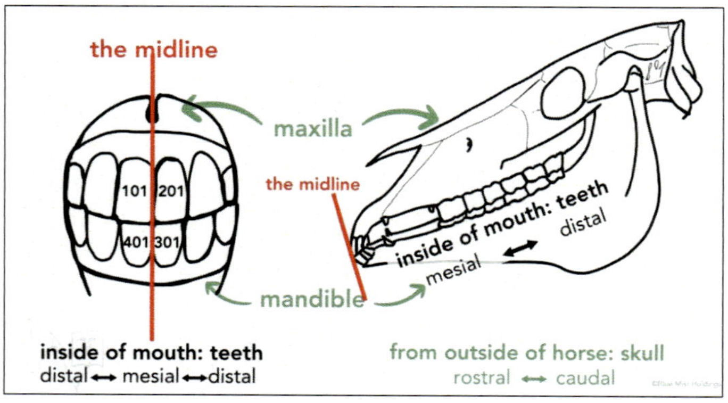

The maxilla and the mandible are the two main portions of the skull. Rostral and caudal are used to describe directions (as shown in green). Once inside the mouth, however, the terms mesial and distal are used instead of rostral and caudal. The midline is shown in red, between the "central incisors", or teeth 101 and 201, and between teeth 301 and 401, via the Modified Triadan System, which will be introduced shortly. Image credit Author.

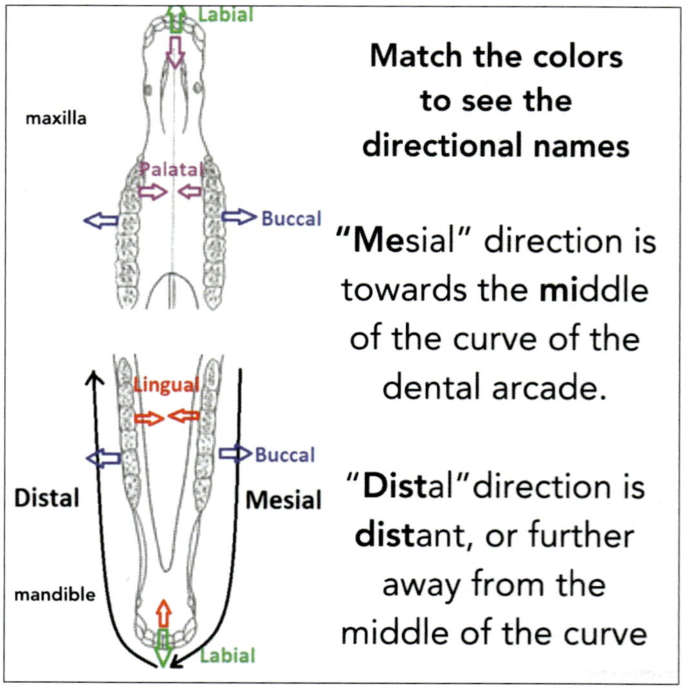

Here's a mnemonic to remember mesial and distal... Original image credit Dr Kirsten Jackson, Dental Vet. Graphic credit Author.

The maxilla and the mandible contain the ***alveoli*** (singular: ***alveolus***), or the tooth sockets. The alveoli are relatively flexible to accommodate the changing shape of teeth which have prolonged eruption. The alveolus is made up of two different types of bone: the lamina dura and the spongy bone. The lamina dura is a thin layer of very radiodense compact bone, which means the thin layer should show up as a hard, white line on radiographs. The Sharpey's fibers, which are important in the prolonged eruption of the teeth, attach to the lamina dura. The spongy bone surrounding the lamina dura and melding with the spongy bone of the mandible and maxilla remains spongy throughout life. It is less radiodense, and therefore blacker on radiographs. Compare the radiograph above right to the mandibular bone cadaver specimen immediately to the right, where the bone overlying the cheek teeth reserve crowns has been removed so you can see the teeth in position.

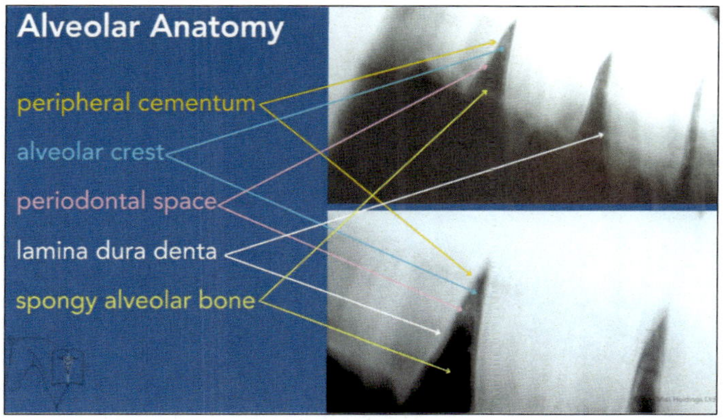

The alveolus is formed from elements of bone, tooth, and periodontal ligament. Image credit Author.

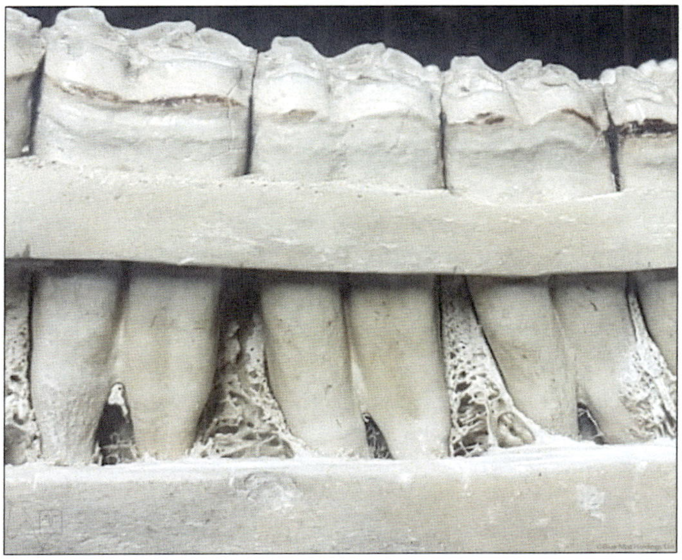

One can clearly see the spongy bone and lamina dura dental on this opened mandibular prep of a skull. Image credit Cathie Heald Greenwell.

Triadan nomenclature: For simplicity, we will be naming the teeth according to the Modified Triadan System (Triadan for short), which uses three numbers to identify each specific tooth. (in human dentistry, only two numbers are used, since people don't usually have more than nine teeth in each arcade, and therefore can use two numbers. The first number denotes the quadrant in which the tooth resides, and the next two numbers denote the position of the tooth, numbered from the most mesial incisor (the central incisor) to the most distal ***cheek tooth***.

In more detail, the four quadrants are named from *our* position as we look into the mouth. See image bottom right.

The first number of a tooth's Triadan name indicates the quadrant in which the tooth resides. Teeth are named from *our* top left (<u>the *horse's* top right</u>), and proceed clockwise as:

100 on *your* top left, then across right to the **200**, then down to the **300**, then across left to the **400**

For the **deciduous** *(baby) teeth*, the numbers differ slightly. Deciduous teeth are also numbered clockwise from our top left again, but start with 500 and progress to 800, or:

500 on *your* top left, then across right to the **600**, then down to the **700**, then across left to the **800.**

The second and third numbers of a tooth's Triadan name start with the '01 at the most mesial teeth, the central incisors. The three incisors are denoted by '01 to '03, the canines by '04, the wolf tooth '05, the cheek teeth by '06-'11 (premolars '06-'08, and the molars as '09-'11). Have a look at the naming protocol in this image.

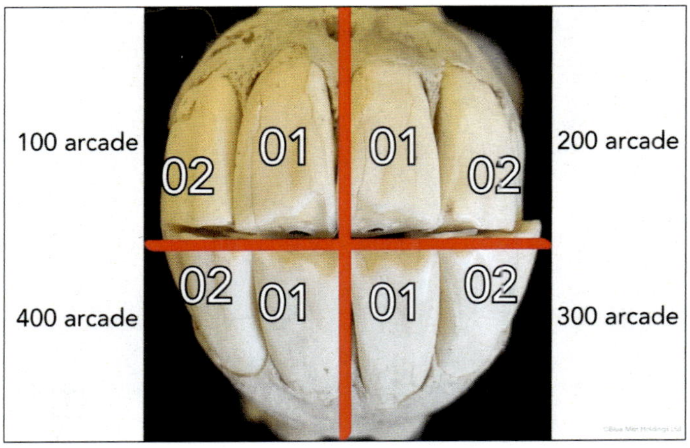

Modified Triadan System used in equids to name the teeth. Image credit Author.

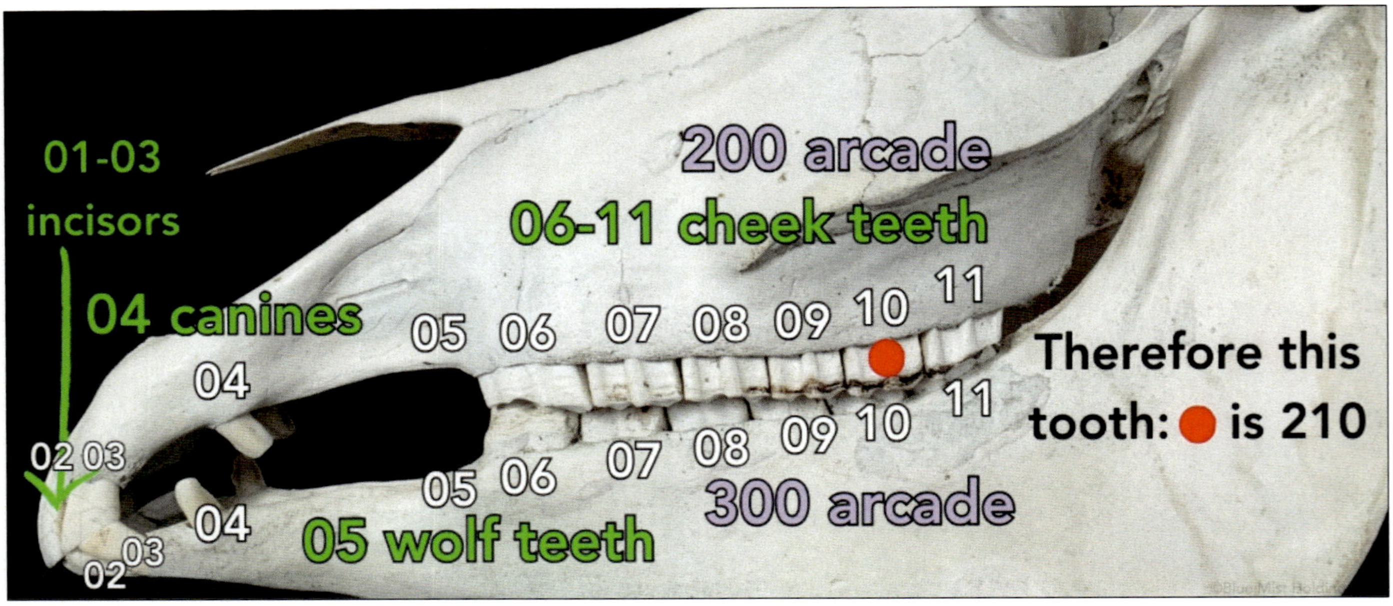

Numbering the teeth distal to the incisors follows the same idea. Image credit Author.

Remember, the first number is the quadrant number from YOU standing in FRONT of the HORSE, facing the horse.

Temporomandibular joint:

The ***temporomandibular joint (TMJ)*** is the jaw joint. It joins the mandible and maxilla, which are also connected by the many strong muscles of ***mastication*** (chewing). This joint has a wide range of sideways motion to to allow a horse to effectively grind hard feedstuffs.

The TMJ also allows the mandible to move rostrally (forward, letting the jaw drop) when the head is lowered.

Types of Teeth and Nearby Structures

EQUIDS HAVE BOTH deciduous teeth and ***permanent*** teeth, as previously mentioned. As the time for exfoliation (shedding/falling out) of a deciduous tooth approaches, the developing and erupting permanent tooth places

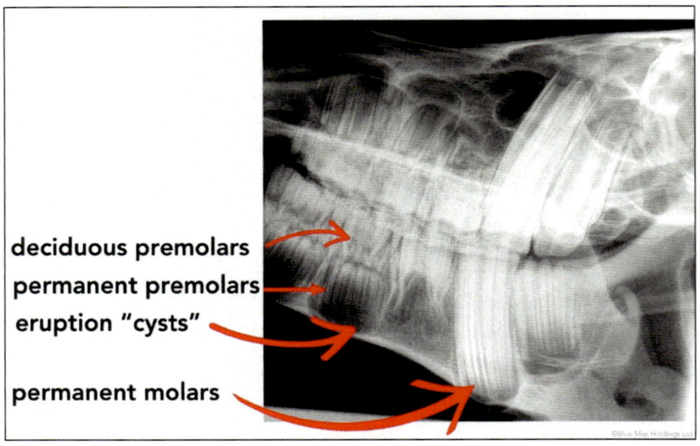

Deciduous and permanent molars and premolars, plus eruption cysts of the permanent premolars are evident in this young Miniature. There is little room in this skull for anything but teeth! Non-miniature horses have significantly more room. Unmarked image credit Dr Amy Ardern, graphic credit Author.

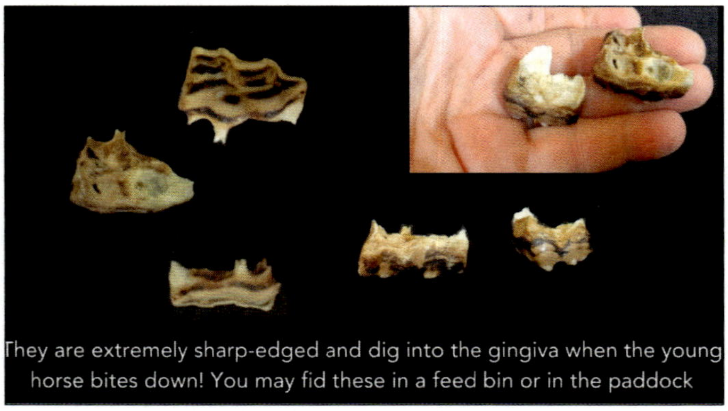

You may find these deciduous "caps" which are normally exfoliated at this time. Image credit Author.

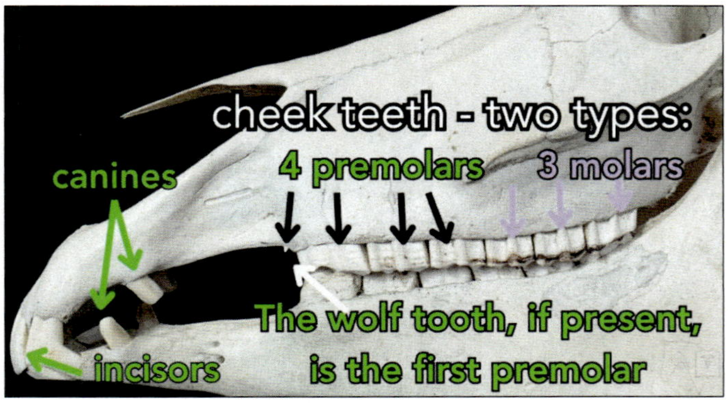

The classes of teeth are illustrated here. While this image shows the older standard names (incisors, canines, premolars, molars), we will be naming teeth using the modified Triadan method in this book for clarity. Image credit Author.

pressure upon the roots of the corresponding deciduous tooth and cause the roots to be resorbed (dissolved and assimilated into the body).

When development proceeds normally, the deciduous tooth (at this stage, called a "cap") falls out and the permanent tooth moves into the correct location vacated by the exfoliated deciduous tooth.

There "should be" a certain number of teeth of each type (incisors, canines, premolars, molars), when development of the ***dentition*** (teeth) goes to plan. Development, however, does not always do this. These variations will be discussed in the following chapters.

From mesial or ***rostral*** (toward the nostrils) to distal or caudal (toward the back of the head) the teeth or anatomical landmarks are called:

Incisors: There should be three of these teeth in each arcade, or twelve incisors in total (three incisors per arcade) x (four arcades) = twelve incisors. There are normally twelve deciduous incisors and later, after the deciduous incisors are shed, twelve permanent incisors. With Triadan numbering, the permanent incisors are named as X(the quadrant)01, X02, or X03 . The 01-03 are the first three incisors starting at the most mesial tooth. In the old nomenclature, the incisors were denoted by "central", "intermediate", and "corner" for incisor '01, '02, and '03, respectively. Remember, the X for the *deciduous* incisor quadrant names, rather than the 1-2-3-4 of the permanent teeth, are 5-6-7 and 8, also in the clockwise direction.

Canines: There should be no canine or one canine in each arcade, or in total, between zero and four canines. With Triadan numbering, the canines are denoted by X(the quadrant)04, or 104, 204, 304, or 404. While canines may be present in any horse, they are more common and often larger in males. They have evolved for fighting, with sharp distal edges for biting their opponent and ripping backwards. If these teeth do not fully erupt through the ***mucosa*** into the ***oral*** cavity, or mouth, they are termed "unerupted canines".

Bars of the mouth (previously called diastema): The area of the mandible and maxilla between the canines and the premolars is devoid of teeth. This has historically been called the diastema, or "bars of the mouth". The bit sits on the tongue in the area defined by the bars. It is now preferred, however, to reserve the term ***diastema/ diastemata*** for a *pathologic* gap between teeth which would normally be packed together in a tight arcade, whether incisors or cheek teeth.

The Tooth Numbers: Incisors

Numbering: XYY

where:
X= quadrant number
YY= tooth number

Incisor here: ●
X = 4 (400 quadrant)
Y = 03
thus ● tooth is named 403

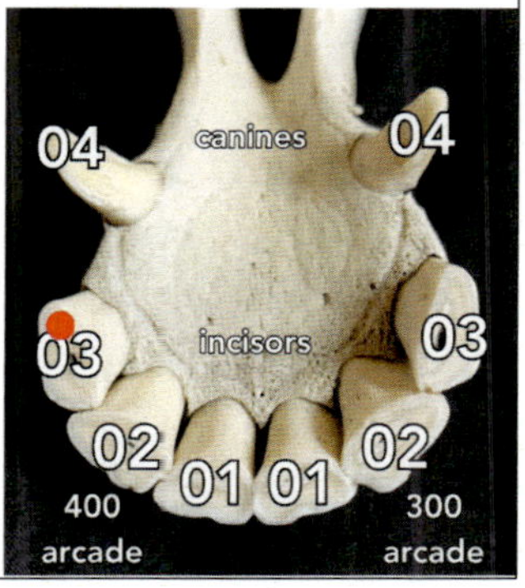

Triadan numbering for incisors. This is a mandible with its mandibular incisors, showing the 300 and 400 incisor arcades, and therefore their Triadan names start with a 3 or a 4, depending upon the arcade wherein they reside. Image credit Author.

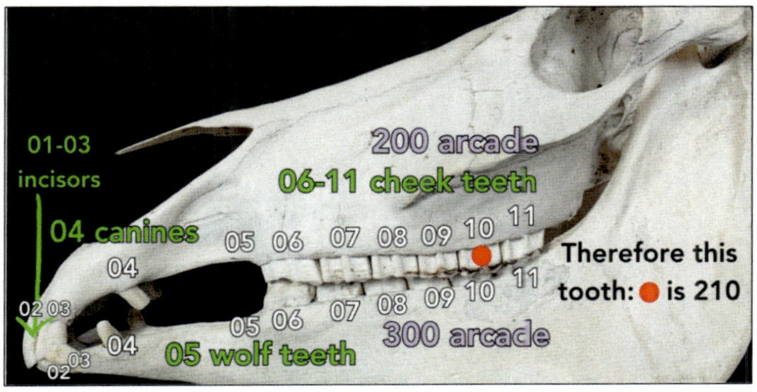

Again we see this image, but with a little more knowledge now. Triadan numbering of the canines and cheek teeth. This image shows the 200 and 300 arcades, and therefore their Triadan name starts with a 2 or a 3, depending upon the arcade wherein they reside. Image credit Author.

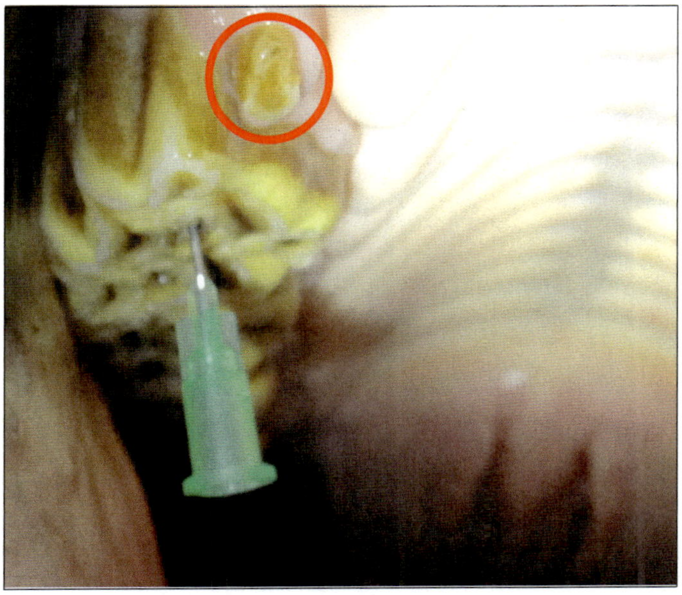

This is a quite large 105 (a wolf tooth, circled) adjacent to the 106, (the first cheek tooth). The needle is placed into a pathologic area, to be discussed in a later chapter. Image credit Dr Denis Verwilghen.

Wolf Teeth: Wolf teeth are small ***vestigial*** teeth which may or may not have a deciduous precursor (Use your glossary and the terms you have learned earlier in this chapter!). They are usually found directly mesial to the much larger maxillary '06s and occasionally the mandibular '06s. With Triadan numbering, they are denoted by X (the quadrant)05, or 105, 205, 305, or 405. They are usually immediately adjacent to the '06s, but sometimes a space separates them. Wolf teeth do not function in mastication (chewing). They may also be called "premolar one", or the "first premolar", which can be confusing because they do not look like the other three premolars (the first three cheek teeth). Another reason to use the Modified Triadan System.

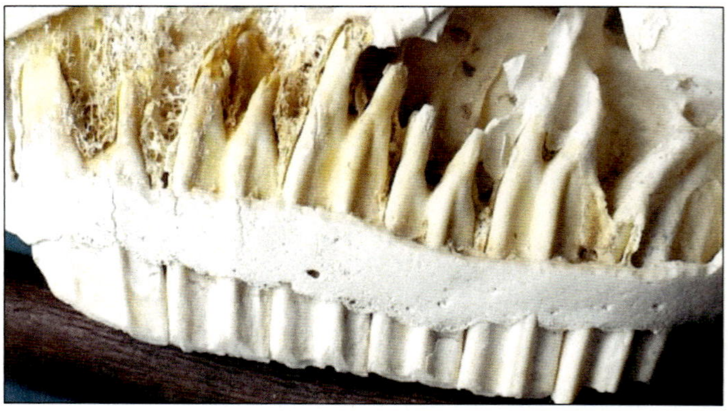

This brilliant skull cutaway shows the apices of the: 206 and 207 (to left) within the maxillary bone, 208 and 209 within the rostral maxillary sinus RMC, and the 211 within the caudal maxillary sinus CMC (to right). The 210 may be in both the RMC and CMC. Note: these vary significantly between horses and by age. Cathie Heald Greenwell.

Cheek Teeth: Cheek teeth are rectangle-shaped, large teeth at the back of the mouth, six to a quadrant. They include most of the premolars and all of the molars, as you will see below. With Triadan numbering, they are denoted by X (the quadrant)06-11, or X06, X07, X08, X09, X10, and X11. Cheek teeth are packed together like bricks in a wall with tight interdental spaces due to the positioning of the apices (root tips), which presses these premolars and the molars toward each other. Remember, for the *deciduous* cheek teeth quadrant names, the X's are 5-6-7 and 8, also in the clockwise direction. The six adjacent teeth in each quadrant are meant to function as a solid unit, essential for grinding hard feedstuffs. With the older nomenclature, the cheek teeth included the second to fourth premolars and all three molars in each quadrant. The X06-X08 (the "premolars") all have deciduous precursors (baby teeth which are shed), while the X09-X11 (the "molars") do not.

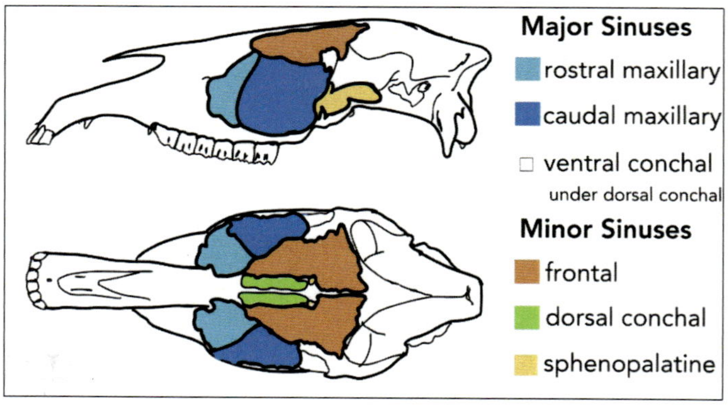

The sinuses of major and minor dental significance. The apices of the caudal cheek teeth reside in the maxillary sinuses for much of a horse's life. Image credit Author.

Premolars: X05, X06, X07, and X08. For those of you familiar with the older nomenclature, the premolars include: the relatively tiny wolf tooth, which is the first premolar, and the first three large, rectangular cheek teeth, or the second to fourth premolars. Each of these three have a deciduous precursor and later, they are replaced by a permanent tooth. The premolars are the first three of the six cheek teeth.

Molars: X09, X10, and X11. For those of you familiar with the older nomenclature, the molars are the last three cheek teeth in each arcade. Molars have only permanent teeth, with no corresponding deciduous precursors. The molars begin to erupt at around one year of age.

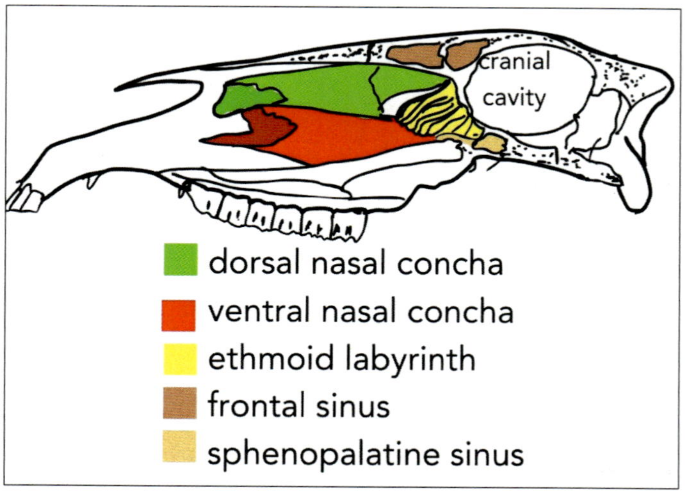

Interior view of the sinuses which may be significant in disease of the head, including the ethmoid labyrinth, or sinuses (yellow). Image credit Author.

Infraorbital canal: The infraorbital canal is a bony tube much like a hard, thick straw lined with soft tissue which begins at the base of the eye socket and ends at a hole in the side of the skull partway down the side of the face called the infraorbital foramen. A nerve and an artery run through the canal.

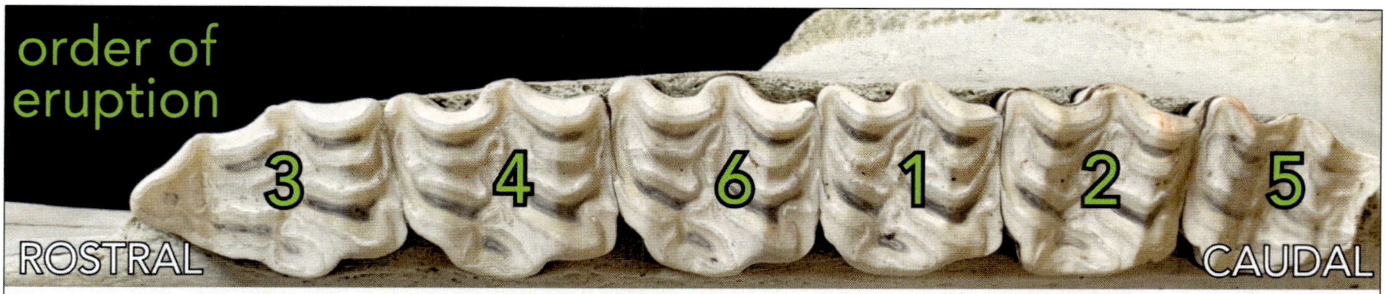

tooth number	206	207	208	209	210	211
approx age	2.5 yr	3 yr	4 yr	9-12 mo	2 yr	3.5 yr

Eruption sequence of permanent cheek teeth and the ages at which the teeth are "meant" to erupt. The green numbers on the teeth are the order in which they must erupt. Image credit Author.

Nasolacrimal duct: Though you likely won't have seen or felt your own nasolacrimal duct, you have probably noticed the effects of their presence when tears have built up in your eyes and suddenly your nose has run with clear liquid. This liquid is ocular (eye) tear fluid which has flowed through the nasolacrimal duct and exited into your nasal passages. It has its own canal: the order of flow inside the nasolacrimal duct is through the: lacrimal puncta - bony lacrimal canal - lacrimal sulcus - nasolacrimal puncta - and out!

Sinuses: Another hidden portion of the head is the sinus network (see top right image). There are several paired (left and right sided) sinuses, many of which directly involve teeth, because tooth roots extend into these sinuses during much of your horse's life. The sinuses with the majority of dental significance include the rostral and ***caudal*** maxillary sinuses, and the ventral conchal sinuses..

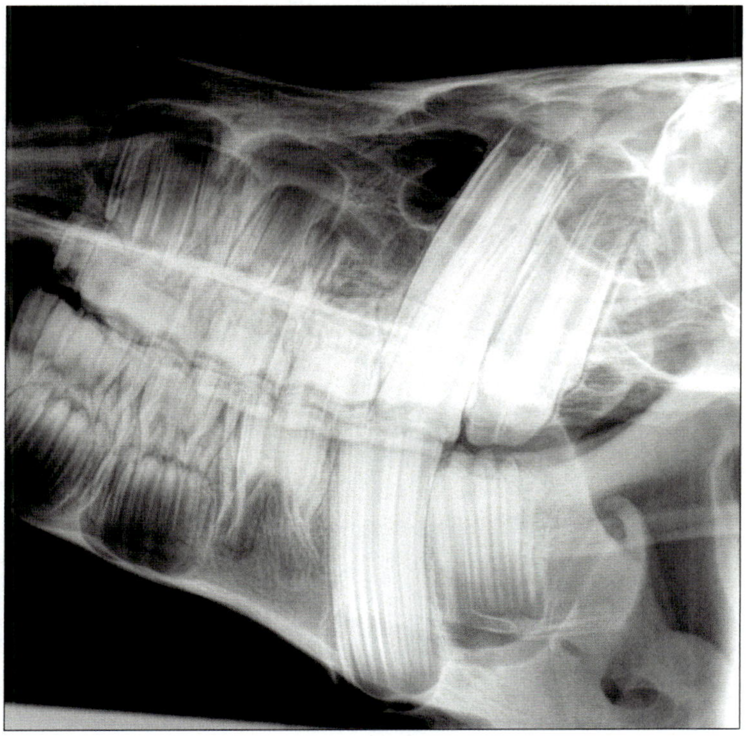

Mini displaying deciduous and permanent teeth.... Her deciduous teeth are all stacked up... and nowhere to go. Image credit Dr Amy Ardern.

What's an Eruption Sequence?

THE ORDER AND the different ages at which teeth erupt have a significant effect upon the ability of certain teeth to erupt into the mouth along their correct "line of eruption", or the path each tooth is meant to follow. Failure of teeth to erupt along this line, or failure to erupt at the correct time, allows development of ***crown elongations*** (overgrowths) and malocclusions (misalignments of maxillary and mandibular teeth) if teeth are not correctly opposed by their corresponding partners in the opposite arcade.

One challenge from even a normal sequence of eruption is the requirement of the ’08s to force their way in between the ’07 and the ’09s. Study the image above for details. The green numbers on the teeth are the order in which they must erupt.

Note that the 208 must erupt last, in between the 207 and the 209. This can cause problems, as you will see later. In this image, it is the 200 arcade, so the tooth is Triadan number 208, but all the other ’08s must erupt in this challenging order.

Could I Have Some Directional Descriptions to Orient Me?

MAKE SURE YOU understand what these words mean. If not, please go back and study the diagrams. It will make the rest of this chapter easier.

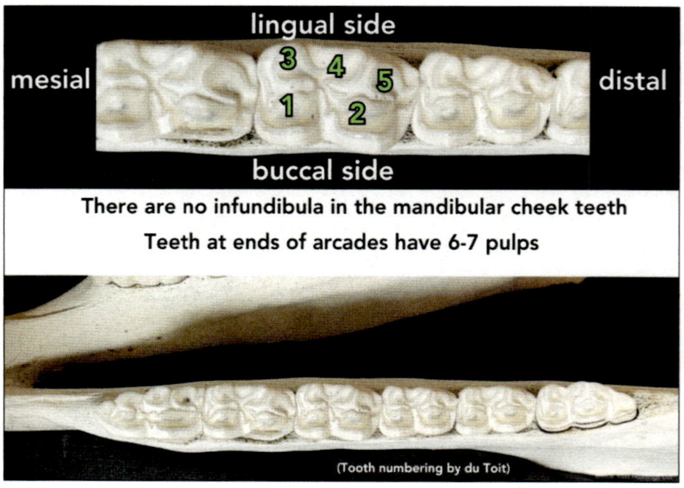

Occlusal surfaces of the mandibular cheek teeth differ from those of the maxillary ones. Image credit Author.

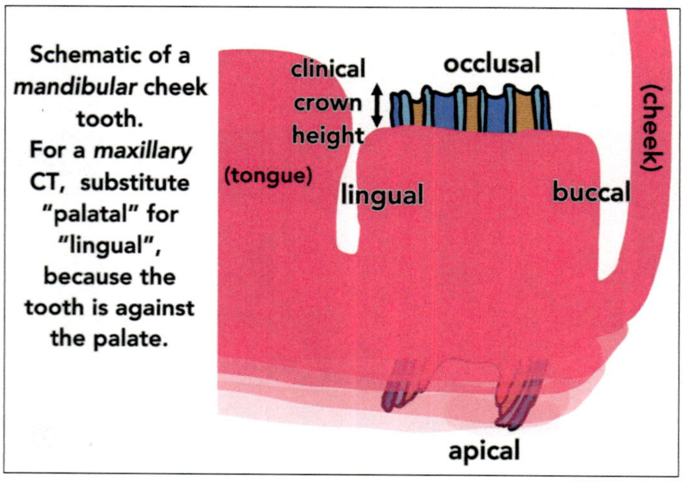

*You can find your way around a tooth if you know **apical, occlusal, buccal, lingual, and palatal**! Image credit Author.*

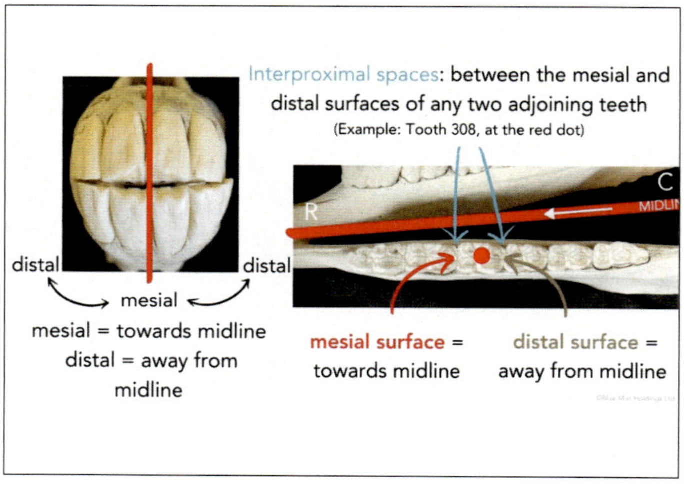

The interproximal spaces are where teeth meet. Image credit Author.

- **mesial:** Toward the midline of the mouth, or the vertical line at the interproximal space between the central incisors.
- **distal:** Away from the midline, toward the ears.
- **occlusal:** The surface of a tooth which occludes, (is in contact) with the opposing tooth when chewing.
- **apical:** The part of a tooth or tissue which is toward the ***apex*** or root, the opposite end from the occlusal surface.
- **buccal:** The portion of a tooth or tissue which is adjacent to the cheek.
- **labial:** The portion of a tooth or tissue which is adjacent to the lips.
- **lingual:** The portion of a tooth or tissue which is adjacent to the tongue.
- **palatal:** The portion of a tooth or tissue adjacent to the palate.

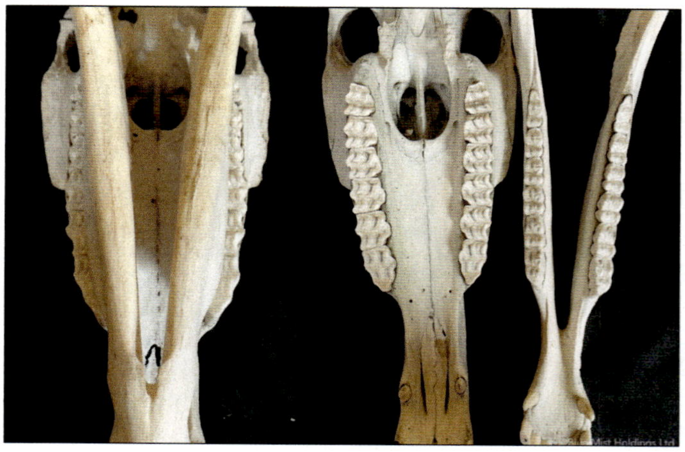

The maxillary arcade sits much further buccally (toward the cheek) than the mandibular one. This is called anisognathia. Image credit Author.

Anisognathism, or "Wow, the Maxilla and Mandible are so Different"!

YOU'LL NOTICE A horse's cheek teeth are not set at the same width in the maxilla vs. the mandible!

This is called anisognathism (an=not, iso=equal, gnath=jaw), or unequal jaws. Horses are anisognathic, which means the arcades of the maxillary cheek teeth are set further apart, or more buccally, than those of the narrower mandibular arcades. To make it even more uneven, the maxillary cheek teeth themselves are wider than the mandibular cheek teeth. When horses grind their food with their horizontal power stroke, the palatal edges of the maxillary (upper) teeth and the buccal edges of the mandibular (lower) teeth undergo the most abrasion and attrition. This leaves the buccal edges of the maxillary teeth and the lingual edges of the mandibular ones to undergo ***crown elongation*** and to become "***sharp enamel points***", or SEPs. The buccal cavity, or the space between the maxillary cheek teeth and the cheeks is very narrow, even when the mouth is closed. When the mouth is opened, the cheeks press more tightly onto the teeth, and if the cheek teeth possess SEPS, they may cut into the cheeks, creating painful buccal ***ulcers*** (painful lacerations in cheek mucosa) especially under halters and bridles. The lingual SEPs can cut into the tongue (and the opposing ***gingiva***, if extremely long). We will discuss these in a later chapter.

The resultant pain may cause the horse to chew abnormally, leading to crown elongations and other malocclusions, causing dental disease. Have you ever seen a horse which chomps their feed in an up and down motion as humans do? They usually only do this when the teeth are unable to move horizontally from side to side, as they should. This tends to occur with severe dental disease.

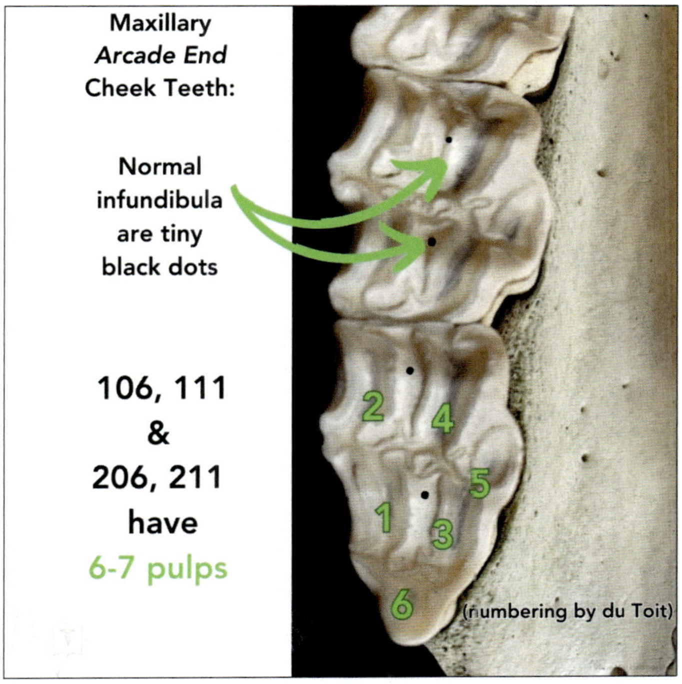

Occlusal surfaces of the maxillary cheek teeth, showing locations of infundibula and numbering for the pulp horns of the end of arcade teeth. Image credit Author.

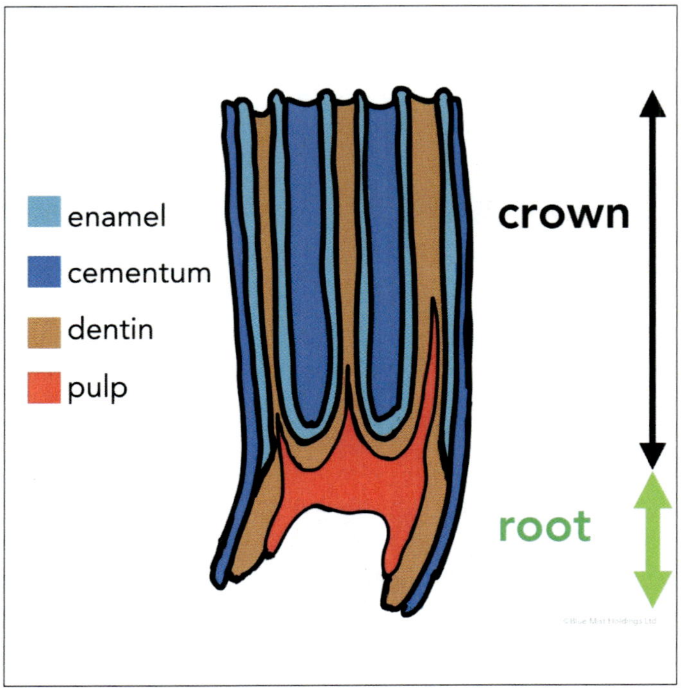

The clinical crown is the part of the tooth which is visible above the gingival margin, while the reserve crown is hidden in the alveolus. Image credit Author.

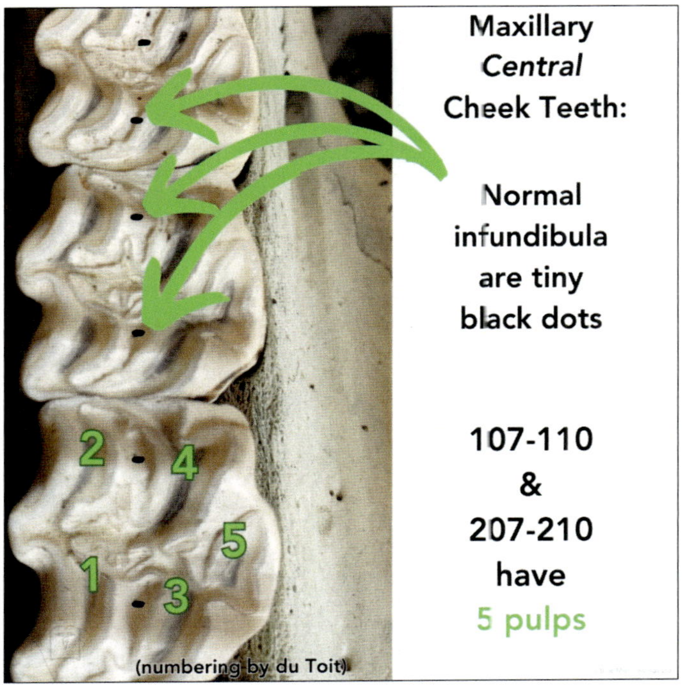

Occlusal surfaces of the maxillary cheek teeth, showing locations of infundibula and numbering for the middle four pulp horns. Image credit Author.

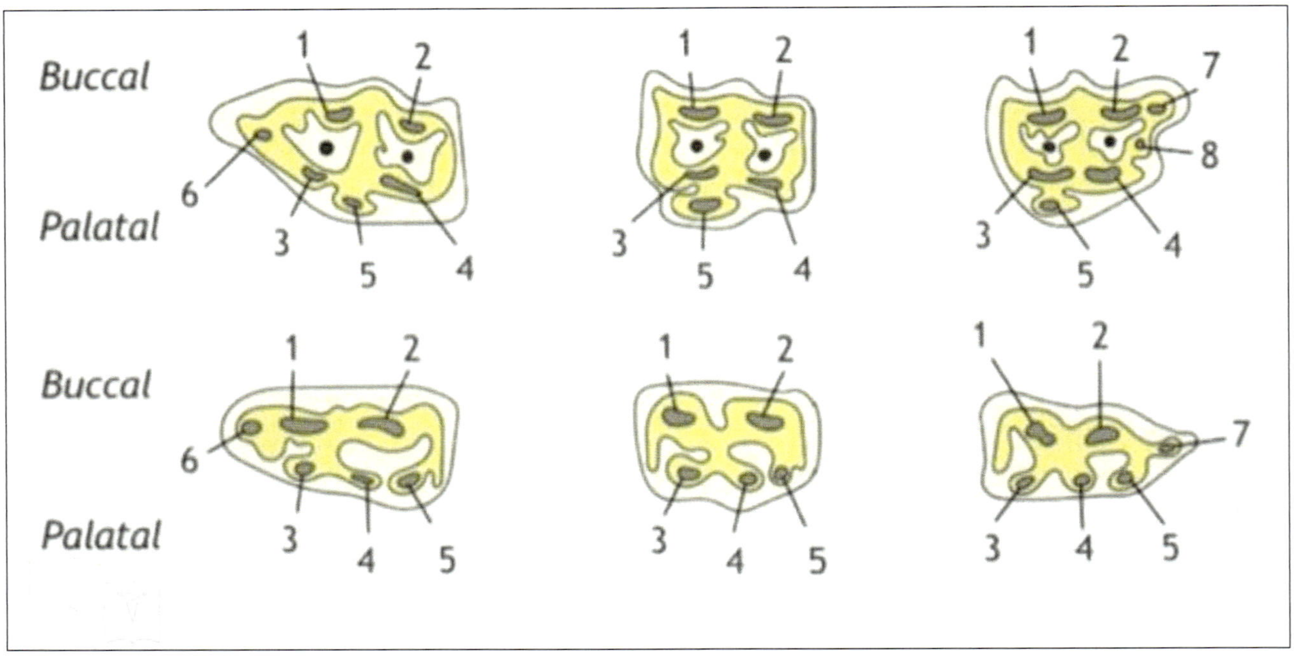

In more colored detail: This diagram shows the occlusal surface of the equine cheek teeth; the upper row shows maxillary cheek teeth (206, 208, and 211) and the lower row shows mandibular teeth (406, 408, and 411). Numbers are individual pulp horns using the pulp numbering system of Du Toit et al. (2008). Redrawn with permission from N. Du Toit. Image credit Dr Pearce C. (2020). Image originally published in Pearce C. Recent developments in equine dentistry. New Zealand Veterinary Journal 68, 178-86, 2020. ©NZVA

Regular ***odontoplasty*** helps prevent development of many malocclusions and helps repair damage previously created by neglect to the dentistry of the horse.

What About the Teeth Themselves?

THE ***CLINICAL CROWN*** is the portion of the hypsodont crown which is exposed to the oral cavity above the gingival margin, or the gums.

The ***reserve crown*** is the portion of the hypsodont crown which lies beneath the gingival margin, or beneath the gumline. You cannot see this part.

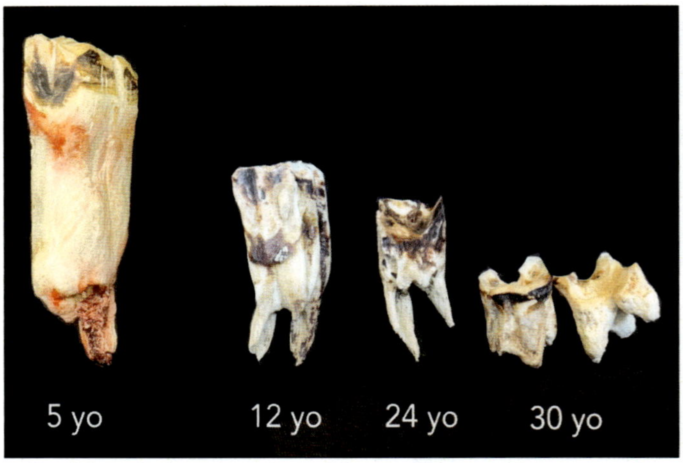

Tooth length changes with age. These teeth are on the same scale. While most of these are pathologic teeth (they were from extractions), the roots are lined up for you to see the extreme length of the reserve crown in a young horse. Image credit Author.

Teeth and their orientation in the mouth

The above and below diagrams illustrate the finer details of the cheek teeth. The numbered brown marks on the one above are showing the pulp horns and their numberings in each tooth, for the the most mesial teeth (left), the center four cheek teeth (center) and the most distal (right), in each arcade.

So, what makes up the tooth?

As we saw in the very beginning of this chapter, while humans have brachydont (short crowned) teeth, horses' hypsodont (long crowned) teeth are quite different from ours. Hypsodont teeth have exposed enamel ridges throughout the tooth to help grind the rough grasses and grains they have evolved to eat.

Dentin, ***cementum,*** and ***enamel*** make up equid teeth. *Dentin* is a mineralized, but relatively soft, ivory-like component of teeth which supports the more brittle enamel. Dentin gradually fills the pulp chamber with secondary dentine as the tooth ages. Cementum (or cement) is a bone-like, relatively flexible, calcified tooth layer. Together with the dentin, cementum supports the more brittle enamel from cracking under the stresses of mastication. There are two types: ***infundibular cementum***, which lines and fills the infundibulum, and ***peripheral cementum***, which covers the periphery of all teeth and makes up a substantial part of the equine crown. Enamel is the hardest calcified dental tissue in the body. It is extremely strong and wear resistant, but unfortunately it is brittle, so it needs support from the softer dentine and cementum to keep the enamel from fragmenting. It covers dentine in the crown of the teeth. Enamel resists staining from feed pigments (so remains white on the occlusal surfaces—see below), but the more porous dentin takes up the pigments and stains a dark brown color. The stained dentin on the occlusal surface of a cheek tooth appears as elongated brown stripes in the images below. The stained secondary dentin is extremely helpful during odontoplasty, as it serves as color coding for how far one may (usually) safely reduce the length of a tooth, as you will see in Chapter 14, Odontoplasty.

Equid teeth, also different from those of humans, exhibit prolonged eruption, which means that their individual permanent teeth continue to erupt for 17 to 30-odd years, unless the teeth or their supporting structures become diseased. The teeth undergo abrasion from grinding rough feeds against the teeth of the opposing

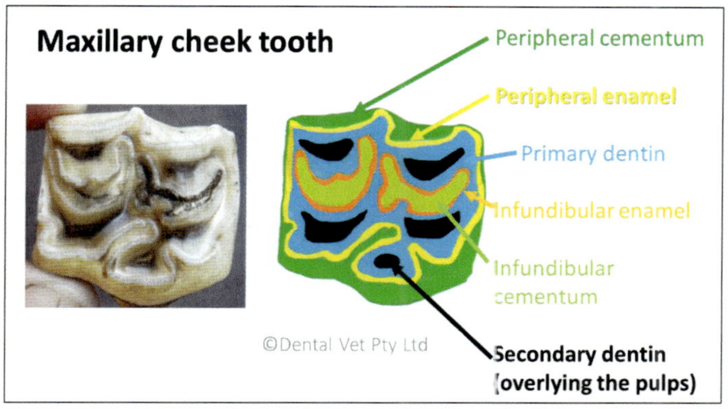

The structures making up a maxillary cheek tooth are illustrated here on this occlusal view. Image credit Dr Kirsten Jackson, Dental Vet.

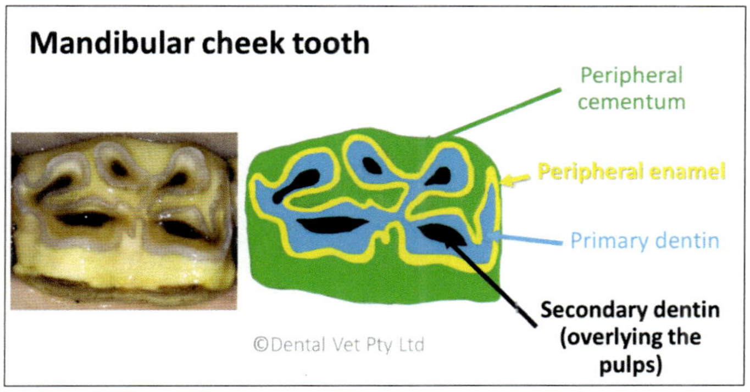

The structures making up a mandibular cheek tooth are illustrated here on this occlusal view. Image credit Dr Kirsten Jackson, Dental Vet.

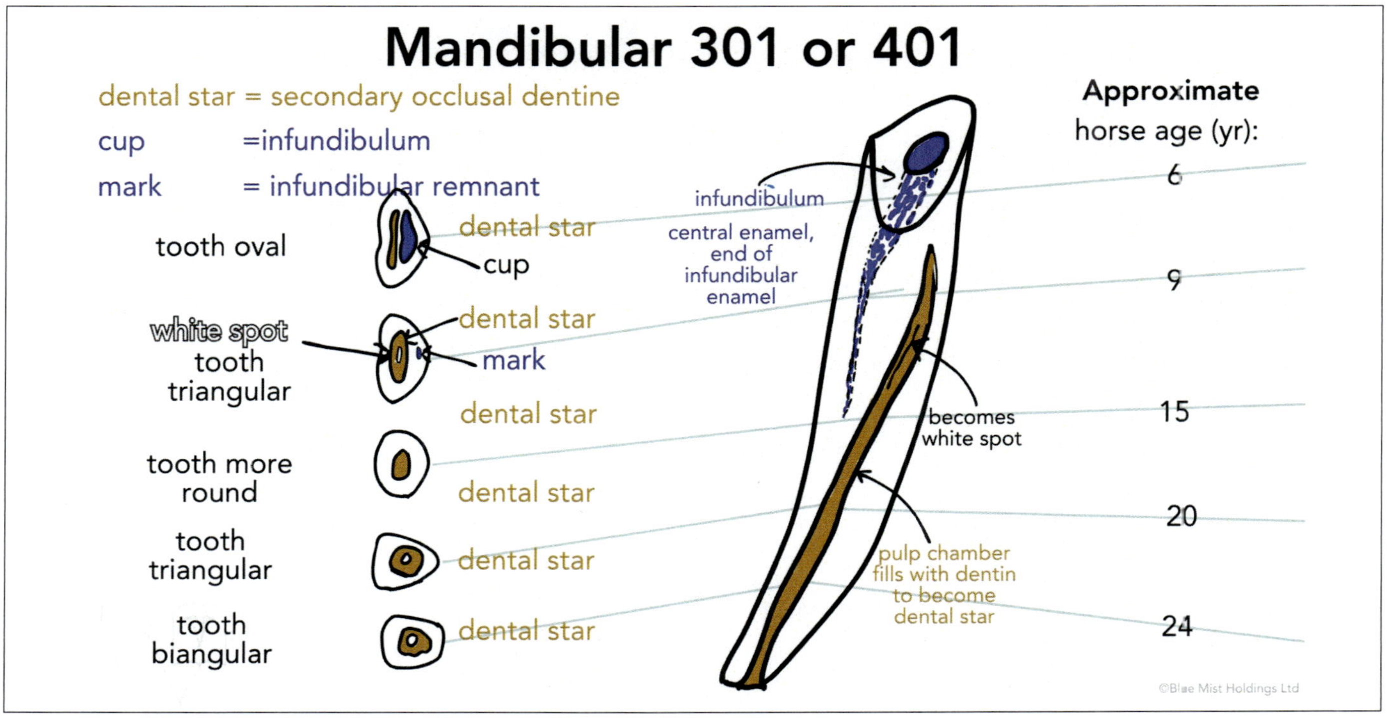

This diagram displays how the different structures appear and disappear as this horse's central incisor ages and the tooth is gradually ground off by attrition. Note the lines are not all parallel because while the (hard) central infundibular enamel is still present on the occlusal surface, attrition is slow. When the tooth is worn past this (mid-teens), the lack of harder enamel causes the tooth to wear more quickly. Image credit Author.

Occlusal Indicator	Actual Structure	Contents
cup	infundibulum	filled with air or feed
mark	remnant of infundibulum	enamel filled with cementum
dental star	remnant of retreating pulp	remnant of retreating pulp

The structures on the occlusal surface of the incisors are frequently used to "age" a horse. Here's what those terms mean. Image credit Author.

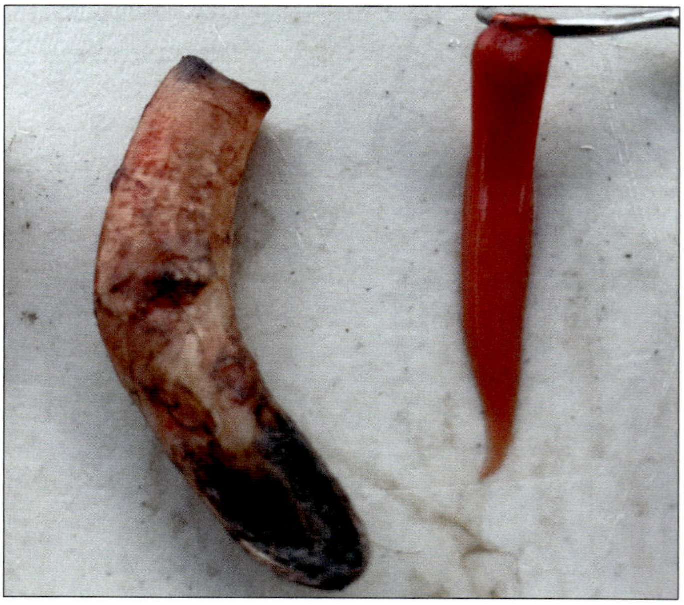

A canine tooth extracted from a cadaver. Note the length of the pulp. This is why we do not cut teeth, whether they are canines, cheek teeth, incisors, or wolf teeth (same goes for camelids!). They can have live pulp tissue from 1-3 mm beneath the occlusal surface, and in unopposed teeth with crown elongations, the occlusal surface to pulp distance tends to be at the low side of that distance. DO NOT CUT TEETH! Image credit Author.

tooth arcade and attrition from grinding against the opposing teeth themselves until the teeth are expired, or worn down past the enamel, leaving only the softer tooth structures of dentin and cementum. After this time, the short stubs of roots topped by the dentinal remnants of the tooth are eventually exfoliated.

In the images to the right, note the distribution of the different components which make up an equid cheek tooth.

The "safe" increment of the occlusal surface and all the other surfaces of the equine tooth to the live tissue of the pulp may be very small, measured in millimeters. You will see in the ***pathology*** sections just why this is VITAL to the life of that tooth, and maybe the life of your horse.

Incisor Cross Section

WHEN I NEEDED to learn the relationship between the anatomic structures of a tooth and the changes seen on the cross-sectional occlusal surface of the tooth as it ages, I drew out this diagram of a mandibular (lower) central incisor (Triadan 301 or 401), shown on the next page. This diagram showed me how the "***dental star***", the "cup" and the "***mark***" relate to the structures as well as the attrition, or wear, of a tooth over its lifetime. It displays the tendencies of the age-related tooth changes, but these ages are not set in stone. The transverse lines indicate levels to which the tooth has been reduced by wear and *roughly* pertain to the horse's age. The equine incisors have a single y-shaped pulp cavity which splits into two pulp horns labially to the infundibulum. It becomes a single cavity as the pulp horns extend toward the apex. The wear of these structures lets us see them in cross section on the occlusal surface, as indicated by the small semi-circular drawings down the tooth to the left. To the left of the tooth diagram is the lingual side. To the right is the labial side. I think of the "dental star" as the "dentinal" star because it is formed of the dentin which fills the gap left when the pulp retreats as the tooth undergoes attrition. As mentioned before, it stains brown due to the pigments in the green feed.

How Did Those Teeth Get There?

EVER WONDER HOW teeth get where they are meant to? Or how they erupt where they shouldn't ever be, and when?

When is all this happening?

Tooth creation starts in the developing fetus inside the uterus of the mare. To give you an idea of *when*, it has been shown that the calcification of the deciduous cheek teeth, one of the later stages of tooth development, occurs by four months of gestation, and the calcification of the first permanent ***tooth buds*** begin at around ten months of gestation. That pretty much covers the whole of gestation and early foal life for development of all the teeth. Considering this timetable, recognize that the nutrition of the mare may have implications in fetal tooth (and other) development.

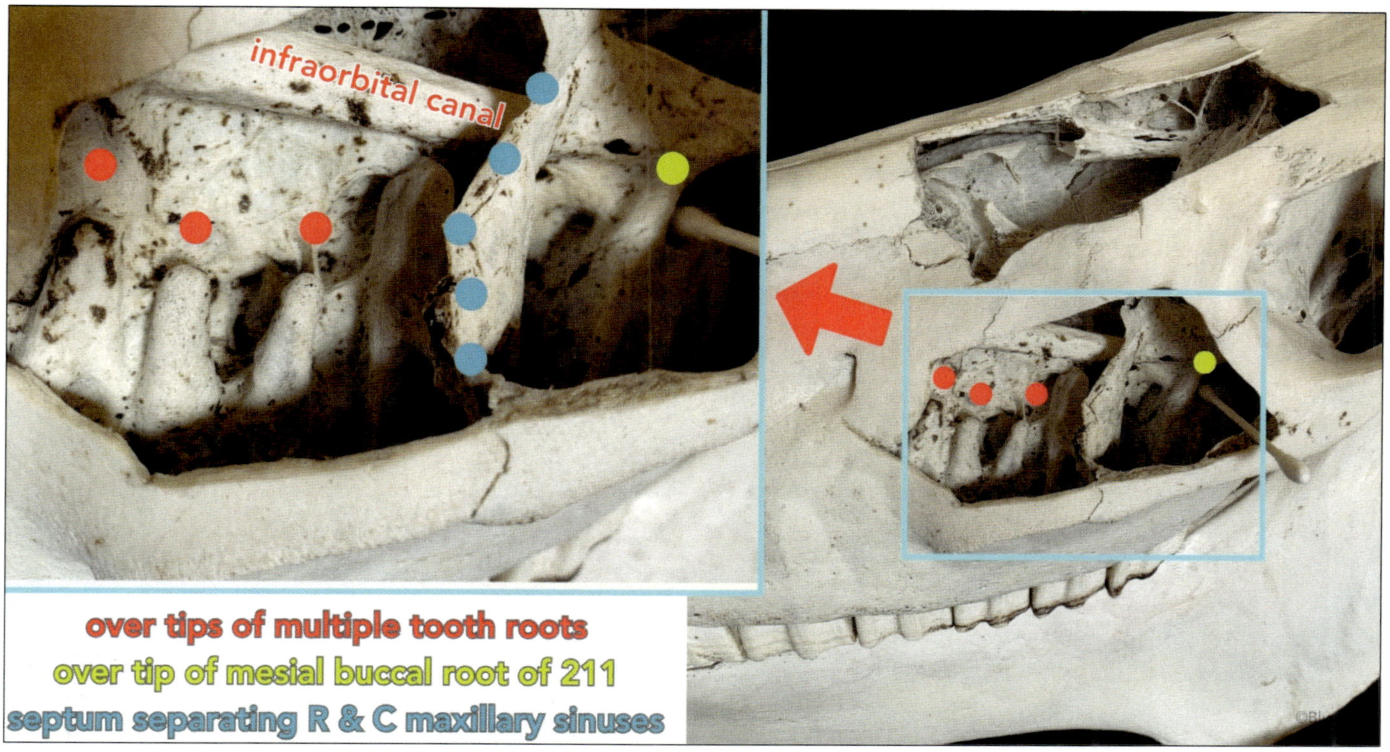

Distal maxillary cheek tooth apices reside in the maxillary sinuses for most of an equid's life. This graphic shows the opened rostral and caudal maxillary sinuses with the infraorbital canal and multiple tooth roots within these sinuses. This horse had only the 211 in the caudal maxillary sinus (the rostral buccal root of the 211 is marked with a yellow dot, just to the left of the cotton bud), while the 210, 209, and part of the 208 in the rostral maxillary sinus (red dots just over the root tips). These two sinuses are separated by the septum, marked with blue dots. Image credit Author.

Tooth development and placement

The incisors and canines are the most similar of all the equid teeth to brachydont teeth (teeth like ours), and they have both deciduous and permanent teeth. Eruption begins at the '01s (centrals), then continues through the '02s (intermediates), and finally the '03s (corners). Incisor and canine roots form at the apical end early in the tooth development and these teeth continue to erupt, and grow, until the horse is approximately 17 years of age. The apices and reserve crowns reside within the maxillary or mandibular bone.

Early development of the cheek teeth differs significantly. The first three cheek teeth, '06s through '08s (the premolars) have deciduous precursors, while the three molars (the '09s through '11s) have only permanent teeth.

The end of a tooth furthest from the occlusal surface is termed the apex. Why not just call that portion of the tooth the "tooth root"? It has to do with the development of the hypsodont roots. When a cheek tooth erupts into the mouth, that tooth is still "growing" and actually lengthening. At this time, the apex of the tooth has not yet turned into a "root". Once the "root" develops at a tooth-age of approximately two years, that growth ceases forever, i.e. the tooth no longer "grows". After this time, the tooth can only "erupt" from the alveolus (tooth socket) into the mouth for the subsequent 25-30 years. For correctness, then, when we speak of an infection of the apical end of the tooth, we call it an ***apical infection.*** This will then encompass both an immature tooth "apex" as well as a mature tooth "root".

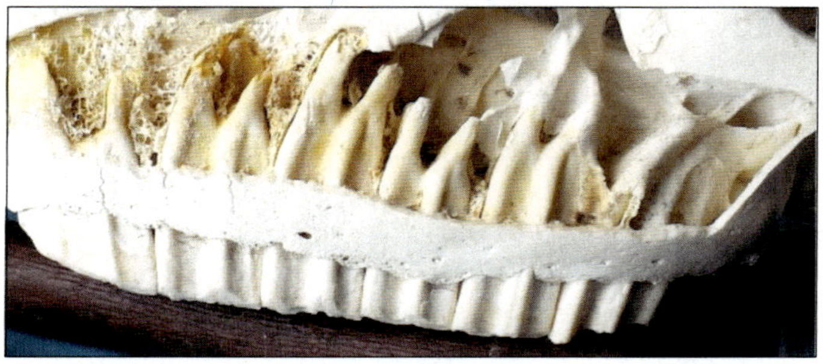

This brilliant cutaway shows the apices of the: 206 and 207 in the maxillary bone (to left), 208 and 209 within the rostral maxillary sinus(RMC), and the 211 within the caudal maxillary sinus CMC (to right). The 210 may be in both the RMC and CMC. Note: these vary significantly between horses and by age. Image credit Cathie Heald Greenwell.

The apices and roots of the mandibular cheek teeth ***usually*** reside in the mandibular bone. The more mesial maxillary cheek teeth (***usually*** the '06s - '07s, and sometimes '08s) reside completely within the maxillary bone, while the more distal maxillary cheek teeth ('08s-'11s) ***usually*** pass through the maxillary bone into the maxillary sinuses.

The placement of the maxillary tooth apices in the sinuses can cause problems for the horse when an apical infection occurs. The infection can break through the thin alveolar wall into the open portion of the sinus and cause a sinus infection with a persistent ***fistula***, or hole, between the mouth and the sinus. These can be difficult to resolve. See Chapter 6, Developmental and Acquired Conditions: Apical Infection.

How Did Teeth Develop in the Fetus and Why Does it Matter to My Horses?

THIS MAY BE more detail than you desire, but it's here for those of you who are interested. Jump to the end for the significance, anyway.

It is an extremely complex series of cellular processes for the development of each individual tooth, the detailing of which takes four pages or more to discuss in veterinary dental textbooks. It helps to have studied cell biology, development, and anatomy to fully comprehend it, but suffice it to say, tooth development is a result of interaction of ectodermal (from outer cell layer) and ectomesenchymal (combined ectodermal and mesenchymal) cells in the developing fetus.

Different classes of teeth originate from different tissues, which is significant in the final destination of each tooth. While this may not seem significant to you, it may be! Why? Here's a brief explanation:

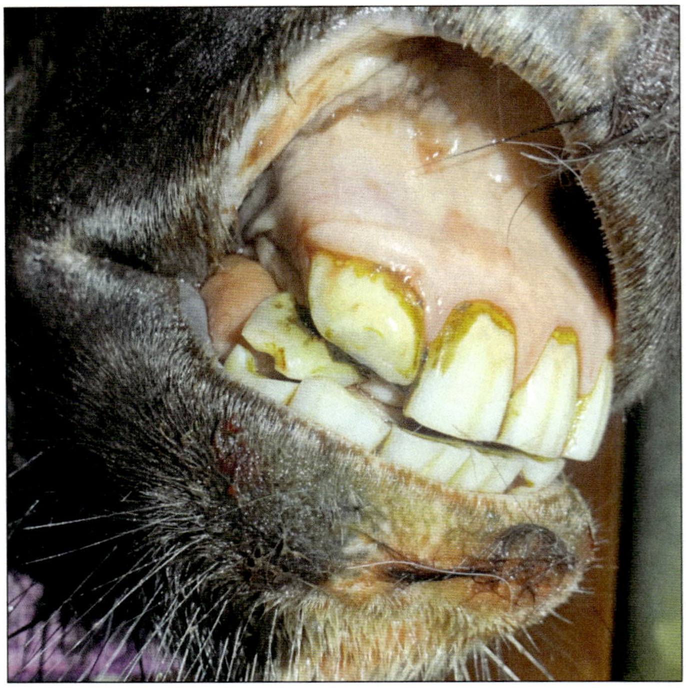

When teeth don't erupt when they should, they can block the correct eruption pathway and cause problems for the horse. It is vital to have regular six-monthly dental examinations during the first five years of life when so many teeth need to erupt into the correct places! Image credit Author.

While all deciduous teeth and permanent molars develop from the enamel organ of the dental lamina, formed by a thickening of the ectoderm (from the outer cell layer) at the outside margin of the fetal mouth, which invaginates (pushes itself into) the underlying mesenchyma (originating from the middle cell layer), the permanent incisors, permanent canines and permanent premolars develop from a lingual or palatal (toward the tongue or roof of the mouth) extension of the dental lamina of the corresponding deciduous tooth, or from an extension of the existing deciduous tooth!

Back to the significance to you: say your horse's deciduous incisor doesn't shed when the permanent needs to erupt. The result may be that the permanent incisor will usually erupt toward the tongue or palate, and the retained deciduous counterpart will usually be displaced out toward the lips, although not every tooth follows "the rules". For those teeth which don't, check out Chapter 6, Developmental and Acquired Conditions: Malocclusions.

What are the Other Oral and Nasal Tissues?

There must be more structures than just teeth and bones! Soft tissues!

Indeed, there are! These may be divided into soft tissues and hard, calcified tissues. The hard tissues have already been discussed earlier in this chapter. The soft tissues make up a significant proportion of the mouth. The soft tissues protect the hard tissues and tend to take the brunt of damage from sharp objects in feedstuffs, dental overgrowths, and malocclusions. The soft tissues of the mouth include the oral mucosa, tongue, blood vessels, nerves, parotid gland and duct, and salivary glands.

Oral Mucosa

The oral ***mucosa*** is a specialized tissue which protects the mouth from cuts, bacterial invasion, and other threats. It lines the mouth and runs from the margins of the lips to the area of the tonsils.

Gingiva

The gingiva is the firmly attached, keratinized oral membrane which immediately surrounds the teeth and the alveolar bone. Near the gingival attachment to the tooth, it is more mobile and called the gingival sulcus. The gingival sulcus is important because in its deepest point, the gingiva attaches to the cementum of the tooth. Even deeper to that lies the periodontal ligament, which holds the tooth in place and is responsible for the prolonged eruption of equid teeth. This area is constantly remodeled, as prolonged eruption is only possible from the constant building of new periodontal ligaments and detachment and reattachment of gingiva to the surfaces of the tooth. When a tooth pulp is infected or the tooth is not alive anymore, one may *or may not* see gingival recession, where the gingiva has receded from the occlusal surface toward the apices, when compared to adjacent teeth.

Tongue

The tongue, like our tongue, helps us eat. It helps draw in food and plays its part in moving the food bolus in its rotational track from the front to the back of the mouth.

Nerves

The nerves are located all over the head. Dental and oral treatments inside the mouth may be accomplished by a combination of ***analgesia*** and ***anesthesia*** to allow thorough treatment of painful conditions such as diastemata and for pain-free dental extraction, including that of the '05s (wolf teeth). There is a difference between analgesia and anesthesia. Analgesia can be defined as a lowered pain state without loss of consciousness, such as a level of pain relief achieved from the use of anti-inflammatories, while anesthesia is a state achieved when there is a loss of the sensations of touch, pain, temperature, and reflexes, with or without loss of consciousness. This can be achieved by veterinary administration of anesthetic regionally (an injection which numbs an area, such as epidural or spinal anesthesia), subcutaneously (to numb the local nerve fibers under the skin), or topically (numbs just the surface via a cream or spray).

General anesthesia is total loss of consciousness from the use of veterinary or medical anesthetics (e.g. a horse lying down on the ground or on a surgical table). Once general anesthesia was used for dental extractions, but for the most part, dental surgery is now performed by veterinarians with the patient under standing sedation plus local and regional analgesia (nerve blocks).The largest of the superficial nerves (on the outside of the head) are the paired facial nerves and their branches, which travel ventrally (down) and rostrally on the sides of the face. These supply the skin and musculature of the face, eyes, lips, etc. There are smaller nerves throughout all the tissues of the head, including the gingiva inside the mouth.

Deep inside the skull, there are large internal nerves, such as the maxillary and mandibular nerves, with many branches supplying all parts of the inside of the mouth, including the tissues around the teeth. Vets, like your own dentist, utilize local anesthetics around these deep nerves to block the sensation of pain to a particular part of the mouth, enabling us to perform dental surgery without pain to the equid. Special, blunt-tipped needles may assist the veterinarian in avoidance of injury to nerves and vessels during these injections, which must be performed with the strictest attention to sterility and a thorough understanding of anatomy and physiology. Many vital structures exist where these nerves reside, and great care must be taken by the veterinarian to prevent injury to the patient.

Salivary Glands

The salivary glands are a system of multiple paired glands which produce saliva, used in the lubrication and digestion of feed. The main salivary glands are the parotid salivary glands, the mandibular salivary glands, and the sublingual salivary glands. These glands can inject over 50 ml per minute of saliva into the mouth when your horse is eating. It is important that operators understand where these glands and their ducts reside to avoid damaging them.

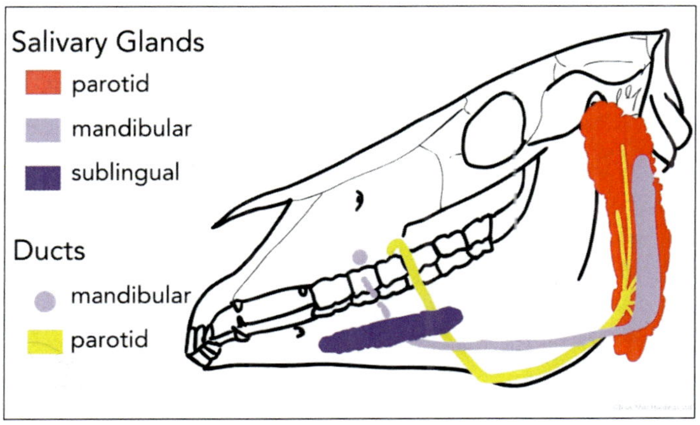

Salivary glands of the horse. Image credit Author.

Blood Vessels

The blood vessels supply nutrition to all the tissues of the head, including the mouth. The skin, gingiva, and oral structures are said to be "highly vascular", which means they have many small blood vessels which assist in healing the many wounds a horse may sustain in its mouth and sinuses, and on its head.

There is a vessel of note inside the mouth called the palatine artery, which runs just inside the maxillary (upper) teeth along the edge of the palate. Those performing dentistry must be highly aware of this artery, as it is easy to cut into this high-pressure artery. High pressure means it bleeds if you hit it. It bleeds profusely if it is not cared for properly. Your vet knows how to do this.

Dental and oral treatments inside the mouth may be accomplished by a combination of analgesia and anesthesia (see above under Nerves) to allow thorough treatment of painful conditions such as diastemata and for pain-free dental extraction, *including* that of the '05s (wolf teeth).

Combined hard and soft tissues: Paranasal sinuses

The paranasal sinuses are a group of paired (left and right) sinuses which surround the nasal cavities.

The major sinuses (with respect to dentistry) include the rostral maxillary sinuses, the caudal maxillary sinuses, and the ventral conchal sinuses. Minor sinuses include the frontal, dorsal conchal, and sphenopalatine. All of these drain directly or indirectly into the nasal cavity. The dental significance of these sinuses is that the apices or roots of cheek teeth '08 through '11 reside inside either the rostral or the caudal maxillary sinuses. What could possibly go wrong? See Chapter 11, Sinus Disease.

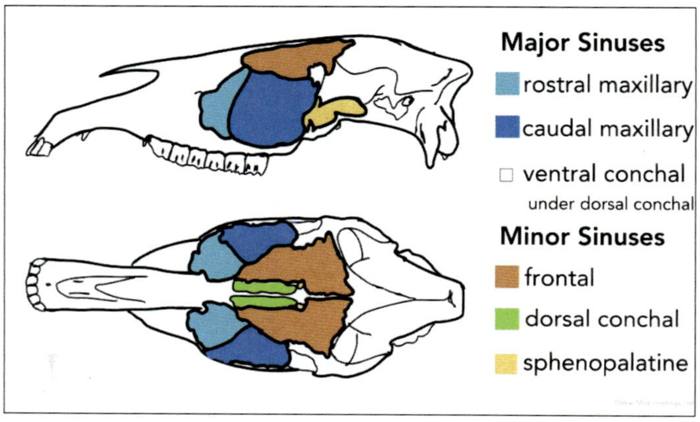

Here are the major and minor sinuses in the skull. The apices of the more caudal cheek teeth reside inside them, along with many other structures. Image credit Author

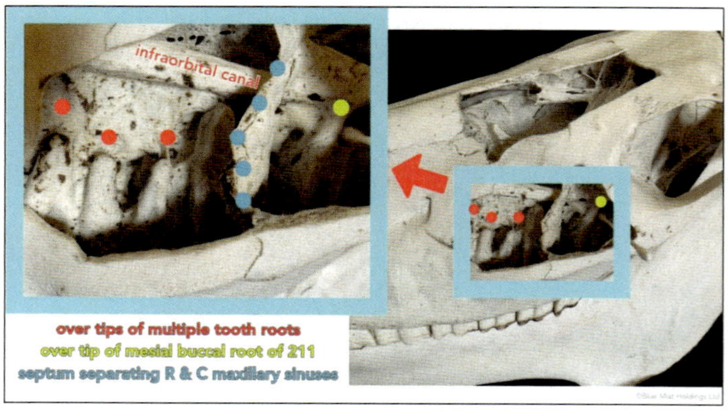

Distal maxillary cheek tooth apices reside in the maxillary sinuses for most of an equid's life. This graphic shows the opened rostral and caudal maxillary sinuses with the infraorbital canal and multiple tooth roots within these sinuses. This horse had only the 211 in the caudal maxillary sinus (the rostral buccal root of the 211 is marked with a yellow dot, just to the left of the cotton bud), while the 210, 209, and part of the 208 in the rostral maxillary sinus (red dots just over the root tips). These two sinuses are separated by the septum, marked with blue dots. See a larger image two pages back. Image credit Author.

CHAPTER FOUR

HOW SHOULD THE MOUTH BE EXAMINED?

"The basis of modern clinical therapy is diagnosis. This presupposes that disease can be accurately identified and then effectively eliminated by the application of appropriate therapy. It would seem, therefore, that information obtained in making a diagnosis is the foundation for successful treatment. Discipline must be exercised in collecting material for a meaningful diagnosis."
—Jack Easley, DVM, MS, DBVP (EqPract), AVDC (Equine)

SO, YOU'VE SEEN the Eight Levels of Dentistry from Chapter 2, right? If you haven't, please go back and read Chapter 2: Eight Levels of Equine Dentistry to see what information can be gleaned from each level. Then we can continue our discussion.

Sedation: Does Effective Dental Care Need It?

Why is sedation important for dentistry?

While sedation of your horse is not essential to ***float*** its teeth, ***veterinary*** sedation *is* necessary for an effective, thorough ***oral*** and dental examination and ***odontoplasty***. You may have understood this from the last chapters.

The relatively small entrance to the mouth, plus the long distance to the ***distal*** (back) teeth requires the practitioner to use long instruments under conditions of poor visibility. Lights are essential here, as is a full mouth speculum, picks, and probes. However, without an intraoral mirror, it's impossible to visualize all surfaces of the teeth and mouth to examine for evidence of ***pathology***. An oroscope improves your examination over a mirror exam as well. If you were to not use sedation, your horse would not be impressed by opening his mouth wide for the speculum, much less the probes, and as for the mirror...

A question for you: *Do you want a mirror in the mouth of your horse if it is not sedated?* Truly? No matter how big and tough your practitioner, when your unsedated horse throws its head or escapes the speculum and crunches down on the mirror or scope, the sequelae are not things I wish to have caused or want to deal with. A handful of broken glass in your horse's mouth is less than ideal, wouldn't you agree? As for the oroscope, the cost alone rules out putting it anywhere near the mouth of an unsedated horse. But more importantly, in terms of the safety of the horse, the practitioner, and especially *you or your child* as the handler, have you ever held up the 20-30+ kg head and neck of a sedated horse? Heavy, isn't it? Imagine the additional weight of a speculum, and an unsedated horse swinging his head around to evade the practitioner... Health and safety-wise, it's not worth considering.

"But my "horse dentist" (lay dental operator) does it all the time without sedation?"

Many veterinarians, EDTs, and lay dental operators filed horses' teeth for years without sedation—I know I did. I also now know we missed a lot of pathology, or disease. Because we didn't *look*. And now that science and dentistry have advanced, what was once acceptable practice is no longer appropriate. We can do better for our horses. You may not be doing their teeth yourself, but you *as the owner* are the one who makes the appointment for your horse's dentistry. My goal is to help you understand what's really going on in your horses' mouths, so you can make informed decisions about the kind of dentistry and the level of care you choose for your equine friend or competition partner.

Neglecting to perform a thorough dental exam on every equid dental appointment is unfair to them. A blanket statement? Let's discuss this. One of the biggest concerns about dentistry consisting of only a "float" with a poor or nonexistent dental examination is that owners may believe: "My horse has had its teeth done, and the problem is not in her mouth". It is sometimes comforting to believe this. Some lay dental operators are quite convincing, and it may cost more money to have sedation and a thorough examination. Unfortunately, an unsedated oral exam may tell if your horse has a very obvious problem in her mouth, but it *cannot* tell you that she *doesn't*. Let me rephrase that.

While one doesn't need sedation to simply float a horse's teeth, only rarely (if ever) could one perform a thorough, detailed dental exam using a full mouth speculum, a light, and a mirror on an unsedated horse. The best your operator can usually get from an unsedated exam is to say that there *is* dental disease, but it would be extremely difficult to correctly say there *isn't* any pathology under most circumstances. Although it may cost more money for a sedated, thorough examination, it will allow your horse's dental problems to be detected, diagnosed and treated before they get the chance to progress to a truly eye-watering pain and expense level.

One simply cannot see with one's fingers or a float, though one does need to ***palpate*** (feel with the hands) the entire inside the mouth by hand. I do it every time. But you also need to *visually* examine every part of the mouth and teeth to ensure your horse has no pathology. As an example, consider a horse with behavioral challenges which could potentially be caused by pain in his mouth. If a suboptimal (incomplete or poor) examination is performed, it is *impossible* to rule out dental pain as a cause of behavioral abnormalities. A thorough examination which can rule out this pathology requires sedation, a full mouth speculum, complete rinsing of the mouth, a strong light, mirror, dental probe, and thorough visual examination of each tooth, oral surface, the skull, and the outside surfaces of the head for pathology... and sufficient operator education to be able to correctly assess the significance of these examination results. Behavioral and health problems attributable to dental pain tend to persist after odontoplasty which follows only a cursory examination, since plenty of pathology may have been missed. Unfortunately, after a "dental treatment" with only a cursory, or no exam, the owner may assume there is no dental pain, since the horse has "had its dentistry" performed. This horse may now be punished or reprimanded for its behavior by the owner or trainer, when in reality the horse is doing its best to avoid oral pain—oral pain which could have been treated after diagnosis via a thorough dental examination. Only by the above-described examinations can it be determined whether behavioral abnormalities are due to oral pain.

What about advanced techniques? Do they require sedation, too?

Yes, more advanced surgical techniques, including treatment of many of the pathologies discussed in Chapters 5 through 13, require precision and extreme care, which necessitates a very still horse. For these, ***perineural anesthesia*** (a "nerve block") is often used in addition to sedation, as it keeps the horse from feeling the pain of the operation and allows the vet to use lower levels of sedation drugs than would otherwise be required.

Do you need to knock my horse out to do an extraction?

Not usually. Today, it is rarely necessary to fully anesthetize a horse under general ***anesthesia*** for dental extractions. Most extraction conditions allow the use of standing sedation with local or perineural anesthesia for intraoral extractions. I perform extractions with standing sedation and perineural anesthesia in my portable ***stocks*** at my clients' homes or at referring veterinary practices. Only in rare cases, when a tooth cannot be extracted intraorally (through the mouth) or when the horse is completely refractory to sedation and perineural anesthesia due to temperament, etc., will they need to be referred for general anesthetic surgery. The exceptions, of course, are when working on non-domesticated animals such as zoo zebras and white rhinos, who are always under general anesthesia for dental treatment.

What About Before and Just After Sedation?

BEFORE SEDATION, IT is extremely important to keep your horse calm (including keeping yourself calm, as they are herd animals and I believe they pick up on your anxiety). The pre-sedation examination should be done in a manner, and preferably in a location, which will avoid upsetting the horse, as excitement can have a detrimental effect on sedation. I spend time talking with the horse and keep him calm, otherwise, sedation becomes a challenge.

After sedation and dentistry, your horse should become more alert within the hour and be keen to eat afterwards. I ask the owners to avoid hay or long grass for at least an hour after horses leave the stocks to prevent choke.

Should they want to eat right away? How about the next day?

Horses should *never* be in pain or unwilling to eat the day of *or* the day after a dental treatment. They should, in fact, be keener to eat than before the dentistry. Unwillingness to eat after dentistry, especially during the week after dentistry, indicates a serious problem which should be addressed immediately by a veterinarian well-trained in modern equine veterinary dentistry, as the dentistry performed may have caused serious, sometimes irreparable, damage. This is VITAL.

What Makes a Dental Exam a "Thorough" One?

PLENTY! More diagnoses get missed by not looking, than by not knowing. If we are going to do the best job possible for your horse, your vet will probably start by stepping back, looking at the horse from a distance, and noting its attitude and body condition. He will ask you about your horse's history, which may include things such as past or current medical problems (which may need a workup before treatment), changes in eating habits and attitude, and tetanus status.

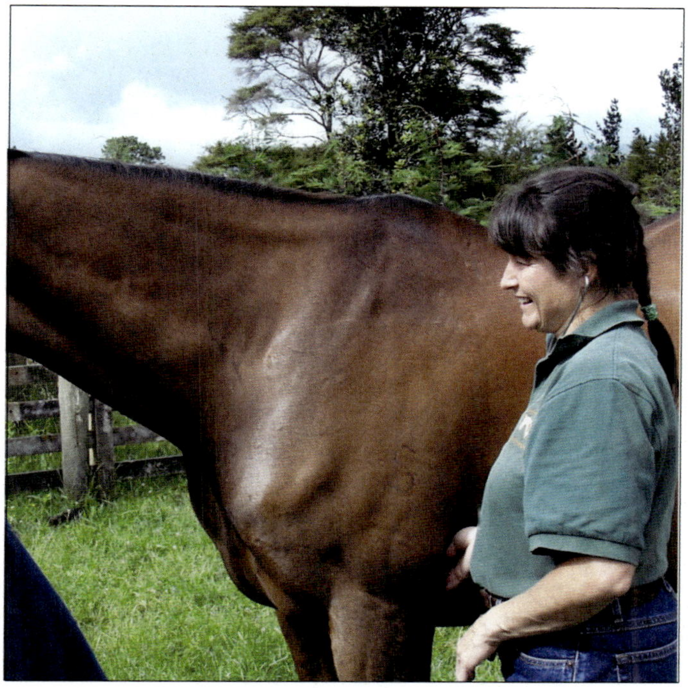

When your veterinarian is preparing for your horse's dentistry, they will auscultate (listen to) its heart, lungs, and trachea as part of a veterinary dental examination, as Dr Elizabeth Thompson is doing here.

Pre-sedation examination

A physical exam will follow, especially checking the trachea, lungs, and heart with a stethoscope, perhaps taking your horse's temperature, and assessing its hydration (may be estimated by pinching the skin to tent it up and observe its return). Heart murmurs, subclinical (not apparent without careful examination) respiratory disease, PPID (see Chapter 12), and other disease conditions will be evident to your veterinarian during this examination. Sedating your horse without a thorough pre-sedation examination is... less than safe. Any of these cardiovascular or systemic (whole body) conditions may mean that your horse reacts differently to the drugs commonly used for sedation – and you don't want to ***exacerbate*** any underlying cardiac conditions. These complications (like seizures, collapse or death or your horse, and severe injuries or death to onlookers or handlers) are especially a problem in horses with underlying health problems, which your vet will pick up on with a good pre-sedation examination. No one else is trained to do this. Sedation of your horse without a veterinary examination may endanger the life of your horse, the life of those people handling the horse, or anyone within proximity of the horse during its sedation. Your veterinarian knows how to do this.

Your horse's examination results, from pre-sedation through to the end of the dental examination and treatment, will be noted in his record.

Your vet will perform an external exam of the head by checking the skull and muscles of the face, neck, jaw, and airflow from the nostrils, looking for asymmetry or swellings, and may percuss (tap and listen for sound quality) different areas of the skull to check for sinus health.

The ***bars of the mouth*** will be palpated, looking for erupted or unerupted (still beneath the ***mucosa***) ***wolf teeth***, unerupted ***canines***, ***lacerations*** (cuts), or bony swellings on the fine ridges of bone making up the bars.

The lips and ***incisors*** will be checked for alignment, health, and any mobility or pain upon palpation. Are all the incisors present? How many ***deciduous***? How many ***permanents***? Are the expected number present, and are they located where they should be? Is there any feed packing between the incisors? Or incisor ***periodontal*** disease?

How about canines and wolf teeth? If wolf teeth are present, your dental practitioner will probably discuss whether or not they should be extracted. Is there ***calculus*** on the canines, or periodontal disease at their base?

The following two tests will tell your practitioner there may be pathology in the back of the mouth before they even enter the mouth:

Lateral Excursion Test

First, the ***mandible*** (lower jaw) may be slowly moved sideways, observing *how many tooth widths* the lower jaw travels until the incisors begin to open due to the ***cheek teeth*** coming into contact with each other and forcing the incisors apart. This is called the "***lateral excursion to molar contact*** test", or "***lateral excursion*** test". This distance should usually be around 1.5 tooth widths. It should never be zero (as would be the case if malocclusions prevent proper horizontal movement) and it should not be more than about that 1.5 tooth widths (as would occur if the teeth had been over-reduced), which would indicate a serious problem for the horse, as its incisors and cheek teeth are in contact all the time, a bad situation for a horse.

Mesio-Distal (Rostro-Caudal) Movement Test

Second, the head can then be moved up to our eye level, then down toward the ground, while the vet watches and feels the forward and backward motion of the mandible with respect to the ***maxilla*** (upper jaw and head), which is called the "***mesiodistal movement*** *test*" (or "***rostro-caudal movement*** *test*"). The incisors are examined from the side while raising and lowering the head. If there is little to no mesiodistal movement, there may likely be malocclusions such as ***crown overgrowths*** preventing it.

The alignment of the incisors can then be compared to the centering of the cheek teeth and noted.

The position of the upper incisors compared to the lower incisors should be viewed with the head still in a *neutral* position, since raising the head moves the mandible caudally, which can give the false impression of ***brachygnathism*** (parrot mouth).

Sedation

If your horse's exam reveals abnormal findings, your vet will discuss the next steps, which may involve working up the problem before proceeding. If all looks otherwise well for floating, now is a good time for sedation. Your veterinarian will use the best combination of sedatives to suit your horse and the procedure about to be performed, then your horse will be sedated and loaded into the stocks, if available.

Stocks? What are they?

Stocks are dental chairs for horses! Portable stocks which are attached to a trailer and tip up and down are now available, which improves the safety and comfort of your horse, handler, and vet on your own farm. Dr Elizabeth Thompson designed the Equi-Still Portable Equine Stocks (NZ) (https://equistillstocks.com/equistill) from necessity and they have sold well internationally from there.

The Equi-Still Portable Equine Stocks shown to right and below are built in New Zealand, modeled by Blue Mist Shemaya, a 16h 3" Warmblood Cross.

The Equi-Still Portable Equine Stocks are available for sale to veterinarians.

Another solid brand of portable stocks are the PortaSafe Stocks, made in Australia by EVDS.

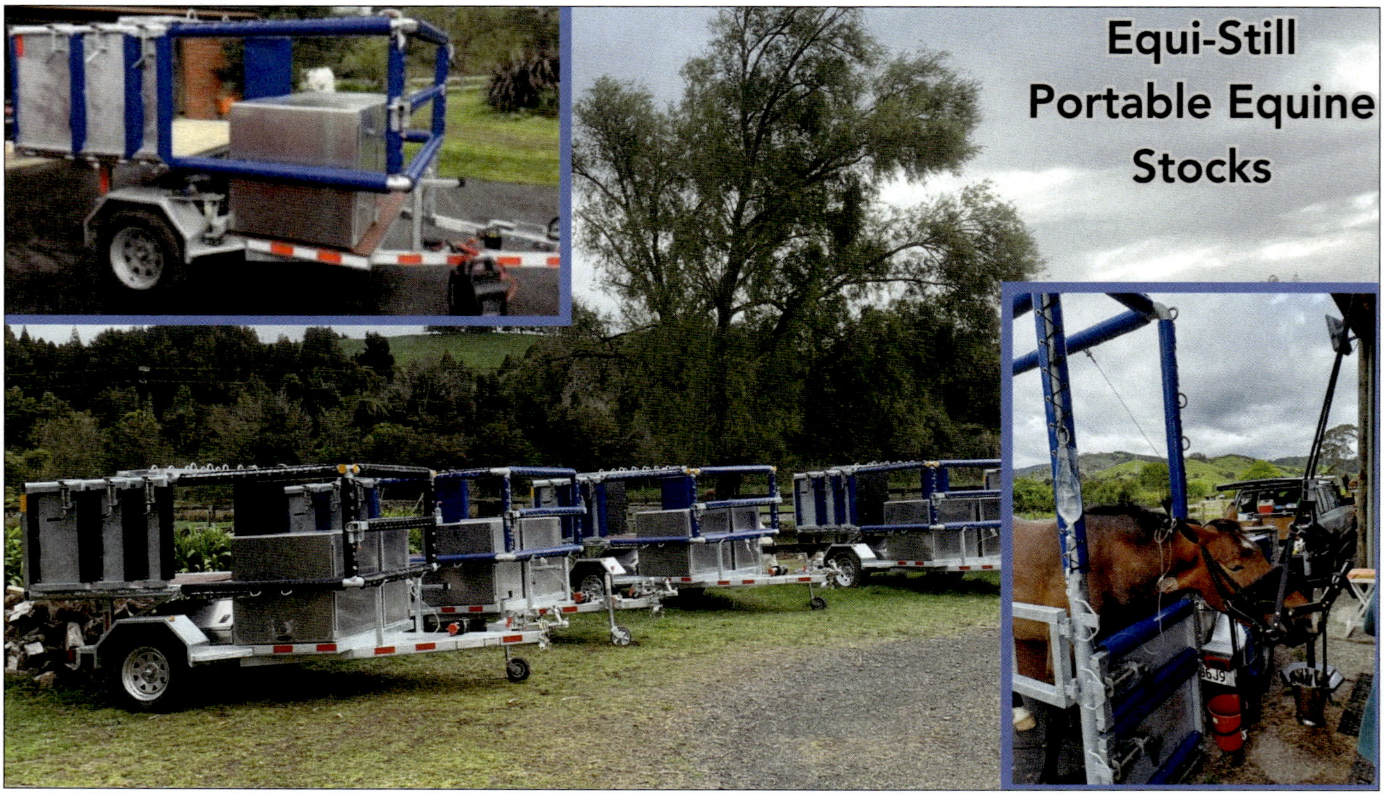

More views of the Equi-Still Stocks, designed by the author for everyone's safety and comfort. Image credits Katrina Price and Matthew Mole, graphic credit Author.

Back to the Examination!

A CLOSE-UP examination of all surfaces of the inside and outside of the lips and the incisors comes next. Are there little pink or red pinpoint lesions on the ***gingiva*** over the incisors? Are there any hard thickenings or draining tracts over the ***reserve crowns*** (the unerupted portion) of the incisors? These are signs which can occur with ***EOTRH*** (Equine Odontoclastic Tooth Resorption and Hypercementosis), which will be discussed at length in Chapter 7, EOTRH. Are the gums receding? Is there calculus accumulation, especially at the gingival margins?

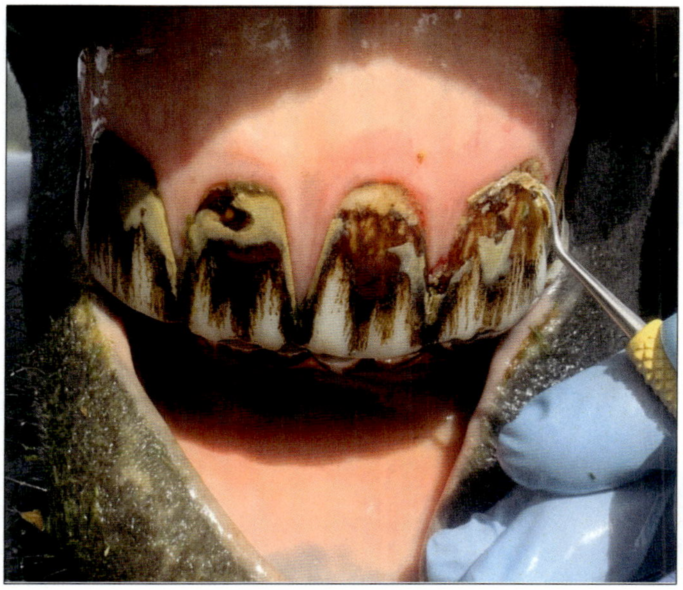

Calculus accumulated at gingival margins of incisors, canines, and all other teeth must be removed and the periodontal areas checked for other signs of periodontal disease and EOTRH. Image credit Author.

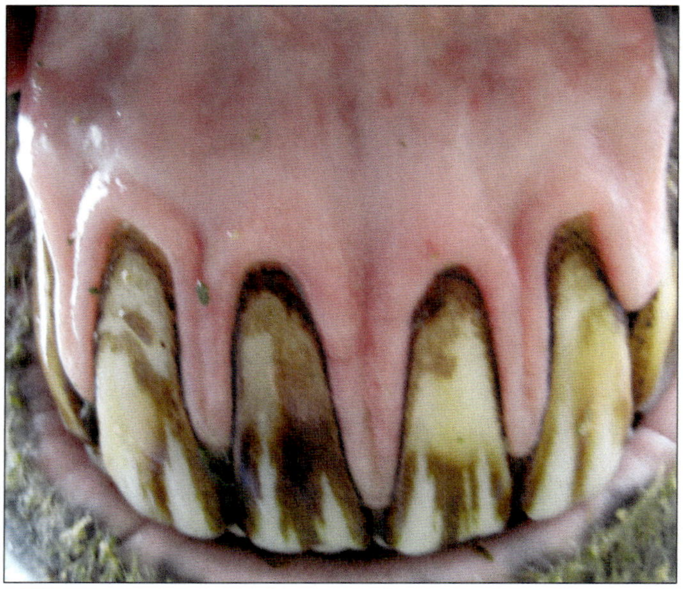

Gingival recession and hyperplasia plus pinpoint red lesions over bulbous tooth roots in this aged mare with EOTRH. Image credit Author.

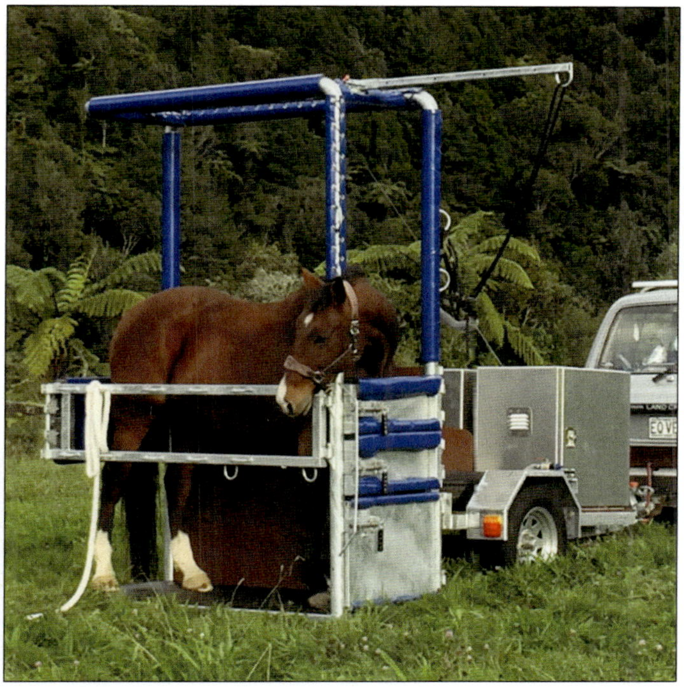

Equi-Still Portable Equine Stocks give your horse a stable, comfortable "dentist chair" to support his body, for his comfort and to support his head so you don't have to. Horses in stocks seem to require less sedation because of this support. Padding in critical locations helps keep them—and you—as safe as possible. A horse outweighs us by around ten times, and a sedated one isn't really always in charge of where his body and feet are going. Image credit Author.

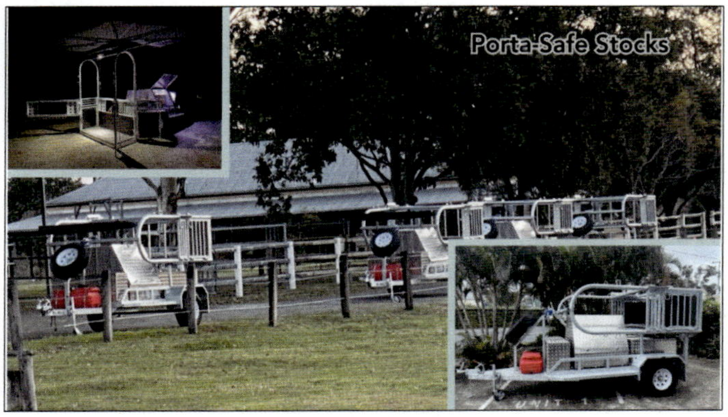

And here are the PortaSafe Stocks. Image credit Dr Oliver Liyou.

Before placing a speculum:

Does the horse resent the incisors or canines being wriggled? It's important to check this before placing a speculum, especially on older horses, as they may have a painful condition of the incisors and/or canines like EOTRH, which will make them resent the speculum plates and object strongly, even through the sedation. If their incisors are painful, there could be problems! (*Equine Odontoclastic Tooth Resorption and Hypercementosis: a very short definition for now: a disease of unknown origin which usually occurs in mid-teen and older horses in which the reserve crowns under the gingiva begin to appear like Swiss Cheese which has tried to fill in all the holes with grit, but please read* Chapter 7, EOTRH.)

It is also important that your operator palpates and manipulates (moves around) the mandible to ensure there are no mandibular fractures which could be exacerbated by placement of a speculum. See Chapter Ten, Head Trauma and Dental Pathology.

An examination of the ***buccal*** sides of the mouth with a cheek retractor displays what the horse is doing with the feed in its mouth. Is she packing feed into one side of her buccal cavity? Is there buccal ***ulceration***? Both? This is a hint of where to seek pathology later.

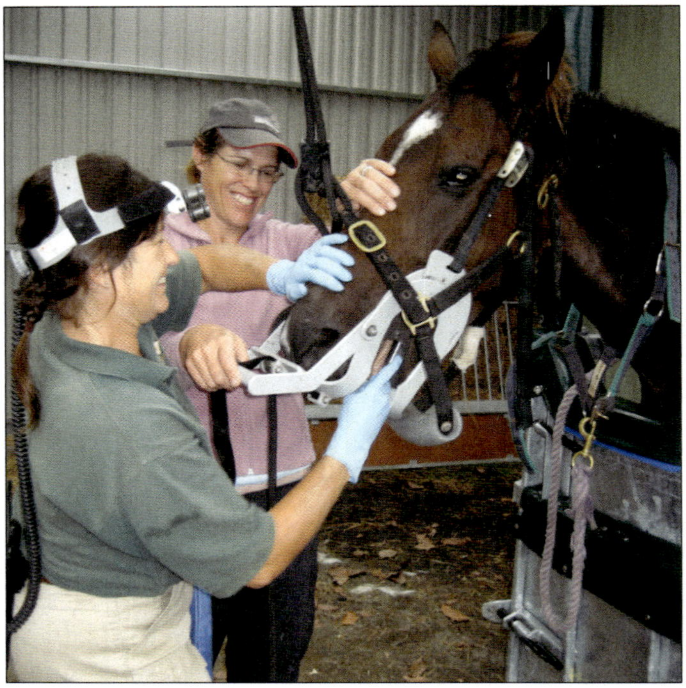

Horse with speculum in place, head supported by Dr Elizabeth Thompson's dental halter and Equi-Still Stocks.

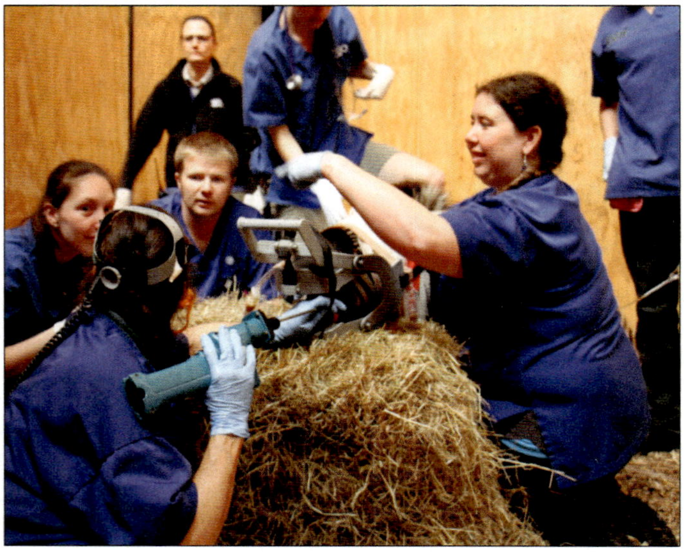

Here is Itika from the Auckland Zoo under general anesthesia for her planned odontoplasty by Dr Elizabeth Thompson, supported by hay bales. The zoo is proactive in their veterinary preventative care and goes to great lengths to ensure the animals' comfort and safety with incredible veterinarians, veterinary technicians, zookeepers, and technical services crew organized into a cohesive, efficient team to give the animals under their care the best life possible. Image credit Vanessa Marsh, used with permission of Auckland Zoo.

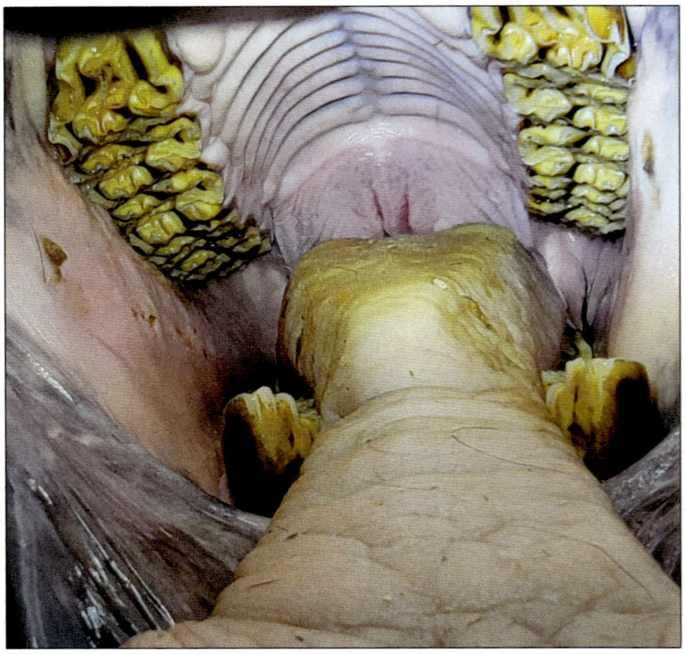

Do you see the buccal ulceration? The 306 and 406 ramps? The diastemata? Image credit Cathie Heald Greenwell.

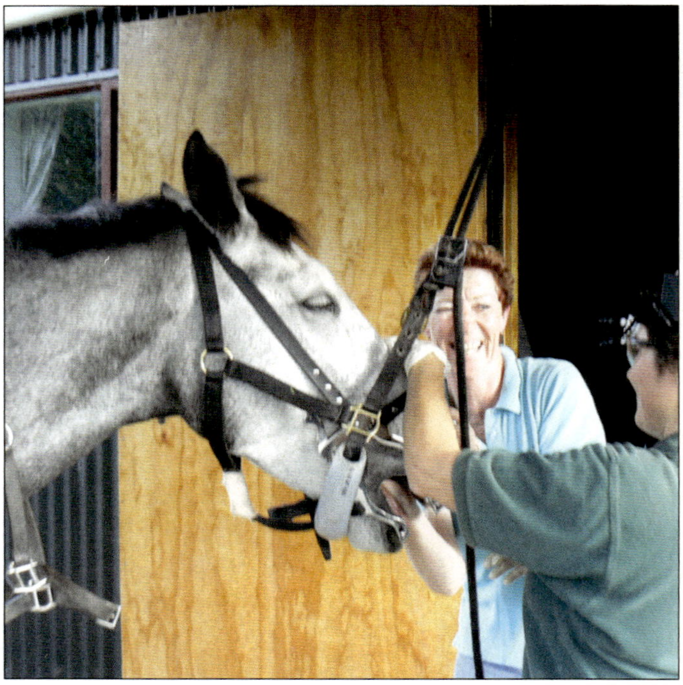

Connie's head is supported by a dental halter while she is manually examined under sedation, prior to her visual examination. Image credit Joan E. Gilchrist.

If the incisors and mandible are deemed fit for placement of a full mouth speculum, it can be placed onto the head at this time and the head supported by a head stand or a dental halter.

Since the head and neck are heavy (say around 30 kilograms, or 60-plus pounds), it's a good idea if they can be supported by a dental halter or a head stand so you don't have to hold them up the whole time. Even more important, if something should frighten your horse (i.e. someone walks behind it... never a good idea while under sedation) you won't be as likely to be trampled if you aren't underneath its head.

The ***bars of the mouth*** can be evaluated visually now, and the presence or absence of wolf teeth confirmed. Based upon the position of the wolf teeth, horse's intended use, and rider needs, if it is deemed that any wolf teeth (usually ***Triadan*** 105/205)

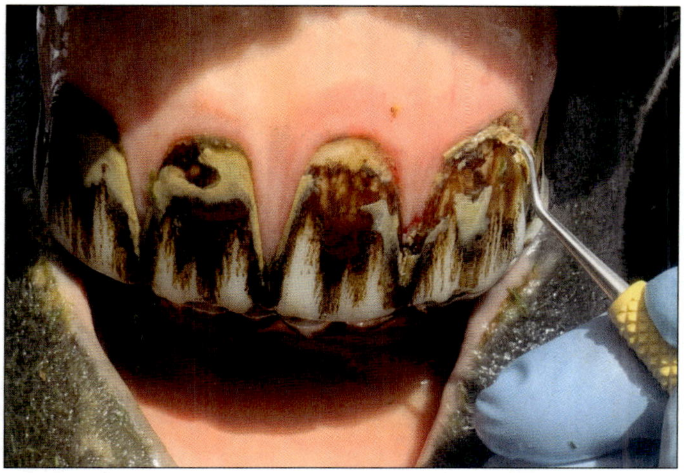

Again, incisors can accumulate calculus at the gingival margins, especially when feed stasis or periodontal disease is present. Dr Elizabeth Thompson removes calculus with a sharp scaler. Image credit Author.

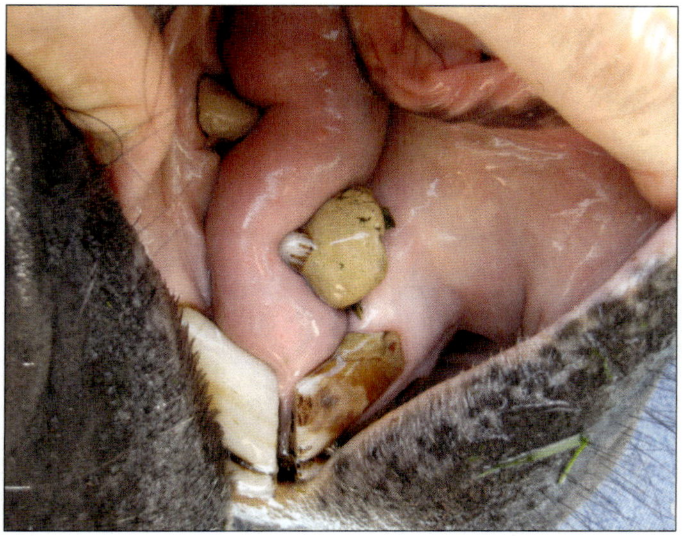

Calculus accumulation on canine teeth with accompanying periodontal disease may be an early sign of EOTRH. Image credit Author.

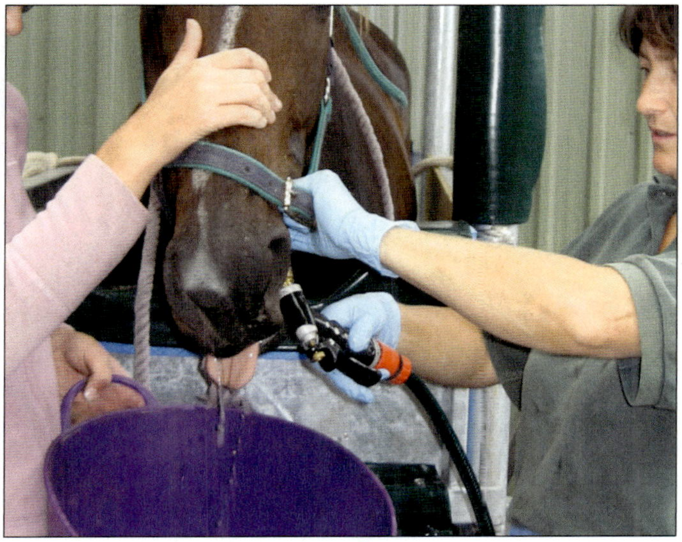

Dr Elizabeth Thompson flushes her patient's mouth prior to intraoral speculum examination.

need extraction, perineural anesthesia (nerve blocks) may be administered now, and the areas surrounding the wolf teeth left to become numb while the odontoplasty (exam and float) progresses. Wolf teeth which are either mandibular (lower jaw), unerupted, or separated from the cheek teeth usually require extraction, while others may or may not need it. See Chapter 15: Veterinary Specific Procedures: Don't All Wolf Teeth Need Extraction?

The incisors can accumulate calculus at the gingival margins, especially in the presence of periodontal disease.

The ***canine*** teeth are distal to the incisors and can accumulate calculus, especially when there is disease present.

Calculus on the canines may be removed at this point, and if there is evidence of periodontal disease, this should be examined further, as it is often where EOTRH first becomes visible. It can be removed with a scaler and may be polished as well, as your dental hygienist would do, and the area examined for signs of periodontal disease and EOTRH.

The mouth will be opened, and a visual exam will confirm where feed is packing, then the head can be lowered and rinsed thoroughly so any pathology can be seen.

Necessary instrumentation for exam

The minimum instrumentation required to perform a thorough dental exam includes 1) a full mouth speculum, 2) a strong head lamp or speculum light, 3) dental mirror, 4) dental picks (1 strong and 1 fine), 5) dental explorer to check infundibula and pulp chambers, 6) long-handled alligator or other forceps to clean feed out of any diastemata, and 7) a periodontal pocket probe to measure the depth of any diastemata.

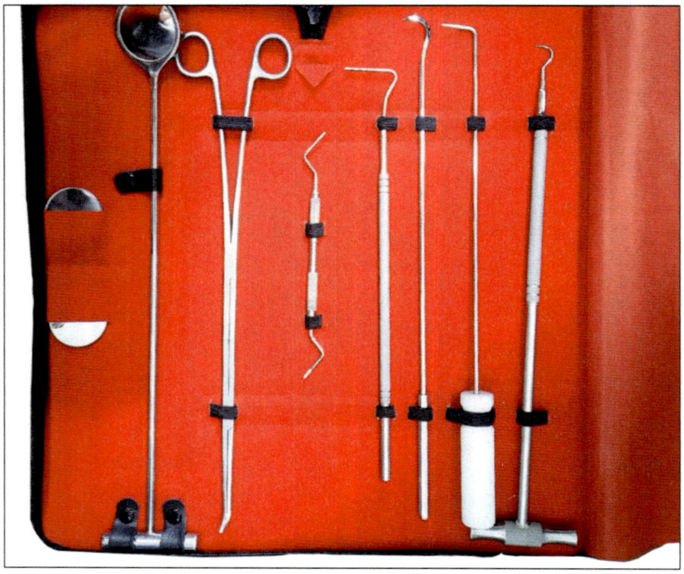

A complete custom Equi-Still Diagnostic Kit. Image credit Author.

How is all this instrumentation used?

Now you will see the necessity of lights, mirrors, probes, and picks in the examination! Without a good head lamp or speculum lamp, the mouth is only a black hole. Remember the Eight Stages of Equine Dentistry? I use a stuffed fleece girth cover over the bridge of the horse's nose to prevent the bright light from my head lamp stimulating the horse, as I want him to stay quiet and asleep. Your vet will use their light and mirror or an oroscope (a dental endoscope) for their visual examination while employing picks and probes to scratch over the pulps on

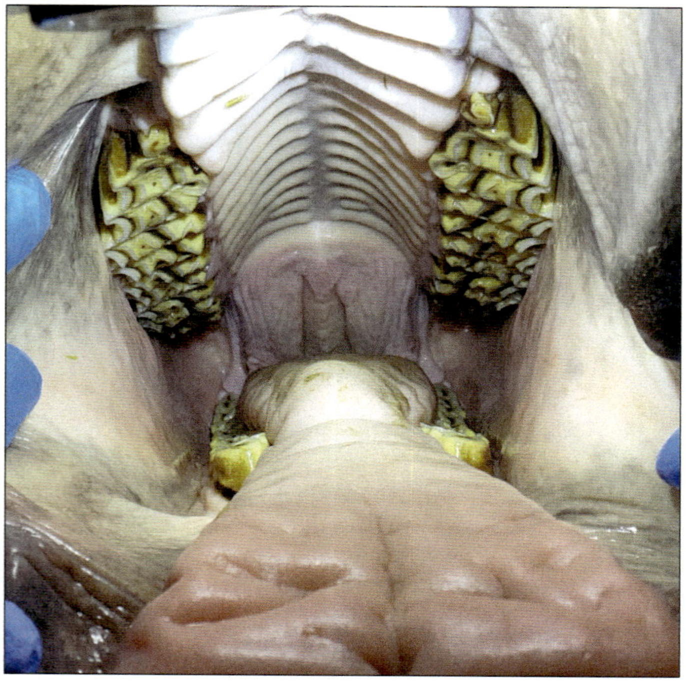

A clean mouth on a horse wearing a full mouth speculum with a bright light. There are two large wolf teeth ***mesial*** *to the 106 and 206. Image credit Dr Elke Pollaris.*

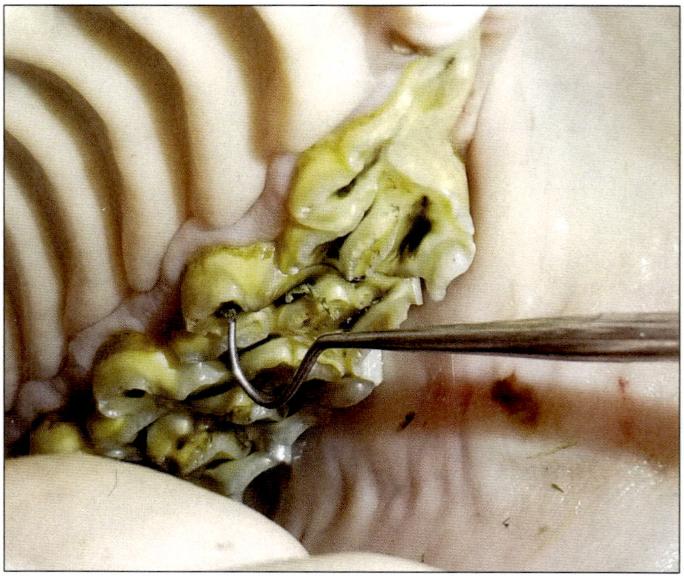

The probe is sticking directly into an open pulp horn on pulp horn #5 of the 207. There is food material inside the pulp horn. This is a serious condition for this tooth. Image credit Cathie Heald Greenwell.

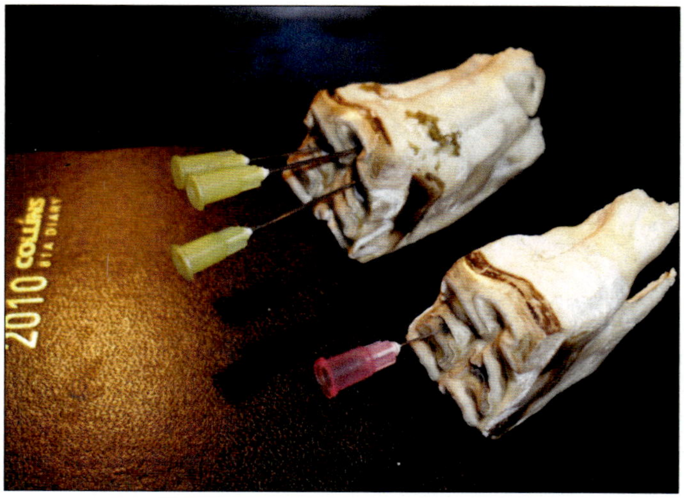

Extracted cheek teeth with nonvital ***pulp exposures*** *from a horse with a unilateral, chronic sinus infection. Although the pulp horns were not able to be probed before or at extraction, four months post-extraction, Dr Elizabeth Thompson found the material filling the pulp horns was soft enough to allow insertion of needles into every pulp. Image credit Author.*

the ***occlusal*** surfaces of each tooth. It should feel like scratching on smooth glass, but if it doesn't, and feels more like scratching a brick, then the protective layer of the tooth may have been disrupted, a problem. If the probe can be inserted into a pulp horn, the pulp cavity might be "open", and bacteria and food material can enter the pulp chamber. Not an ideal situation.

However, even if a tooth is dead, one cannot always place a probe or an endodontic file into a pulp in a live horse. Sometimes the only sign that a tooth is dead or infected is that the pulp is a slightly different color, black instead of the normal dark brown. On the previous page are two dead teeth which were extracted from one patient in which I couldn't probe the pulps in the live horse, or even at extraction. However, four months later, I could place needles into every pulp horn on both teeth.

Your dental operator will evaluate the gingiva (gums) near each tooth and the mucosa inside the cheeks, the palate (the ridged flat part at the top of the mouth), beneath the tongue, and the entire tongue itself. The teeth will be counted to check for absent or extra teeth, and any malocclusions or abnormalities will be noted for diagnosis and treatment.

Accurate and complete records are vital to monitor treatment progress, or your horse's response from visit to visit. The bars of the mouth and canines are again checked for health, presence of wolf teeth (including seeking mandibular wolf teeth or unerupted wolf teeth). Table angles are evaluated. The cheek teeth are examined for ***sharp enamel points***, ***hooks***, ramps, steps, infundibular and ***peripheral caries***, waves, diastemata, periodontal pockets, misaligned teeth, any other abnormalities.

All these surfaces may then be palpated for any irregularities. Some pathology may initially be easier to feel than to see with a mirror, such as very small feed-impacted (or filled) diastemata. An oroscope will give the operator a thorough look at the whole mouth.

Evaluating diastemata

Any ***diastemata*** with feed impaction found may now be evaluated and decisions made with you about any necessary therapeutics. If decision is made to treat, administering local anesthesia at this point is indicated, as treatment of diastemata is painful for the horse. As you can see to the right, a mirror or oroscope is essential.

Odontoplasty (examination-guided "floating", or filing of necessary teeth) follows, then checking and rechecking the teeth. This will be covered in Chapter 14, Odontoplasty. Some vets let owners see and feel the teeth before or after odontoplasty. Once you have felt the sharp enamel points and buccal ulcers, you'll never forget.

By the time the odontoplasty is completed, the local anesthesia should have taken effect. Next, picks and forceps will be used to clear the larger pieces of feed material from the periodontal pockets. Impacted food may be removed with picks, forceps, pressurized water picks, and/or K-files. A pressurized water pick speeds up the process and does an excellent job in the final evacuation of pockets, though they must be evaluated after flushing to ensure all feed material has been removed. The pockets will then be measured for depth with a periodontal probe and recorded in the horse's chart. Your vet will decide if further diastema treatment is necessary at this time.

Your vet will most likely recheck the mouth after finishing the odontoplasty and diastema treatment via mirror or oroscope, and by hand. This may seem like a long list of things to check in your horse's mouth, but for an experienced and well-

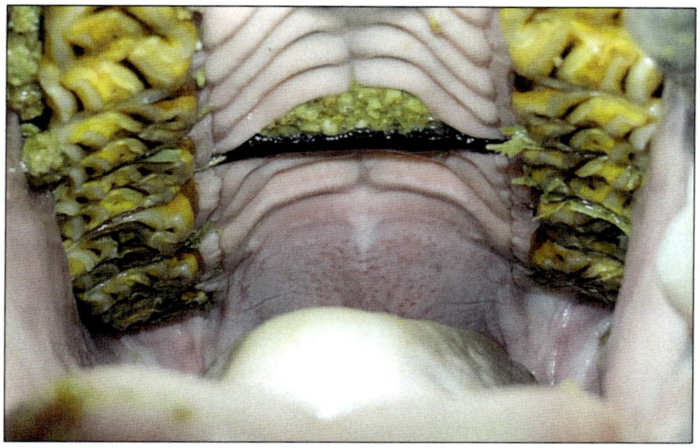

*Sometimes the unexpected appears: This horse had a stick jammed between two teeth of his maxillary **arcades**. By the looks of it, the stick had been there for quite some time. Image credit Dr Kirsten Jackson, Dental Vet.*

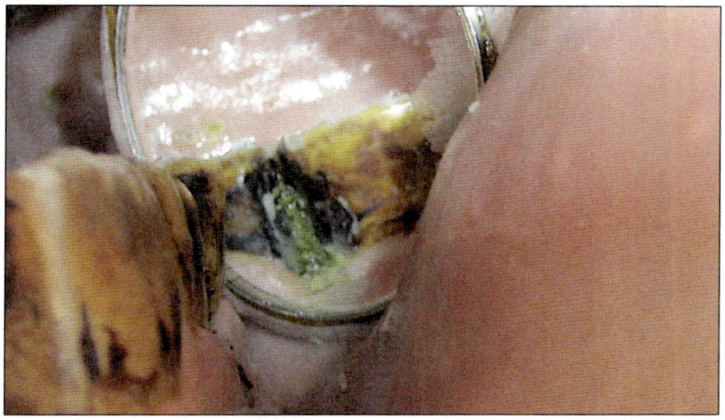

Feed filled diastema is visible well with mirror and light. This needs treatment by your veterinarian, with pain relief and not merely sedation, as it extremely painful to your horse. Image credit Author.

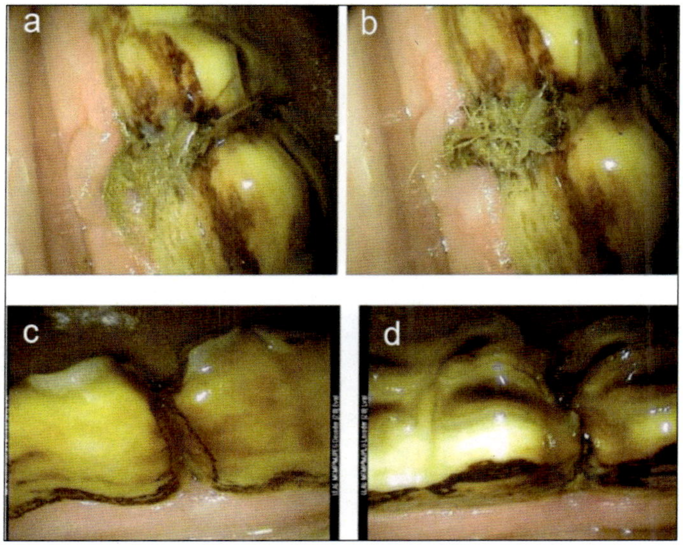

*These oroscopic images of 307 and 308 show a narrow diastema with food impaction in the **interproximal space** and periodontal disease. The lower images show the same teeth three months after partial occlusal widening (not full diastema drilling). Image credit Dr Pearce C. (2020). Image originally published in Pearce C. Recent developments in equine dentistry. New Zealand Veterinary Journal 68, 178-86, 2020. ©NZVA*

trained operator, it is second nature. Luckily, with power floating instruments, the relatively long time previously needed for odontoplasty is shortened, leaving more time for the vitally important, thorough examination.

After a sedated dental examination and treatment, it's a good idea to keep the horse away from hay or long grass to prevent an episode of "choke". I've always been careful to advise owners to withhold hay for an hour after the horses exit the stocks, but hadn't previously worried about grass. Clearly, I needed to put it into this book, because I had my first patient with post-dentistry choke last month. This horse usually lived on very short grass and while waking up from sedation, it was hand-grazing some grass. It turned out to be very long grass. Bad idea. Ten minutes later, the owner asked if her horse was meant to have "green stuff" (a.k.a. chewed up grass in saliva) coming from her nose, or "choke". That would be "no". Fifteen minutes later, the mare coughed up this twisted ***quid*** of long grass coated in saliva. Take-home message: no hay *nor* grass for at least an hour after the horse leaves the stocks, which will then be more than an hour after sedation!

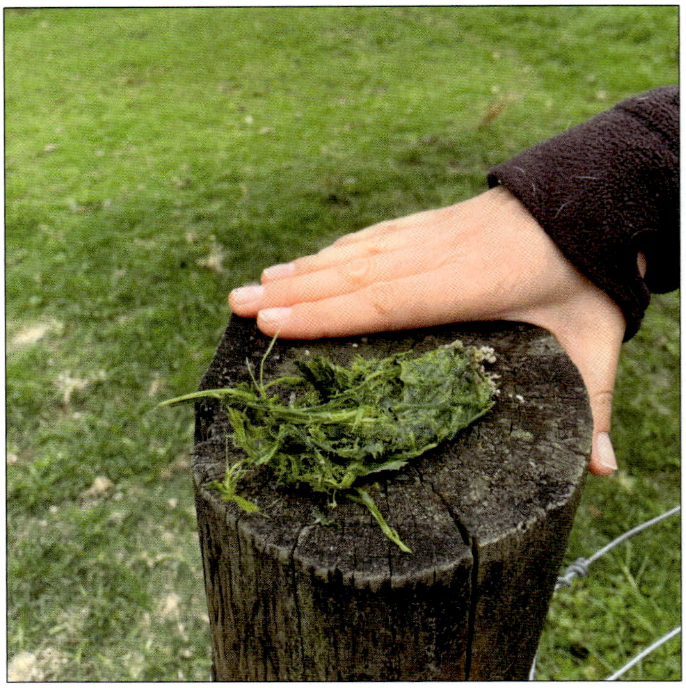

Wad of long grass coated in saliva coughed up by a horse which had already left Dr Elizabeth Thompson's stocks after a normal sedated dentistry. Message: no hay NOR grass until an hour after leaving the stocks! Image credit Author.

Treatment of diastemata is an important part of keeping your horse pain-free and preventing more serious dental disease. However, remember that diastema treatment is "working below the gumline", and in many locales, this is defined as a significant surgical procedure and falls under the realm of the practice of veterinary medicine. Check with your regulatory agencies if you're not using a veterinarian for your dentistry to ensure your operator is legally allowed to perform these operations, along with the sedation. In New Zealand, both the operator and the owner are liable for large fines if a non-veterinarian performs these or other acts of veterinary medicine.

How Can I "Age" My Horses?

WHILE SOME PEOPLE seem to think "a real horseman can age a horse", one of the most important things to remember about the aging of horses is that *horses rarely read that book, either...* and although in the first five years of age, when incisor and ***cheek tooth eruption*** give you a fair idea of age, estimating their age is an educated guess. Many factors influence the teeth and wear, which alter the appearance of the incisors, and thus the apparent age of an equid. These factors (for example: feed quality and type, breed, environmental conditions, disease, injury, and heredity) make examination of the teeth for age determination an inexact science. Historically, horse traders took advantage of these age-related changes by altering occlusal tables to make horses appear younger than they were.

Here are a few terms which will help the following discussion make more sense.

hypsodont: Long crowned teeth which erupt throughout the animal's life until the teeth expire.

dietary abrasive forces: Forces generated by rough feedstuffs grinding against the teeth in chewing. These forces result in increased ***abrasion*** of the occlusal surfaces of the teeth.

tooth growth: Actual growth of the tooth from its ***apical*** end. Incisors actually grow for approximately seventeen years. The cheek teeth grow until two years after the tooth is erupted into the mouth, then it ceases growth and tooth "lengthening" over time is actually only through eruption, until the tooth expires.

tooth eruption: a progressive protrusion of the tooth out of its ***alveolus*** (socket), which is normal in hypsodonts.

How can I tell a horse's age?

As discussed in Chapter 3, Anatomy: What is an Eruption Sequence?, the cheek teeth erupt sequentially at fairly consistent ages, but outside of dental examinations, it's difficult to see into the back of the mouth, and not recommended to prevent injuries!

An experienced practitioner can give a fair approximation of a horse's age by comparing the angulation of the incisors from the side and the appearance of the occlusal surfaces. On these surfaces, they can compare the "cups" (infundibula), the "***dental star***" (***dentin*** which has filled in the retreating pulp chamber), and the shape of the tooth to documented "normals" for the different ages. Understand, however, that a definitive age cannot be given in horses by their teeth because of variations caused by their diets,

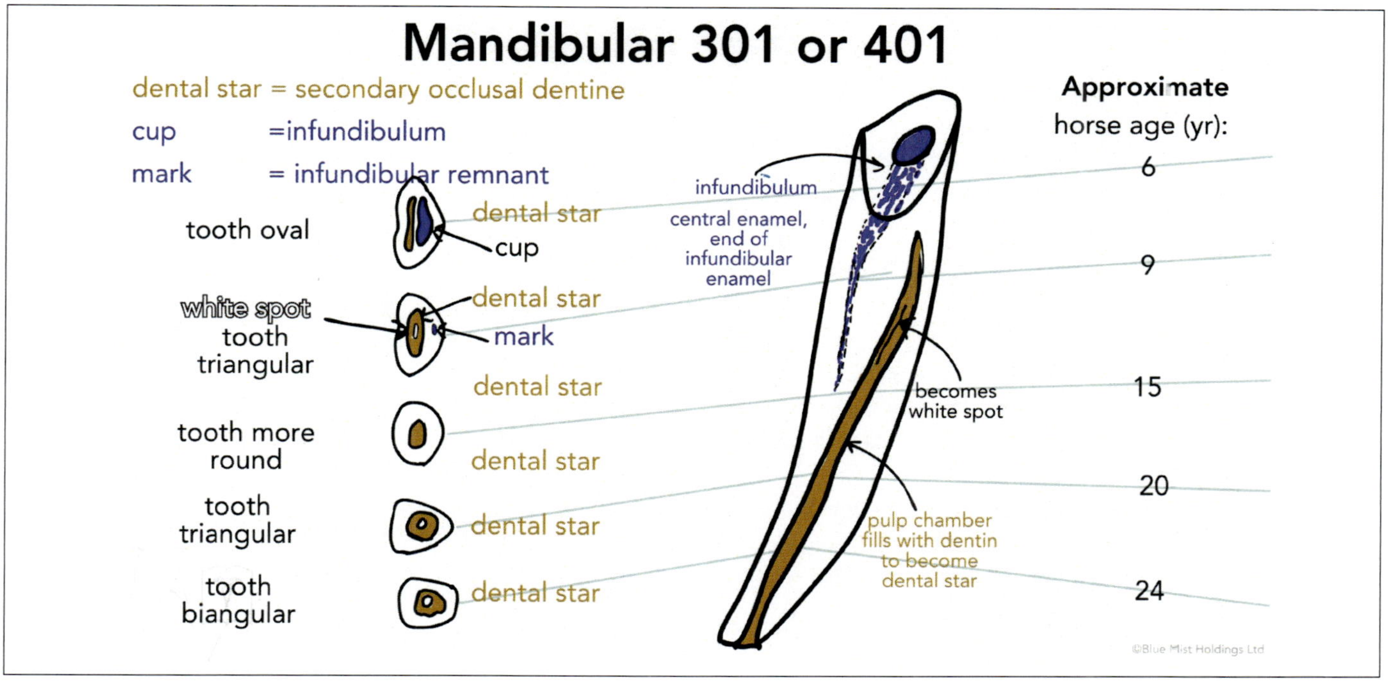

This diagram displays how the different structures appear and disappear as this horse's '01, or central incisor ages and is gradually ground off by attrition. Image credit Author.

their breed, etc., and the appearance of the structures just mentioned becomes less reliable in estimating age as a horse grows older.

When you understand that dietary abrasive forces cause ***attrition*** or wear, resulting in gradual exposure of these structures as they are ground away, you'll see that increased wear from coarse, gritty feed, sandy paddocks, etc. may give the impression that horses are older than they are. There is also a large degree of breed influence as well as individual variation. Some breeds have later or earlier eruption, and if you have miniatures, things get even more uncertain, as their eruption is often delayed by several years from the equine Standardbred average.

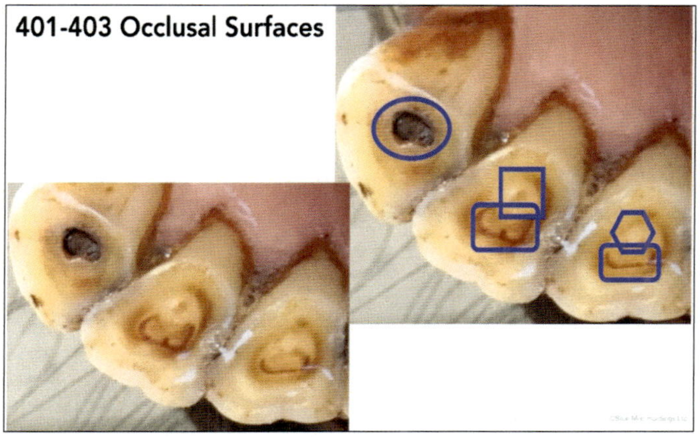

Incisors 401-403 on a teenaged horse. This illustrates how different the teeth can look between the three, as each tooth differs in age by approximately 1 year. Unmarked Image credit Dr Kirsten Jackson, Dental Vet, graphic credit Author.

In analysis of the available studies, the only thing that appears consistent is that horses within certain breeds tend to have some consistency in the age at which these tooth changes occur. So, if you want to sound like you really know what you're talking about, let people know this.

In Chapter 3, Anatomy of the Mouth, you will find a discussion about the anatomical structures of the tooth and the changes seen on the cross-sectional occlusal surface of the tooth as it ages. If you haven't seen Chapter 3, Anatomy: Incisor Cross Section yet, please read it now.

Each of the teeth in a quadrant of the mandibular incisor arcade will appear very different until the horse is in their late teens and showing only the dental star on all of the teeth. Remember that the permanent incisors erupt at approximately 2.5, 3.5, and 4.5 years? It makes sense, then, as you go from the '01s (centrals) toward the '03s (corners), each tooth differs from the next by a year or so in age, and thus will appear quite different from the adjacent teeth because it shows different structures on the occlusal surface due to the ages of each individual tooth. Looking at a set of real incisors and comparing this to the chart on the next page may help.

I think of the dental star the "dentinal" star because the star is formed from the secondary occlusal dentine. Dentin or dentine stains brown due to the pigments in the green feed. The dentinal star appears on the central ('01) incisor in the mandible (in Standardbred horses) at around 5-6 years of age.

This horse's 401-403 (below right) show nice examples of a disappearing *cup* on the 403 (circle), the *enamel ring* with some *cementum* on the 402 (the square), the dental stars (rectangles) and then the ***mark***, a tiny dot of *enamel* on the 401 (hexagon) This is a perfect example of different stages, if not ages! It reminds us that a horse's teeth don't always match the charts.

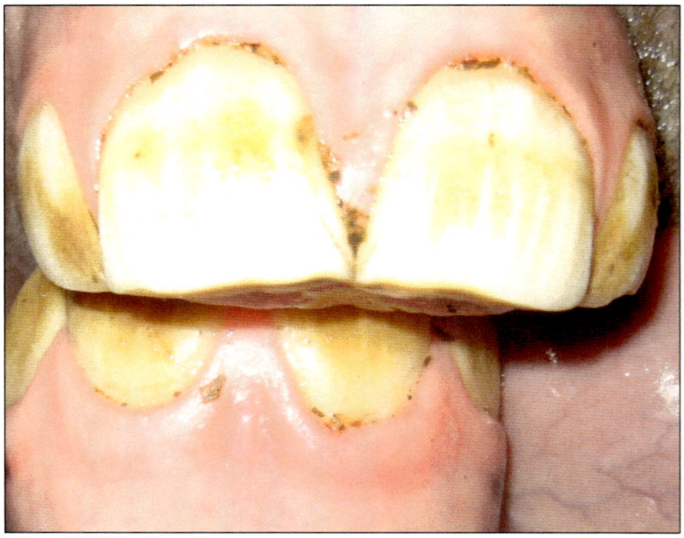

*Examining one of Dr Elizabeth Thompson's yearling patients with **prognathism** (overbite). Image credit Author.*

What are approximate eruption ages?

A tooth is said to first "erupt" when it cuts through the gingiva and first appears in the mouth. The term can be a little confusing because this same tooth will continue to "erupt", or progressively protrude into the mouth until the tooth ***expires***.

Incisors:

Deciduous (baby teeth): The easiest way to remember very young foal aging is to think of the deciduous incisors, from the '01s (centrals) toward the '03s (corners), which erupt at approximately: six days, six weeks, six months. Not perfect, but it's close.

Permanents: from'01s (centrals) toward the '03s (corners), incisors one through three, are denoted by "I1-3". The published average ages for eruption of these teeth from '01 (I1), through the '02 (I2) to the '03 (I3) are 2.5, 3.5 and 4.5 years, respectively.

However, as an example of how these eruption ages vary between breeds, a study in Europe showed the differences by breed of this:

Belgian Draft Horses: I 1-3: ± 3, ± 4, ± 5 years of age
Standardbred Horses: I 1-3: ± 3 ± 4, ± 5 years of age
Arabians Horses: I 1-3: ± 3.5, ± 4.5, ± 5.5 years of age
Mini-Shetland Ponies: I 1-3: ≥ 3, ± 4, ± 5 years of age

Wolf Teeth:

Permanent only: wolf teeth usually erupt around 6-18 months, if they erupt at all.

Canines:

Deciduous '04s: tooth is usually only a tiny spicule, which may not erupt fully, if they erupt at all.

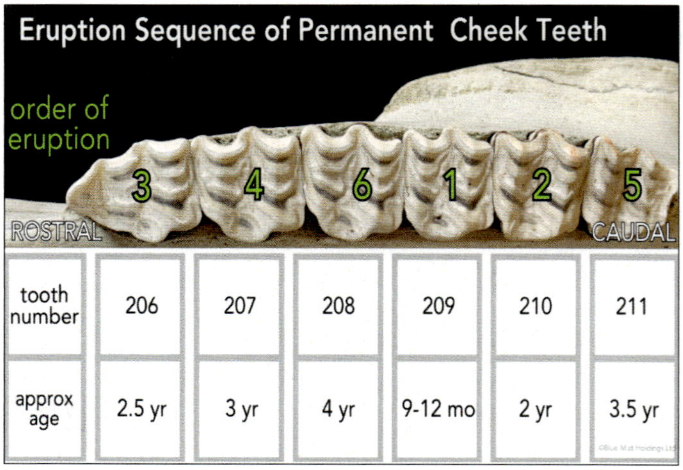

The order of eruption of equid cheek teeth. Image credit Author.

Permanent '04s: usually erupt between 4-6 years old, if at all; some remain unerupted and some are not present at all.

Cheek Teeth:

See the diagram (right) for approximate eruption times of the cheek teeth. The order of eruption is marked in green on the teeth themselves.

Premolars

Deciduous: '06s - '08s

Permanents: '06s - '08s

Molars (no deciduous molars)

Permanents only: '09s - '11s

In summary, old habits die hard regarding aging horses. While the ancient established methods of aging horses may be an inexact science, aging by teeth still provides us with a practical tool for roughly estimating the ages of equids. Advances are still taking place, now that scientists are studying aging and taking into account breed, location, feedstuffs, and the like. See more detailed discussions on this topic in Bibliography and Further Reading.

Special Dental Exams: Prepurchase Exams

AS MENTIONED PREVIOUSLY, horses may show few signs, or many, of dental disease. It can be a cause of subtle, unexplained lameness and in these cases, a thorough dental examination is indicated.

While the presence or absence of thorough dental examinations during a prepurchase examination is up for debate in different countries, I feel they should be included. Many horses have been purchased after prepurchase examinations which did not include an oral exam. Unfortunately, it is not rare to discover severe dental disease, including cheek tooth fractures and other severe dental issues after purchasing a horse and getting it home. This is seriously disheartening to a new owner, not to mention expensive.

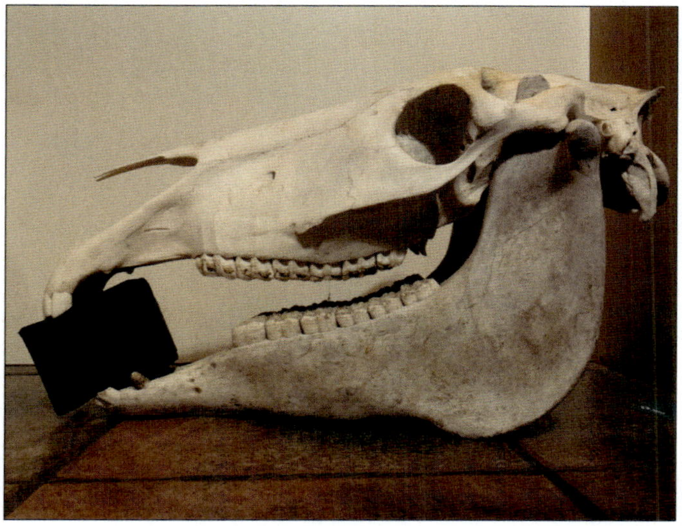

Block between incisors maximizes separation of cheek teeth arcades on "oblique" radiographs, or those taken at approximately 30-45 degrees to the horizontal. Image credit Author.

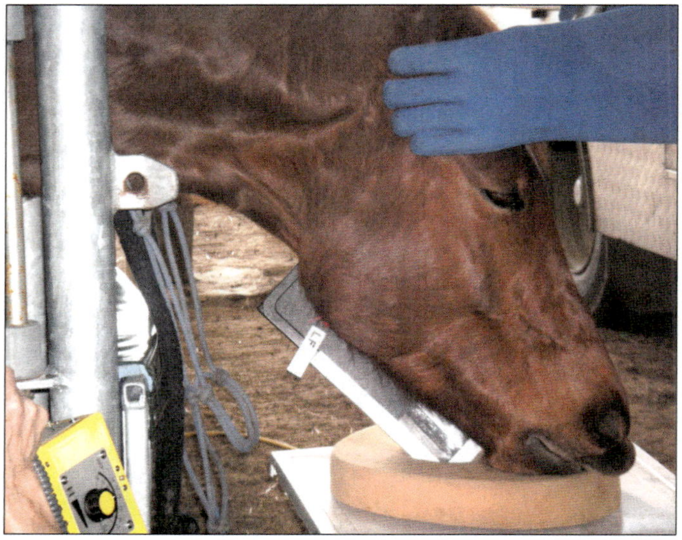

Dr Elizabeth Thompson explains the setup she will use for taking mandibular cheek tooth radiographs to the owner of this sedated horse. The patient is in the stocks with safety equipment ready, and appropriate labeling equipment is already on the receiver. Although lead-lined gloves are available, all hands will be away from the x-ray field before the radiographs are taken! Image credit Author.

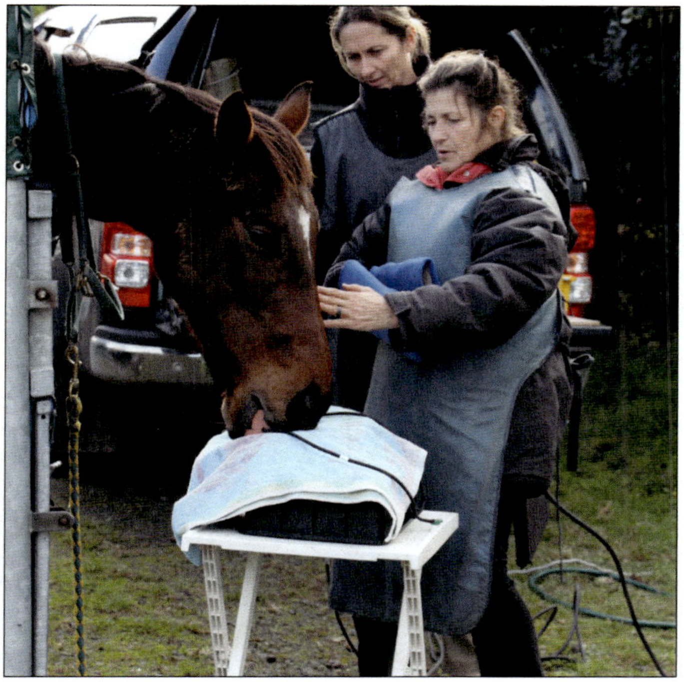

This horse is ready for its dental radiography examination by Dr Orla Roan and Dr Elizabeth Thompson. Image credit Matthew Mole.

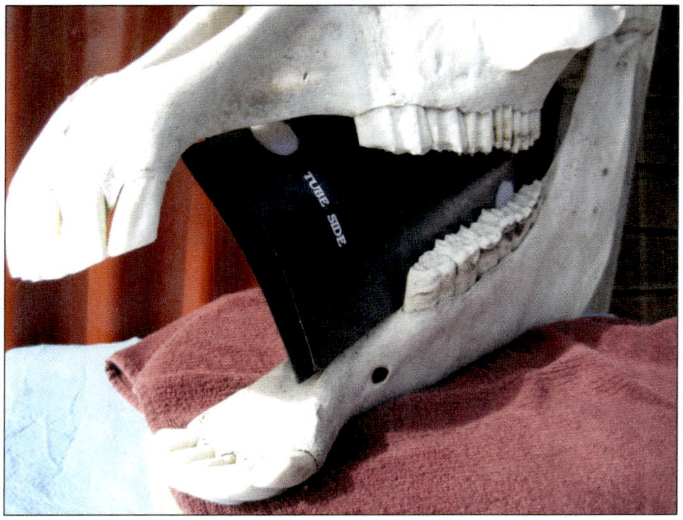

Intraoral radiography can eliminate the overlap of the opposing arcades and give a much clearer image, but it not very practical at best. This is a plain film intraoral cassette inside this skull's mouth. Unfortunately, some digital systems do not yet have equine intraoral plates. Image credit Author.

Special Exams: Advanced Diagnostic Instrumentation

AS DENTISTRY PROGRESSES, so does the equipment available for diagnostic and therapeutic use. These diagnostic tools range from radiography (X-Rays) through to oroscopy, sinus endoscopy, CT, MRI, and nuclear scintigraphy. Oral flushing instruments are useful both for cleaning the mouth to allow a proper examination, and for therapy of diseases such as diastemata.

All of these instruments have their benefits and drawbacks. Some of them are difficult to access due to location or cost, but your vet may already have sufficient equipment in their practice to perform some or most of these diagnostics.

Radiography

Most practices can perform effective dental radiography in the field. Stocks help keep the horse from moving forward, while a padded portable table gives the sedated horse a good surface to rest its muzzle while radiographs are taken.

Separation of the incisor arcades via a block or radiolucent speculum plates offers the best visualization of individual teeth on radiographs and gives your veterinarian the best opportunity to provide you with a correct diagnosis.

Separating the incisors is essential because of the overlap of teeth when taken from one side of the horse to the other (extra oral technique). Unlike a dentist (your own dentist) who usually uses *intra*oral techniques with the sensor or film inside your mouth and thus has little to no overlap of teeth, most veterinarians do not have intraoral sensors or plates which will eliminate this overlap. Further, intraoral radiography is not practical when taking a comprehensive radiographic study of a horse's whole mouth, especially with young horses, which may have cheek teeth too long to be viewed on a single intraoral plate or receiver.

Radiographs plus the clinical signs exhibited by your horse allow a vet to diagnose tooth death, long standing infection, fractures, sinus infections, and other diseases of the head. Radiographs which meet the criteria of effectively showing everything needed to diagnose disease are termed "diagnostic".

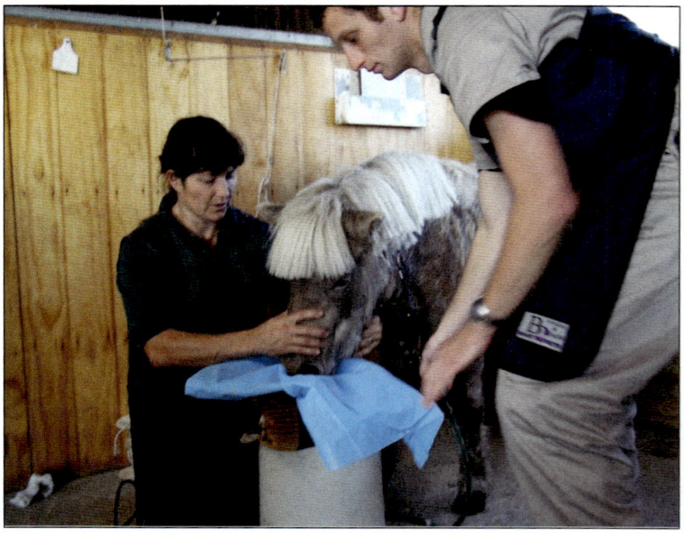

Working with miniatures can be challenging. Dr Elizabeth Thompson finds that good kneepads help.

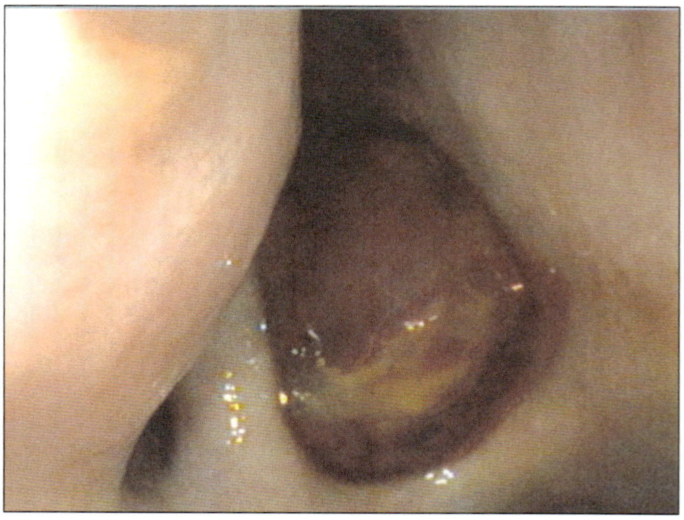

Trans nasal endoscopy showing a large red bleeding mass at the level of the ethmoid. This is a typical image seen for an ethmoidal hematoma. Image credit Dr Denis Verwilghen.

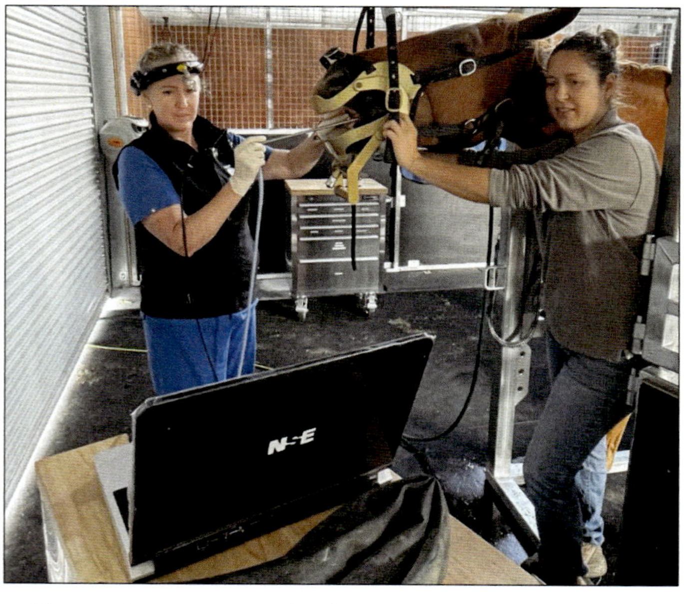

The use of oroscopes, or oral endoscopes, is becoming the standard of practice for equine dental veterinarians. The visualization with a quality oroscope is exquisite. Image credit Dr Olivia James.

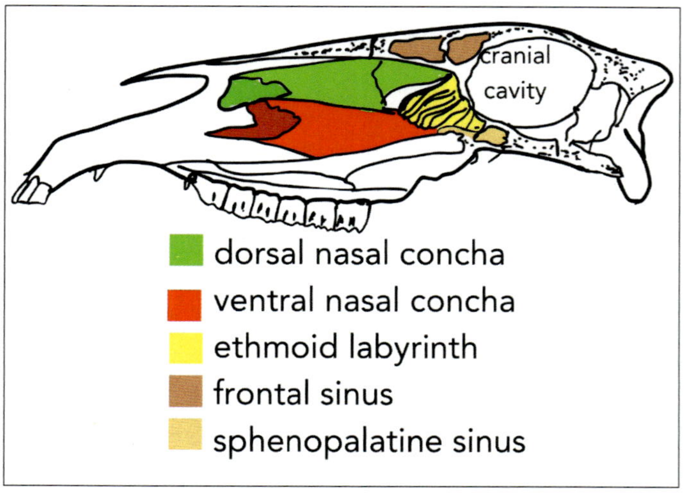

Interior view of the sinuses which may be significant in disease of the head, including the ethmoid labyrinth, or sinuses (yellow). Image credit Author.

Taking "diagnostic" dental radiographs which may be used to decide the next steps for your horse require significant training and practice. Differing equid sizes may require creative thinking, such as working with miniatures vs. draft horses.

Often the information from the radiographs is still sketchy, no matter how excellent the images. Correct interpretation of dental radiographs also requires still more training and practice, but they may be sent to other veterinarians for their opinions or referral. X-Rays are truly your best friend in equine dentistry.

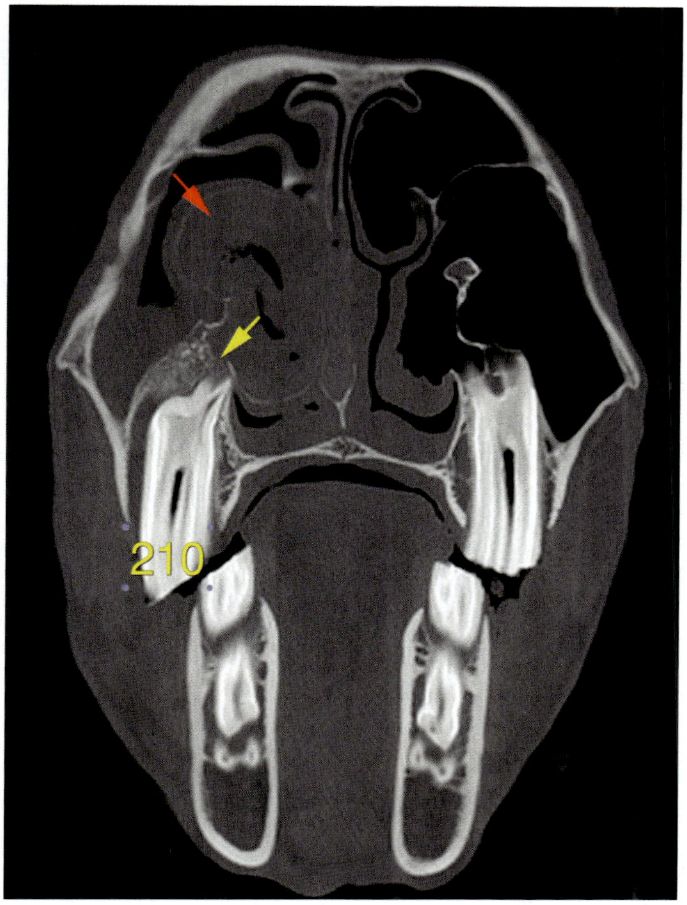

A CT image in a transverse (cross) section clearly shows blunting of the roots from an apical infection of 210 (yellow arrow) and filling of sinuses by an infectious mass. Image credit Dr Denis Verwilghen.

Oroscopy, or oral endoscopy

Oral endoscopy with a flexible endoscope is available in most practices with the endoscopes they already possess. The best instrument for oral endoscopy is an actual oroscope, which is a slim, rigid endoscope with an appropriately angled lens, connected to a computer or other digital device. They are now readily available at a reasonable price, so they are becoming standard of practice in equine dentistry. A mirror is essential, but an oroscope makes dental life worth living.

Sinus endoscopy

A practice's (sterile) gastroscope or oroscope may be used to visualize structures inside ***sinuses*** as needed during the performance of sinus surgery, but new rigid sinus endoscopes are in use by more and more specialist equine veterinary practitioners for sinus surgery.

CT, MRI, and nuclear scintigraphy

Computed Tomography (CT), Magnetic Resonance Imaging (MRI) and nuclear scintigraphy can help identify hard-to-find

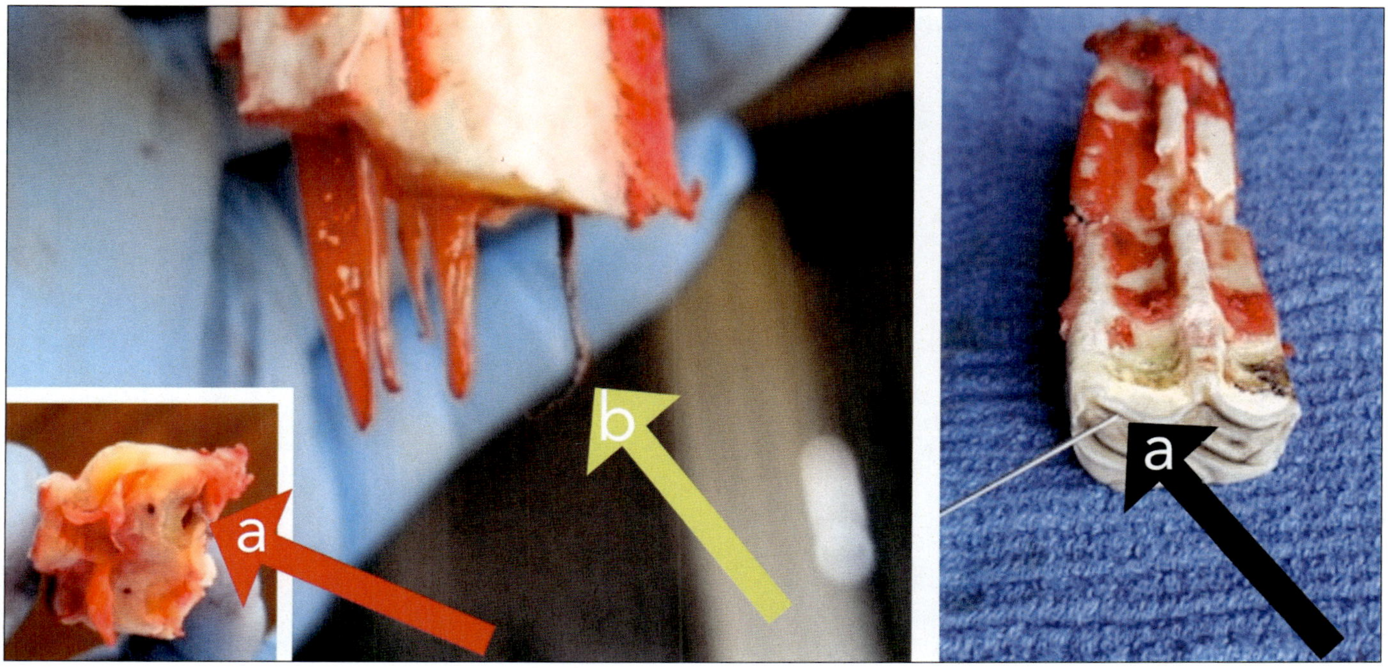

The CT of this patient showed gas pockets in pulp horn #2. See the dark area of the tooth around this pulp horn (red arrow labelled a), where the shriveled black pulp (seen at the yellow arrow b) used to reside. The other plump, healthy red ***tissues*** *parallel to it are more healthy pulps. In the right-hand image, a metal probe is in the open pulp horn on the occlusal surface (black arrow a) of the tooth. Unmarked image credit Cathie Heald Greenwell, graphic credit Author.*

problems in the skull and individual teeth but are not yet readily available in all locations. The size of a horse can also be an issue. All of them are fairly pricey, but these modalities offer information which nothing else currently can.

Running an MRI on a horse's big head usually takes over an hour of general anesthesia, so it is less frequently used than the more rapid CT. MRI tends to mostly be useful only for individual teeth which have already been extracted, and not still in the horse's mouth. These challenges limit MRI's usefulness, especially now that CT is more readily available.

Nuclear scintigraphy was once the go-to before we had CT and MRI, as it could help localize an inflammatory or cancerous reaction, but again, CT is taking over the stage for many reasons, including health and environmental concerns around the chemicals used for nuclear scintigraphy.

CT for head and dental issues, however, is becoming more widely used. It is relatively quick, and depending upon the system used, may be performed with the horse under standing sedation. It can pinpoint elusive pathologies which are radiographically "inconclusive", or difficult or impossible to visualize on radiographs. To the right is a CT of a horse with an apical infection and a sinus mass.

As previously mentioned, some horses with ***chronic*** nasal
discharge may have one or more black (rather than brown) pulp horns, but some horses don't show even this... However, on CT examination, they can be found, as shown above. This horse had a CT, and it revealed some gas in one of the pulp horns... and look what they found? The shriveled black tissue (marked by the the yellow arrow) is the affected pulp. The other plump, pink tissues are normal pulp horns. ***Purulent*** material was running from the nostril on the same side as this tooth, due to this pulp infection. This tooth was cut during extraction because the horse was so young, and therefore the tooth was extremely long. The only way to intraorally extract the tooth was to section it in a transverse plane (cutting across the tooth) by a sectioning burr, as was mentioned in Chapter 2. This is the ONLY use for a sectioning burr, cut-off wheel, molar shears or molar cutters, as you will hear again!

CHAPTER FIVE

WHAT ARE SOME DENTAL CONDITIONS WHICH AFFECT EQUIDS?

WHEN PEOPLE DISCUSS diseases, they often use the words ***acute*** and ***chronic.*** These words say nothing about the severity of the disease, but rather of the timing or stage of a disease process.

An acute condition is one in its early, or immediate stages. Depending upon the condition, this may be over a period of minutes to months in duration. A human example of this is a just-fractured wrist, or an early case of appendicitis.

A chronic condition is one which has continued past the acute stage. Depending upon the condition, this may be anywhere from weeks to months in duration, or continuing indefinitely. A human example of this is chronic arthritis in a person's knee joint which has been ongoing for years.

What Other Diseases are Caused Indirectly From Poor Dentition?

IF A HORSE has what we call poor dentition, or has teeth in poor condition, he may have difficulty effectively ***masticating*** (chewing) his feed. As an indirect result of this, there are several disease conditions which may occur.

Choke

Many painful dental conditions cause affected horses to chew abnormally, (e.g. ***sharp enamel points***, ***mucosal*** ulcers, ***diastemata***, ramps, ***hooks***, excessive transverse ridges (ETRs), waves, steps, and fractures). This leads to ineffective mastication of long stems in their feed and may result in these long stems being swallowed without adequate chewing. The horse may struggle to ingest this resultant "quid" or wad of twisted-up hay or grass and may spit it out ("***quidding***") or somehow swallow it. If the wad is too large to make it through the esophagus, it may cause a blockage, or a "choke", where the esophagus becomes blocked. While this is not blockage of the airway, as choking would be in people, it's uncomfortable for the horse and stressful to the owner, as large quantities of feed-stained, bubbly saliva drain from the mouth and nostrils, as it cannot go down the (blocked) esophagus. Choke can also occur from ***hard feed***, especially in older equids, so be sure to follow the manufacturer's recommended instructions for soaking any pelleted or flaked dry feed (e.g. sugar beet). If they are not fully soaked, these feeds may expand in the esophagus and result in choke. In addition to dental causes, other conditions may cause choke, such as neurological dysfunction. Your ***veterinarian*** can diagnose and treat your horse's choke! Contact your veterinarian if choke occurs, because even if a choke clears on its own, during the episode the horse may have inhaled the feed-laced saliva and need further veterinary treatment to prevent or treat pneumonia.

Colic

Dental problems that prevent proper chewing due to pain are risk factors for colic. As above, improperly chewed feed can encourage formation of blockages of the gut which cause colic. Contact your veterinarian at the first sign of colic. There may be a higher incidence of colic in horses with poor dental condition in the autumn or winter, when it is more common to feed supplemental hay. This coincides with the times when horses are restricted in their exercise due to weather, mud, etc. Dental causes of colic may be prevented by at least yearly veterinary dental examination and as-needed therapy. Unfortunately, over the last few millennia, we haven't selected for good dentition when we bred equids, so we need to take care of them!

"Chipmunk Cheeks"

Often people comment about their pony's "cute chipmunk cheeks", but its cause is less than amusing. Horses and ponies which pack partially chewed feed in their ***buccal*** cavity, between their ***cheek teeth*** and cheeks frequently have painful ***oral*** conditions. Dental ***pathology*** which can result in an equid showing these cheek lumps may include:

- Sharp enamel points and ***crown elongations*** (tooth ***overgrowths***) from lack of effective ***odontoplasty***, with resultant pain and ***ulceration*** of the mucosa or tongue
- ***Periodontal*** disease, which progresses with the help of the feed- and bacteria-produced acid in the packed-in wads of feed
- Fractured or loose teeth
- Missing teeth and overgrowth of their opposing teeth. This restricts the normal jaw movement, and the crown elongations may progress to the extent that the tooth protrudes into the soft ***tissue*** (or even the bony tissue) of the opposite jaw.
- "***Dental drift***" of teeth after loss or extraction of a tooth, and neglecting the six monthly-for-life post-extraction odontoplasty requirement
- ***Pulp exposure*** and pain causing incorrect chewing of feed materials
- Foreign body in the back of the mouth or tongue (stick, piece of wire, etc.) preventing the equid from chewing correctly
- ***Supernumerary*** teeth, which are usually not opposed by teeth in the opposite jaw, leading to overgrowths (as above)
- Any other disease which causes oral pain

How about "Get-A-Life", Bit-Related Injuries?

AS THE GREAT UK equine surgeon Tim Greet said, the "get a life" injuries are some of the worst things a rider can do to a horse. What are these? Injuries caused by riders jerking or hauling on their horse's mouth or by improper fit and/or use of bits, especially overly aggressive bits, and tongue ties. See Chapter 5, "Get-A-Life", Bit-Related Injuries. These riders need to "get a life" and stop injuring their horses.

Not only can riders create soft tissue injuries such as tearing the tender commissures (corners) of the mouth or the ***gingiva*** (gums) overlying the bone, but they may also injure the hard tissues such as the bone of the ***mandible,*** or teeth. The sharp-edged mandibular bone of the ***bars of the mouth***, between the ***canines*** and ***wolf teeth*** or cheek teeth, is covered by a thin layer of highly sensitive gingiva. Heavy hands can not only damage, bruise, or cut the gingiva, but also damage the bone beneath it, or damage teeth.

Until the past few decades, this sort of injury has been relegated to an occasional mention here or there, but now veterinarians around the world are researching the topic of bit-related injuries, especially with respect to competition horses and equine welfare.

Damage to the mouth may include:

- injury of the commissures (corners) of the mouth and/or the buccal (cheek) mucosa.
- injury of the mucosa, periosteum, and/or the bone of the bars of the mouth.

The periosteum is the thin layer of connective tissue covering the bone which supplies the underlying bone with its nutrition. Injury here may result in the formation of osteophytes, (bony lumps) or "roughening" of the bone under the gingiva, which may be painful the next time the mandible comes into contact with a bit.

A bit which is fitted too wide will significantly increase the risk of developing a soft tissue or bony lesion because more bit movement is possible in the mouth. Especially with jointed bits, the rider can easily pull the "joint" of a snaffle in between the commissures and towards the mesial part of the mandibular 06.

- fracture or loosening of teeth.

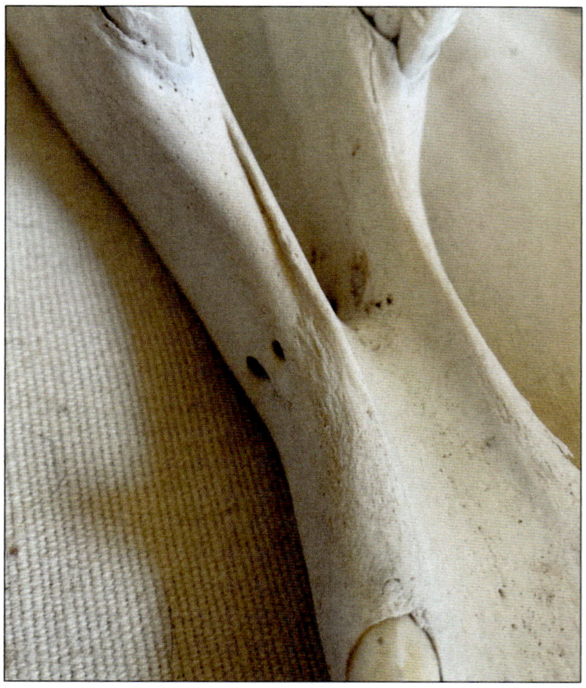

The sharp edges of mandibular bone below the sensitive mucosa of the bars of the mouth. Pressure over the bars can damage the bone and cause severe pain. Image credit Author.

- fracture, with or without ***osteomyelitis*** (bone infection) of the mandible.
- tongue ***lacerations***.

While these injuries may happen during a ride or event, accidents such as when a rider falls and the reins remain in their hands, many of these injuries simply need not happen. Hence the "get a life" title. These injuries may occur during competition from a bit, or from the use of tongue ties in racing.

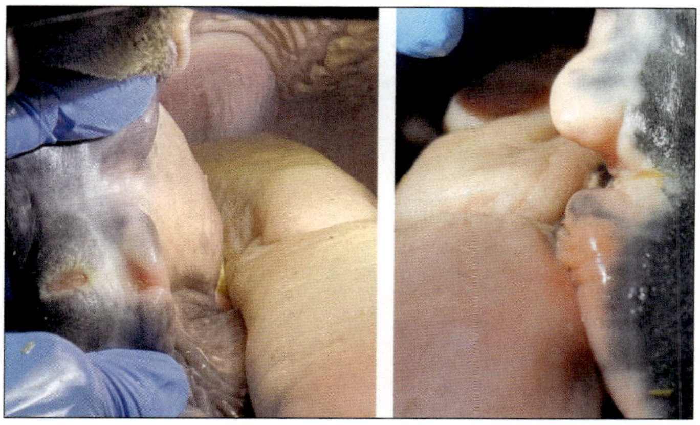

These bit injuries are chronic, or long-standing injuries which have repeatedly happened over a long time period. This is a totally unnecessary cause of pain for this horse. Image credit Dr Elke Pollaris.

- ***Bit related injuries in competition***

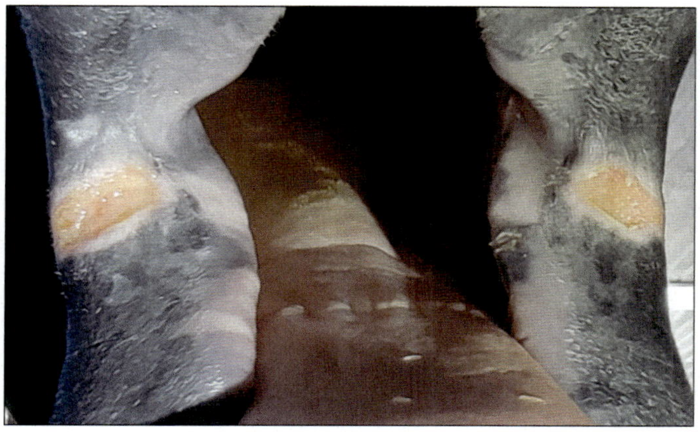

Bitting injuries to commissures of mouth. Image credit Cathie Heald Greenwell.

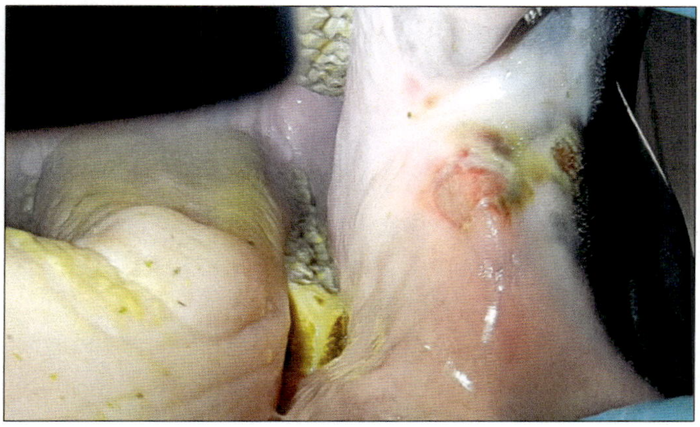

Severe bitting injury to the commissure of this mouth. Image credit Cathie Heald Greenwell.

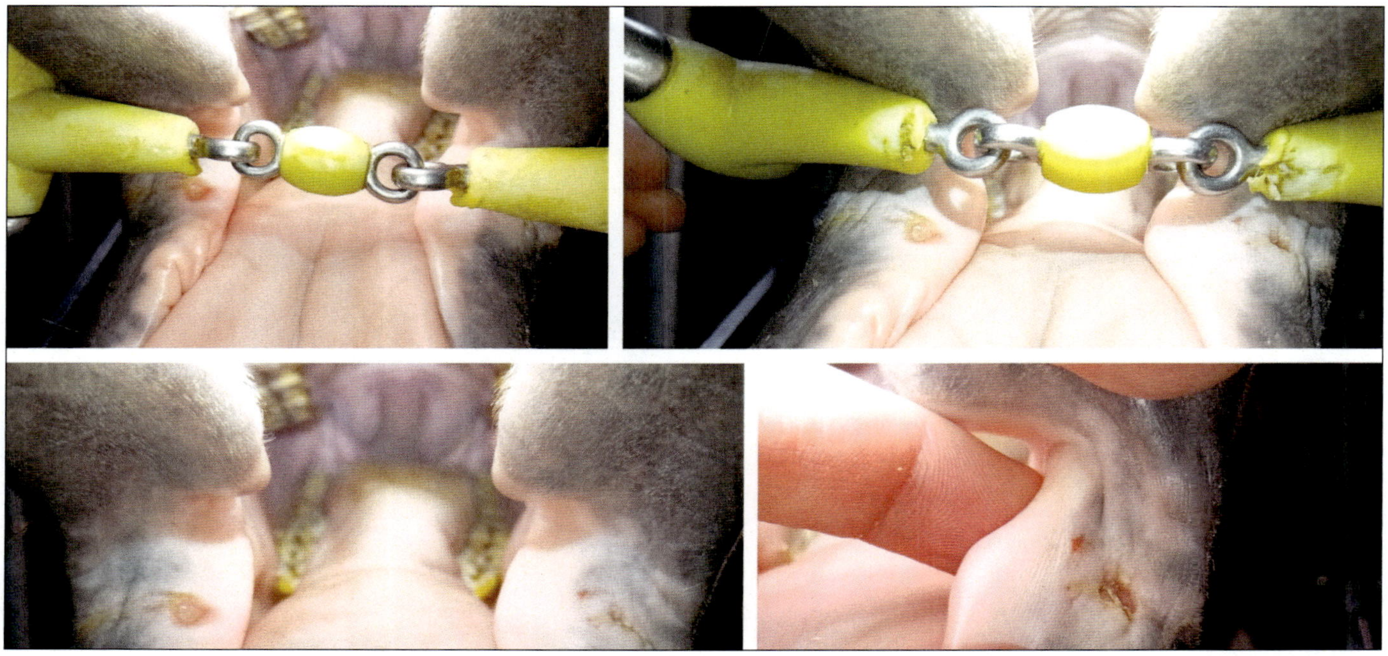

This sequence shows how a combination of a double-linked snaffle and chewing damage to a plastic bit can cause severe and painful injuries to the commissures. A double-jointed mouthpiece lets the bit rest at a very tight angle, which squeezes the mucosa and contributes to the degree of damage. Note in the first image that the physical damage to the plastic-coated bit is not so apparent as it is when the bit is rotated bottom-side-up. The chewed portions of the plastic bit are very sharp and contributed to the mucosal lesions. Note that a smooth double jointed bit can also cause a lot of damage, as can a single jointed bit when it is too wide for the horse. Image credit Dr Elke Pollaris.

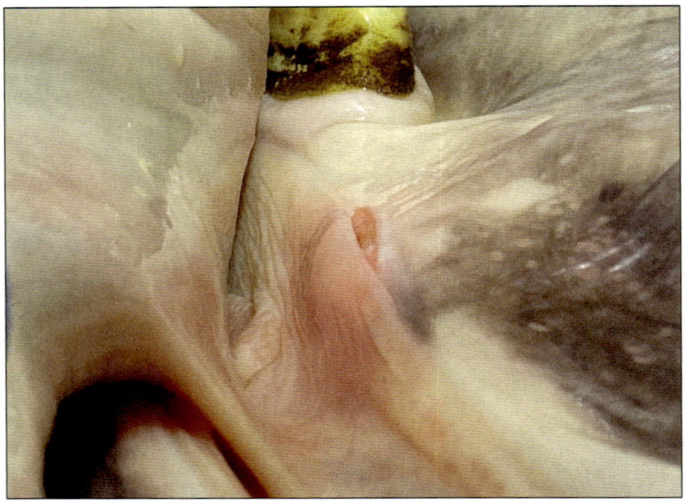

More bit trauma to the soft tissue (and likely also to the periosteum and underlying bone of the bars). Image credit Dr Elke Pollaris.

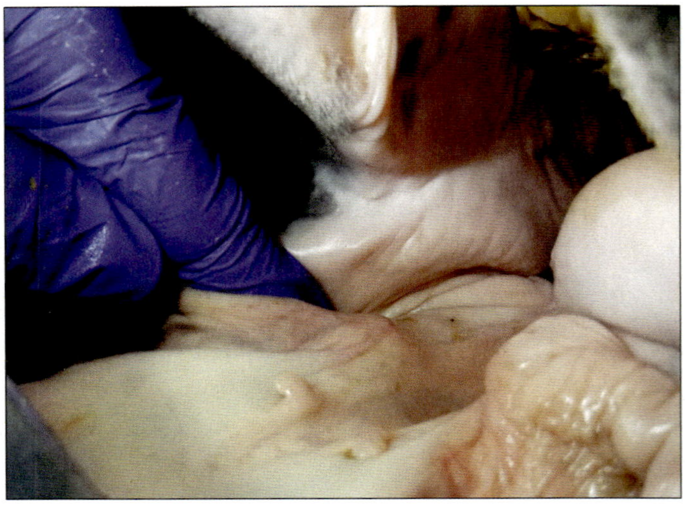

Bony osteophyte from bit injury to the mucosa and periosteum. Image credit Cathie Heald Greenwell.

Researchers have recently been looking at various combinations of clinical signs and lesions in bit-related injuries in horses. These articles may be found in Bibliography and Further Reading. The researchers have been evaluating many different aspects of this topic, including presence and severity of lesions in the general population (one group found around 30-50%!), and across various equine disciplines: before competition, at prelim level of competition, and at finals level of competition. In general, researchers are finding moderate lesions present at low levels pre-competition, more severe lesions at prelim levels, and the most severe *acute* lesions with increased frequency at finals levels. One group found the risk of acute bit-related injury after an event was 52%. More severe commissure injuries were associated with thin or thick bits (compared to middle sized (14-17 mm) bits). Bar lesions were more common in horses with unjointed bits (one study found 40%, another found 67%) vs basic double jointed (10%), formed double-jointed (8%), or single-jointed (5%) bits. Further, mares were found to be at higher risk of moderate or severe lesions than geldings. Several researchers found overly wide bits caused more bar lesions, likely because they moved around excessively and didn't sit properly. Some found curb bits with ports caused bar lesions more frequently as well.

These findings are being used to make recommendations on monitoring these injuries at events with the aim of decreasing painful bit-induced injury and to improve equine welfare.

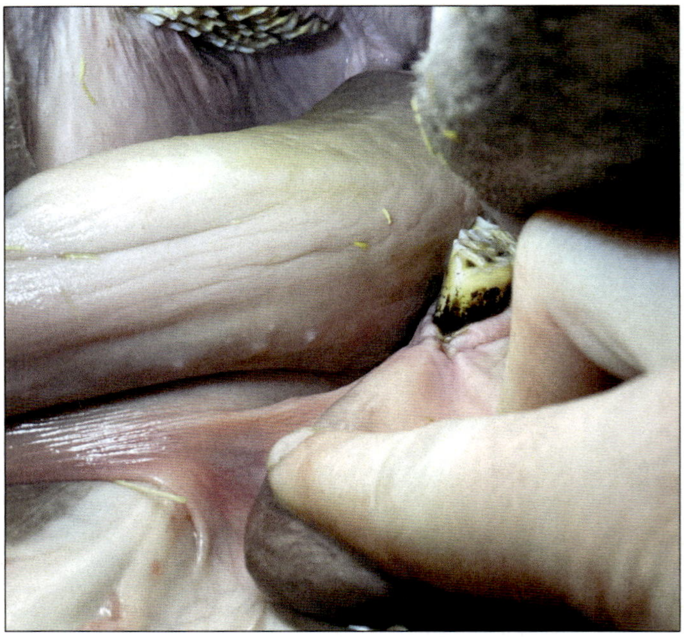

*Trauma to the soft tissues of the bars from a bit **mesial** to the 306. Image credit Dr Elke Pollaris.*

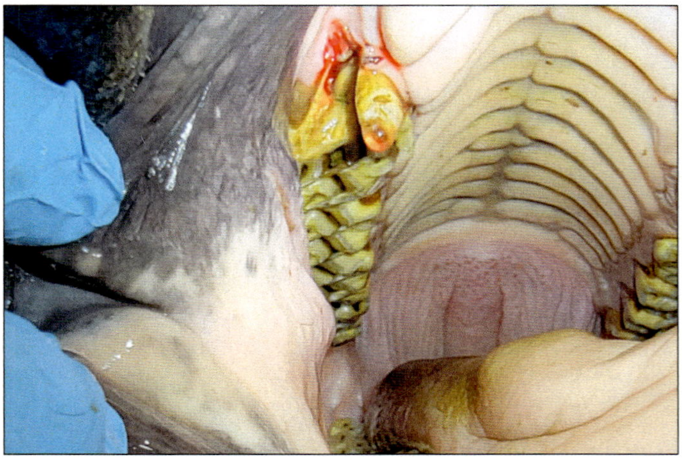

Fractured 106. Image credit Cathie Heald Greenwell.

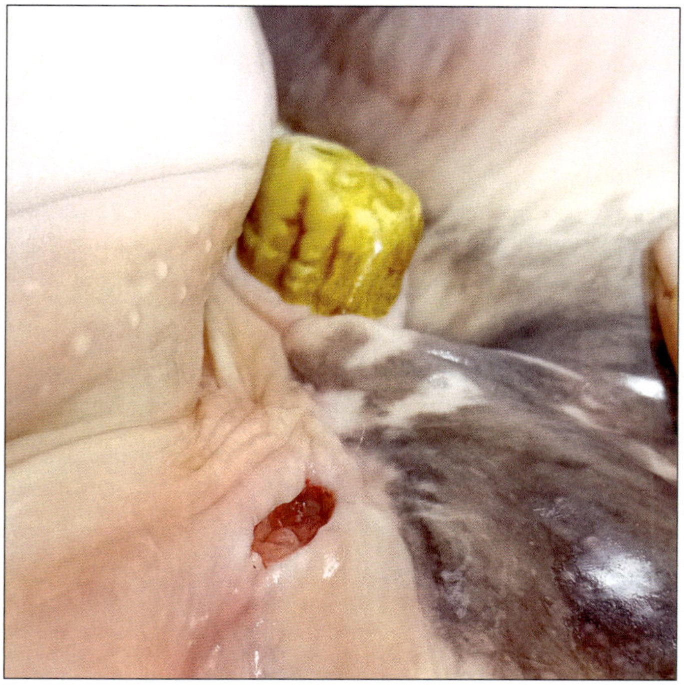

Open wound on the bars of the mouth associated with a sequestrum ((like the one in the image below). The initial damage was likely due to a previous bit injury. Image credit Dr Elke Pollaris.

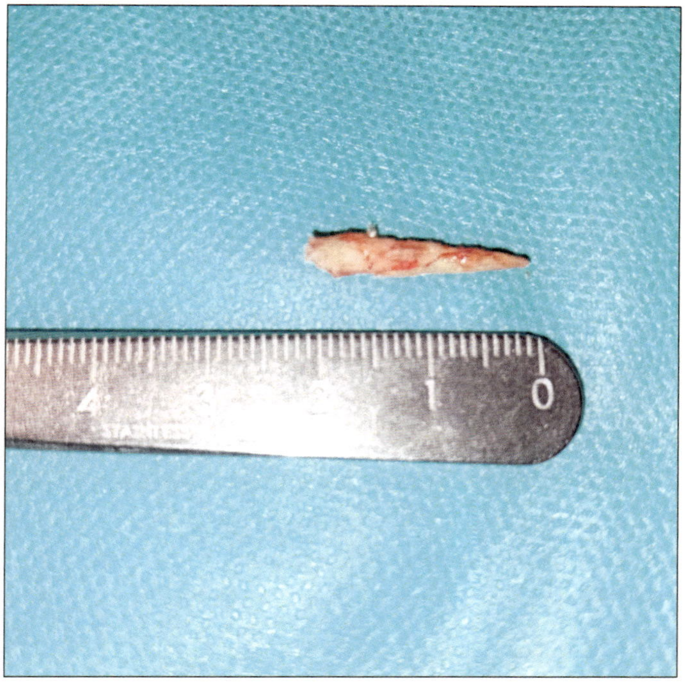

A sequestrum, or a piece of bone which has died due to damage to the layer of nutrition-providing periosteum lying on the bone's surface. This sequestrum was surgically removed from the bars of the mouth and was likely due to a previous bit injury. Image credit Dr Elke Pollaris.

- ***Use of tongue ties in racing and other***

The use of "tongue ties" in Thoroughbred and Standardbred racehorses is a contentious issue and the research is not clear on the necessity of this practice, but it seems to indicate that tongue ties frequently create adverse behavioural effects, as one might expect from tying one's tongue to one's mandible... For those not familiar with the practice, here is a short summary of some of the available research. The use of tongue ties (TT), (which may be defined as a fixation of the tongue to the mandible by tying a band of something like leather, rubber, lycra, or neoprene tightly around the

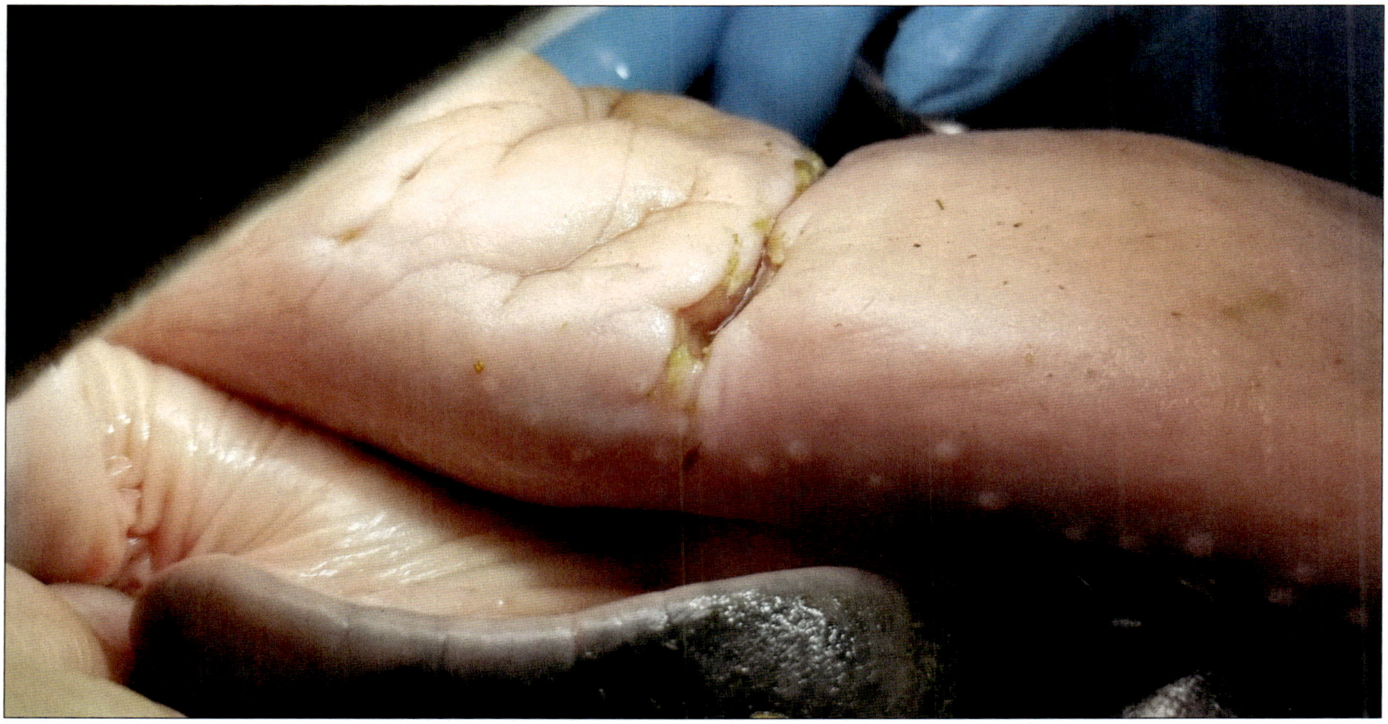

Tongue lacerated from a tongue tie. Image credit Cathie Heald Greenwell.

tongue and then around the mandible) is permitted under the rules of racing and is widespread in both Thoroughbred and Standardbred (harness) racing in many countries. TTs are used by racing trainers to improve racing performance, with the idea that the TT will 1- prevent the horse from getting their tongue over the bit during a race (and improve rider/driver control) and 2- improve airflow in horses which may otherwise have breathing difficulty, displaced soft palate, etc. Research has shown an array of results. The papers are in the Bibliography. While one paper indicates that a certain population of horses benefit from TT in terms of airway improvement, another has shown that TT did not increase the pharyngeal or laryngeal diameter (diameter of the airway through the pharynx and larynx) and there was no evidence of improved upper airway function. The authors indicated that the results of this study did not support the use of tongue ties to enhance upper airway function. Other studies showed that application of TT caused adverse behavioral effects (increased head tossing/ shaking, ears laid back, and gaping of the mouth), and physiological changes suggestive of a stress response, while another study showed obvious adverse behavior effects, but only slight evidence of an increased systemic stress response. A pilot study using a survey indicated that over half of the respondents had encountered either a physical or behavioural complication due to TT use and that complications seemed to be associated with the length of time the TT are in place and how it is checked for tightness.

For whatever reason TT are used, they can cause problems like lacerations of the tongue and other soft tissues. How common are these injuries? Are they all reported? One cannot be sure, but see the image above.

CHAPTER SIX

WHAT ARE DEVELOPMENTAL AND ACQUIRED DENTAL CONDITIONS?

DENTAL DISEASE CONDITIONS may be divided into disorders which develop from the time a fetus is still in the uterus of the dam or during ***eruption*** of the foal's teeth (developmental conditions), versus those which occur after this time (acquired conditions). The developmental disorders will be shown first.

What Developmental Disorders Occur Before Eruption?

IN CHAPTER 3, Anatomy of the Mouth: How Did Those Teeth Get There?, we learned how tooth germs, or the precursors of teeth, develop during fetal development inside the mare's uterus. When anything happens to interfere with this development or placement of pre-erupted or erupting teeth, malocclusions may result. Different developmental malocclusions are a result of different "errors", if you will, either before or during eruption.

Heterotopic or ectopic teeth

Heterotopic or ectopic (misplaced) teeth are caused by inappropriate positioning of erupting teeth. These can cause serious problems for the horse, because they allow the development of food packing and ***periodontal*** disease, which leads to severe problems if not corrected early enough.

In some cases, ***deciduous*** teeth fail to shed because ***permanent teeth*** deeper in the jaw are following an incorrect path and not doing their part in the ***exfoliation*** (shedding) of the deciduous teeth. Ideally, the dental sac of a permanent tooth will put pressure on the roots of the deciduous tooth, causing root resorption of the deciduous tooth and causing its exfoliation. If the eruption path of the permanent tooth is not on the same path as that of the deciduous tooth, it cannot assist the loss of its deciduous precursor, and the permanent tooth cannot erupt in its correct path. As a result, the permanent tooth will have to erupt beside, behind, or in front of the deciduous one. This causes ***crown elongation*** problems because the newly erupted tooth is not usually opposed by a tooth in the opposite ***arcade***.

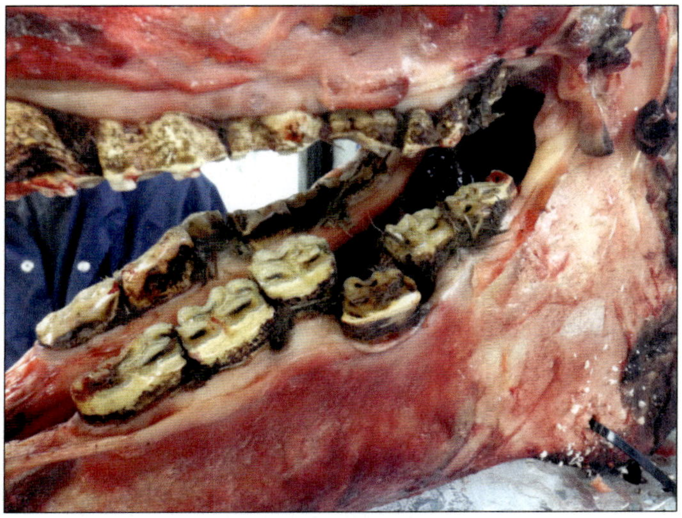

As this cadaver shows, heterotopic teeth can lead to serious trouble, causing development of severe periodontal disease, including erosion of the mandible (at 309) and focal crown elongations. Image credit Dr Denis Verwilghen.

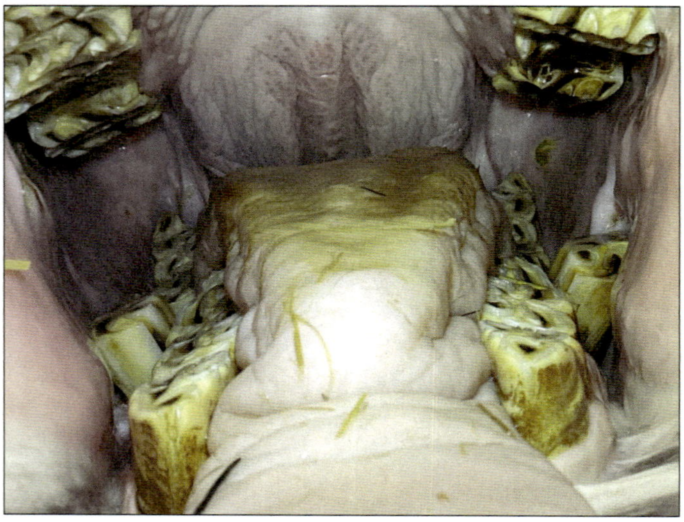

These malpositioned mandibular cheek teeth are causing this horse serious problems, including buccal ulceration, focal crown elongations, and probably periodontal disease. Image credit Dr Elke Pollaris.

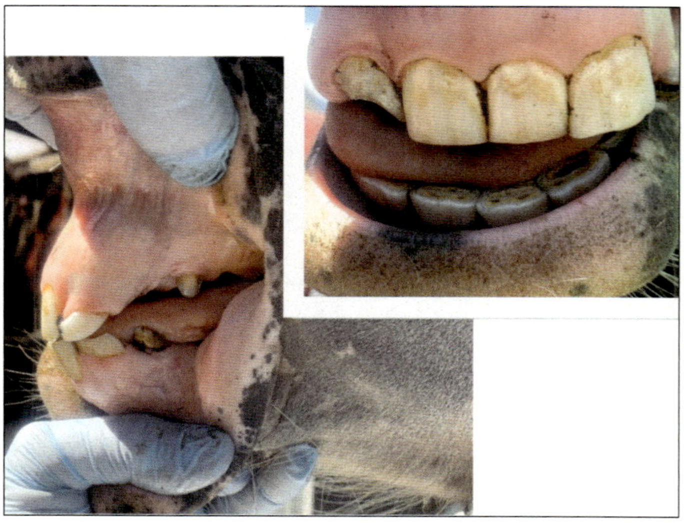

This miniature's ectopic maxillary corner incisors are rotated and have painful pulp exposures and periodontal disease. Image credit Author.

Hypodontia or Oligodontia

Defined as too few, or missing teeth, this condition may be a result of a damaged tooth germ never developing or a result of a tooth germ not migrating successfully to its correct destination, thus, no tooth will be present to erupt. Oligodontia may be associated with other epidermal defects such as poor hair or hoof development, and radiographs may be necessary to confirm the diagnosis of oligodontia or hypodontia. Either way, the resultant missing tooth becomes a problem because it is no longer present to prevent ***crown elongation*** of the opposing tooth. The elongation of the existing tooth into the gap left behind will cause severe, painful problems with ***mastication*** (chewing). This will only get worse until effective treatment is provided to gradually reduce the focal overgrowth by odontoplasty every two to three months to gradually reduce the tooth to the level of the rest of the teeth, then six-

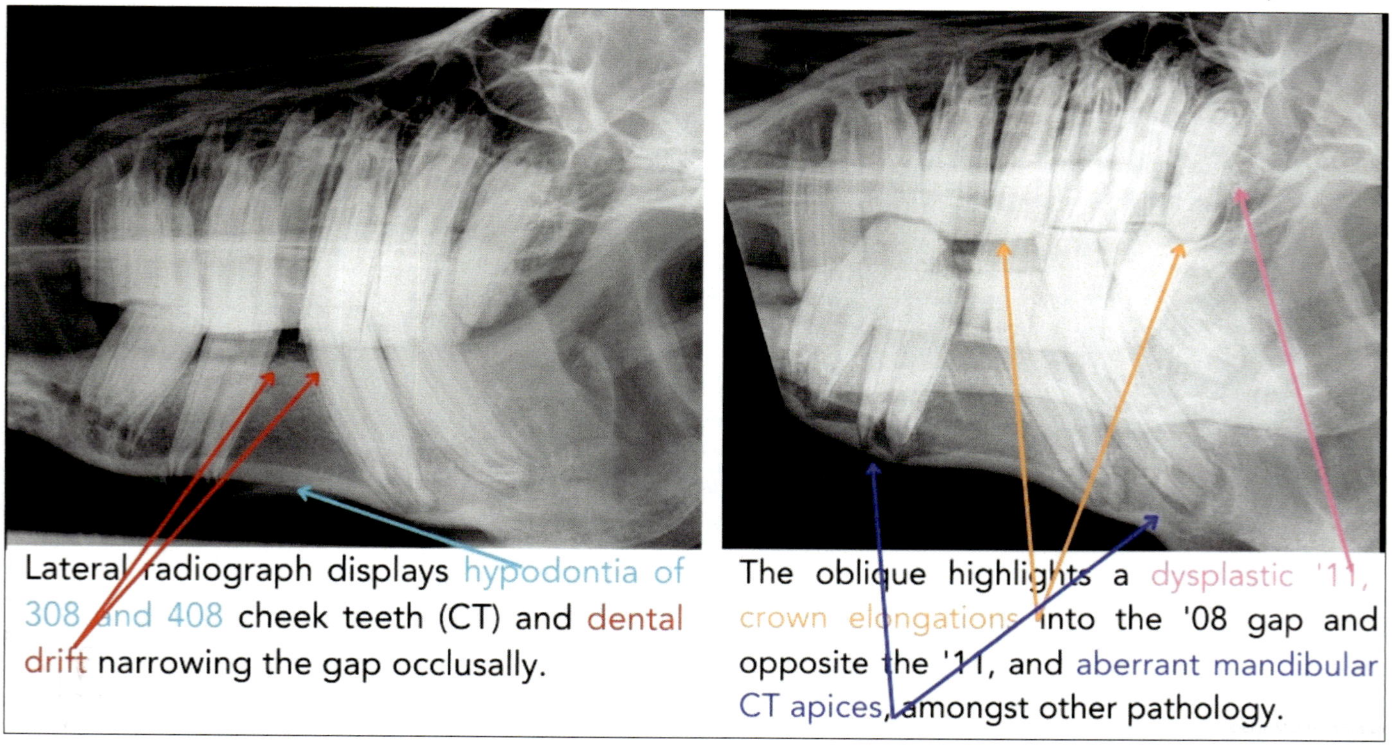

Two views of a mature miniature displaying oligodontia (308 and 408), opposing crown elongations, one dysplastic '11, and dental drift into the location of the absent lower '08s. The mandibular apices would not look normal for a non-miniature horse, but they commonly appear irregular and blunted like this in "normal" miniatures. Image credit Author.

monthly odontoplasty will be required for the remainder of the horse's life.

Oligodontia or hypodontia is common in miniature horses. The latest study indicated it occurred in 19% of the 100 miniature horses evaluated. See Chapter 12, Special Equids: Geriatrics and Miniatures: Miniatures.

Polyodontia (Supernumerary Teeth)

If there are more teeth than there should be in any category of teeth, the extra teeth are called "supernumerary". These relatively rare teeth are thought to arise as a result of an accidental split of the dental buds during tooth development, and they tend to result in an extra, abnormally shaped tooth. They cause the same focal overgrowth problems discussed above for oligodontia if they have no opposing tooth..

Unless they are somehow opposed by another supernumerary tooth or have had careful, regular odontoplasty, the supernumerary tooth or teeth will overgrow into the opposing jaw or soft ***tissues*** and cause severe pain and difficulty in mastication.

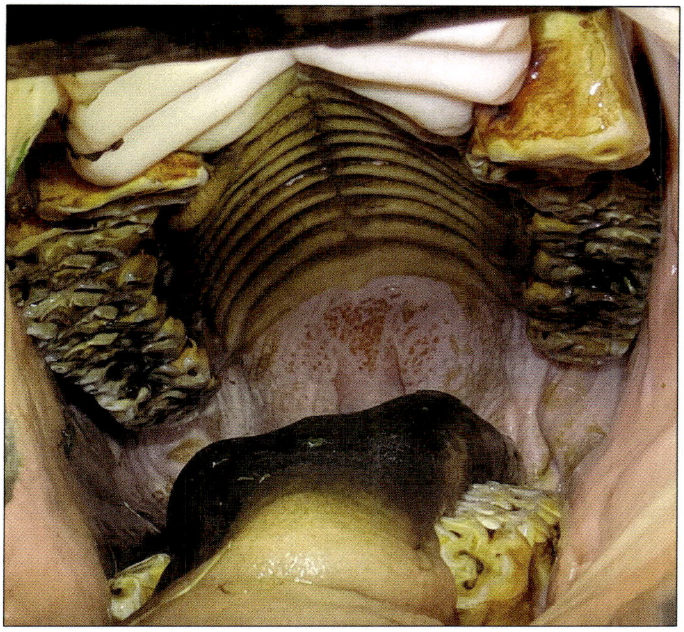

Bilateral polyodontia. Usually, the supernumerary tooth develops behind the last maxillary cheek tooth, but these supernumerary '06s developed at the front of the arcade. Image credit Dr Elke Pollaris.

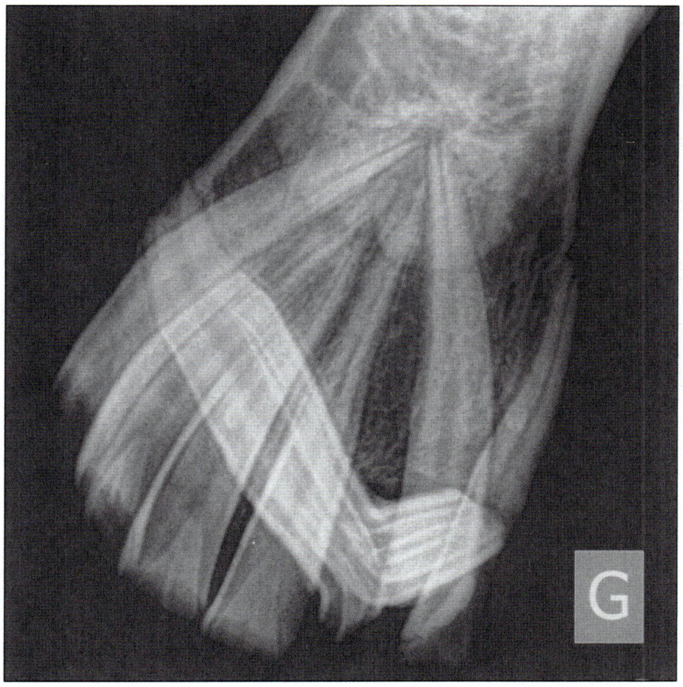

This supernumerary tooth has caused incisor displacement. Without X-rays, it would not have been possible to identify the orientation of this tooth. Following X-ray, it was decided not to attempt extraction as this would have disrupted the entire incisor arcade. Image credit Dr Denis Verwilghen.

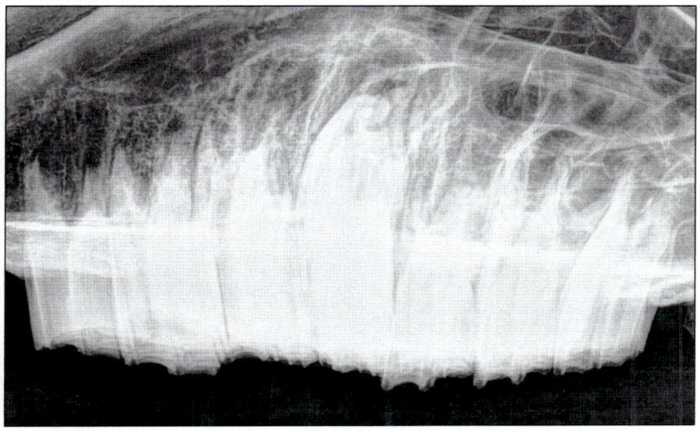

Polyodontia: a supernumerary tooth in the maxillary arcade. Count them: (hint: there should be six in that arcade). Image credit Dr Denis Verwilghen.

Extraction of the supernumerary tooth is the best long-term treatment. Temporary relief may be offered by carefully reducing the length of the overgrown teeth over time, but not by cutting or chopping the tooth, which will likely result in pulp exposure or tooth fractures with pulp exposure, both conditions extremely painful and potentially life-limiting. These teeth tend to occur ***distal*** to the maxillary cheek teeth rows, where extraction is difficult.

Temporal Teratomas and Dentigerous Cysts

Temporal teratomas, also known as "ear teeth" or temporal odontomas, are a particular type of teratomas caused by a rare congenital malformation which results in disorganized dental tissue surrounded by a cystic structure in the cranial or temporal region (near the base of the ear). These are hard masses which usually contain dental structures

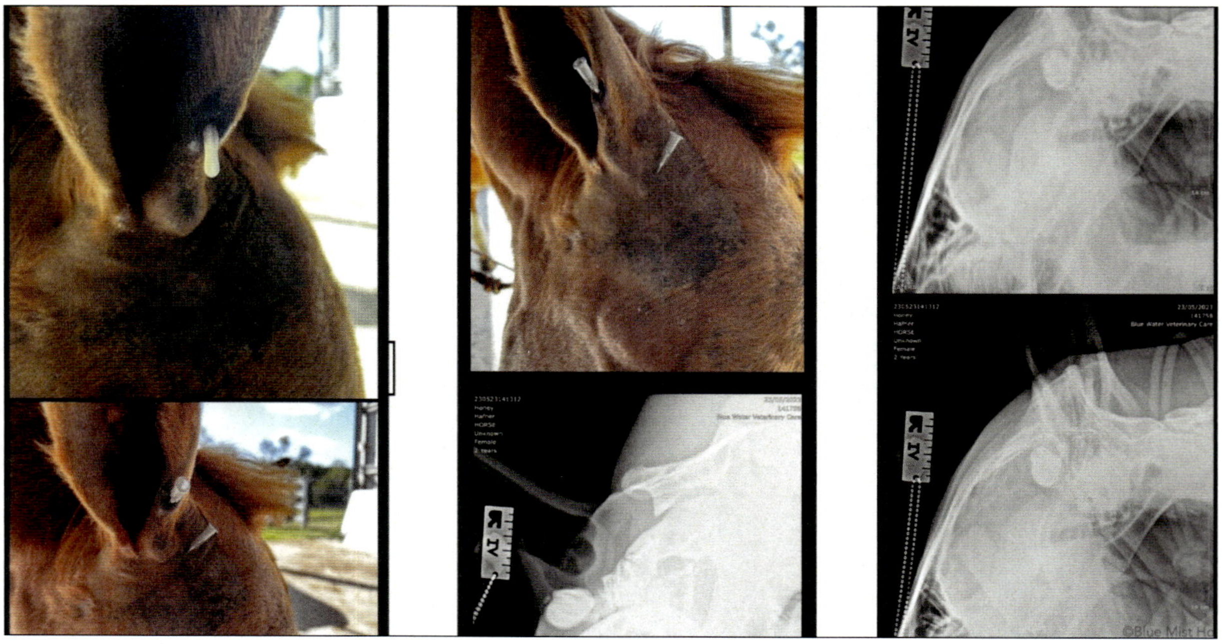

This horse had one draining tract just below the ear. These are called temporal teratomas, or sometimes referred to as "ear teeth" because they contain dental material such as whole teeth and parts of teeth within a cystic structure. That cystic structure may also contain cystic fluid. Image credit Dr Ashleigh Fisher.

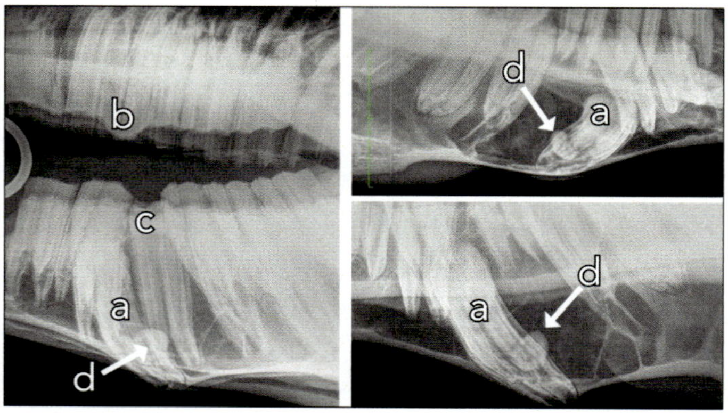

Mandibular dentigerous cyst:(a) note the abnormal placement and shape of the '08 with the large cementoma attached; at (b) note the increased crown height of the maxillary '07 and '08, down into the gap (c) between the mandibular '07 and '09; (d) is one of the cementomas. Image Credit Dr Olivia James, Radiology credit Dr Georgina O'Neill.

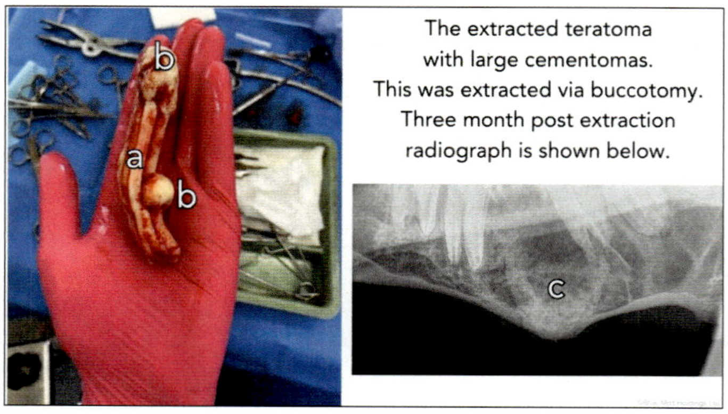

(a) The extracted tooth with a (b) large cementoma at the apex and another 2/3 of the way along the tooth. The three-month followup radiograph shows (c) the alveolar area is filling up nicely. Image Credit Dr Olivia James, Radiology credit Dr Georgina O'Neill.

like teeth and/or salivary gland tissues. They may have liquid draining from them, which is often the reason owners call to request an examination on their young horses. I have only seen this condition once in my ***veterinary*** career.

They used to all be called "dentigerous cysts", but because some of these lack a cystic structure, this has been found to be incorrect for some of them. Some of these are still called a true dentigerous cyst, due to their true cyst lining containing cystic fluid. These may also arise in other parts of the head or mouth, such as shown to the right.

In the Chapter 3, Anatomy of the Mouth, we discussed tooth development. In the embryo, the cells which form the teeth and the cells destined to become part of the ear are formed from the same tissues. Abnormal migration of these cells likely causes this condition.

Surgical removal of the abnormal temporal teratoma tissues by your veterinarian is usually curative.

Central Infundibular Cemental Hypoplasia

In this condition, insufficient or poor quality cementum has been laid down inside the infundibulum of incisors and/or maxillary cheek teeth to completely fill the infundibulum due to inadequate nutrition of cementocytes (the cells which create the cementum). If the infundibulum is incompletely filled with cementum, it instead becomes packed with rotting feed material, a bad situation for a tooth. Cemental hypoplasia may be caused by compromised infundibular blood supply (cut off the blood supply) to the cementocytes during tooth development.

For example, in the normal situation for a developing permanent cheek tooth, blood vessels enter the ***occlusal*** surface of the tooth and nourish the cementocytes so they can make enough cementum to completely fill the infundibulum. This happens only if the deciduous tooth is in place and protecting the vessels on the top of the developing permanent tooth from the hostile environment of the mouth. When the deciduous tooth is shed, the soft tissues overlying the erupting permanent tooth, including those vessels supplying the cementocytes, are destroyed the first time a horse chews some feed, and cementum deposition essentially stops. Some researchers have found an accessory, temporary blood supply close to the distal infundibulum, which may allow continued blood supply from the apical end of the tooth. This may allow continued deposition of cementum into the distal infundibulum (closest to the blood supply) and could account for the relatively lower prevalence of distal ***infundibular caries***, compared to mesial infundibular caries. Find these papers in the Bibliography and Further Reading.

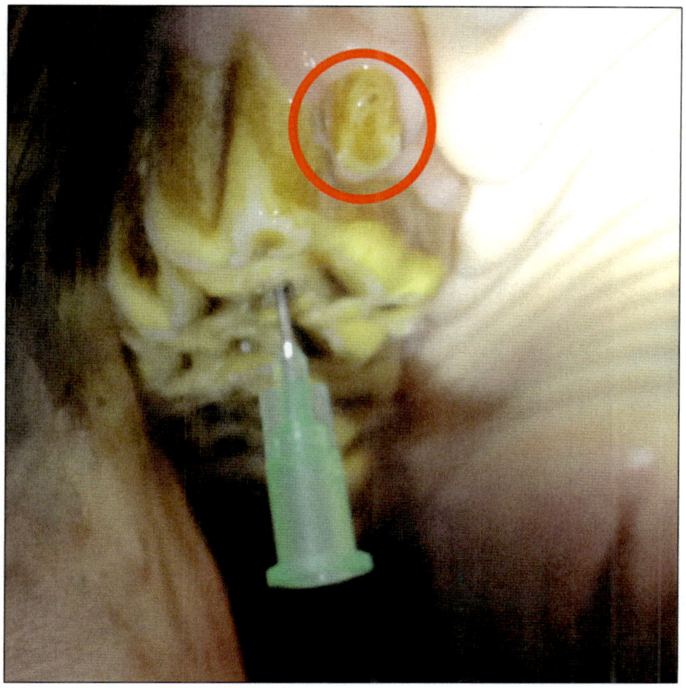

Here is a large wolf tooth and mesial infundibular hypoplasia of the 106. Note the how deep the needle can be inserted within the tooth. A worn-off wolf tooth is circled. Image credit Dr Denis Verwilghen.

The significance of this condition to you as a horse owner is that "premature" (too-early) removal of "caps", the thin remnant of the deciduous teeth, can cause this condition. Deciduous tooth caps should only be extracted if the permanent tooth is already visible beneath the cap, or if other teeth in the corresponding quadruplet have shed.

Determining that a cap should be removed by a certain age because "most horses lose them by this age" and removing it only because of this determination is faulty logic and puts your horse's teeth at unnecessary risk. Occasionally caps become fixed in place for too long, and then they become known as "retained deciduous teeth".

Which Developmental Disorders Occur at Eruption Time?

Vertical impaction

Impaction of teeth occurs when they try to erupt into too small a space, such as where cheek teeth are packed too tightly into their row or arcade. This is common in miniatures and small ponies. As a result of the eruption sequence, the '08s and '09s must erupt into tight locations between already-in-place permanent teeth. Sometimes one or both of these teeth cannot properly erupt into the mouth.

Sometimes they can enter the mouth, but they are rotated (often both the left and right exhibit this change, when it occurs) or lie outside of the normal eruption path,

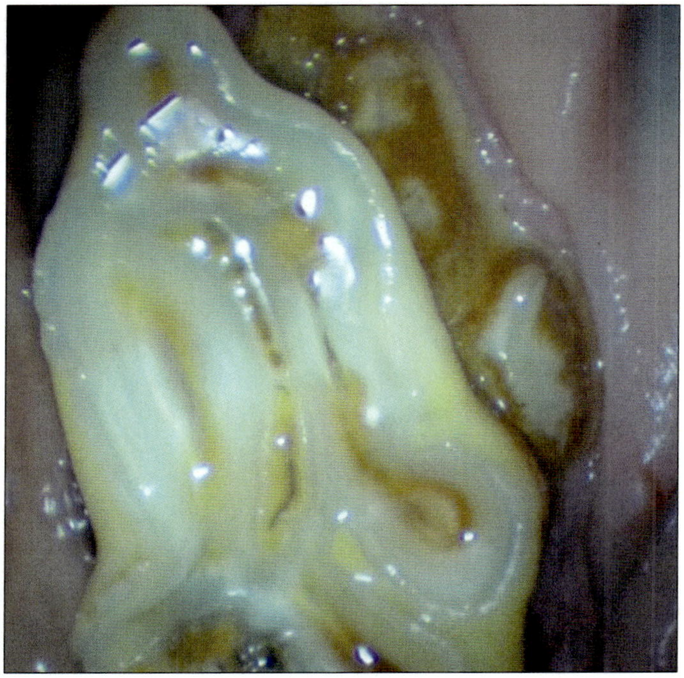

Here is a deciduous '06 which is overlying the erupting permanent '06. This "cap" is ready to be extracted. Image credit Dr Kirsten Jackson, Dental Vet.

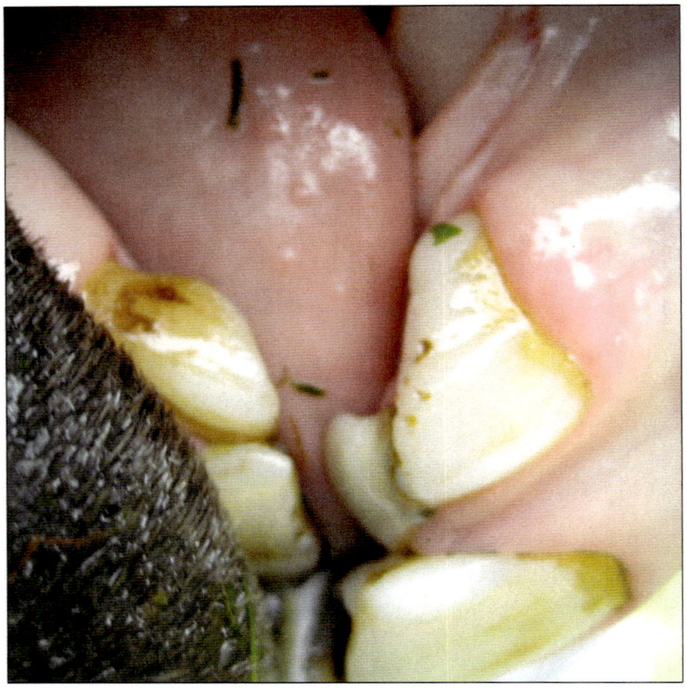

Retained deciduous incisor cap is shown here. Image credit Author.

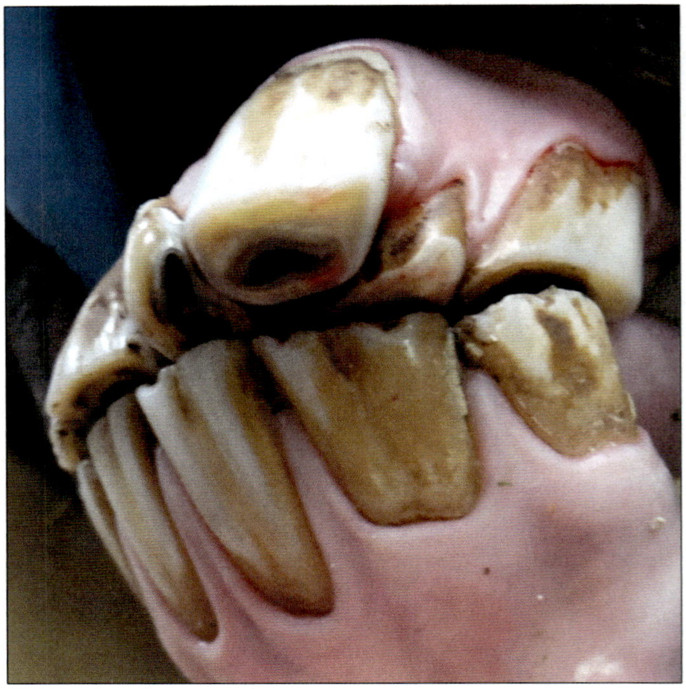

Retained 602 in this miniature horse may have caused the 102 and 202 to erupt along the incorrect pathway. Image credit Dr Tracy Tinsley.

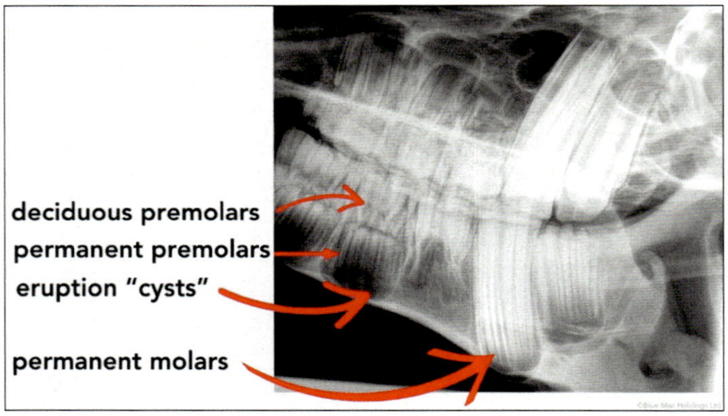

A miniature version of trying to fit all the erupting teeth in sequence. Unmarked image credit Dr Amy Ardern, graphic credit Author.

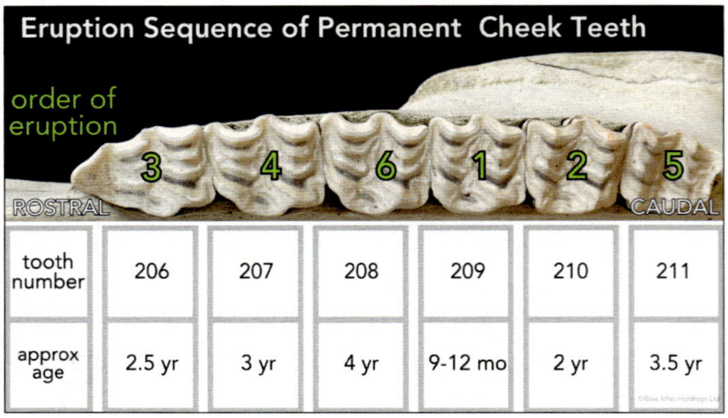

Eruption sequence of cheek teeth and the ages at which the teeth are "meant" to erupt. Image credit Author.

resulting in crown elongations, as discussed above. Normal cheek teeth, as mentioned in Chapter 3, Anatomy of the Mouth, are meant to fit tightly together, leaving no room for feed impaction between them. Both of the above sequelae tend to result in gaps between the normal and displaced or rotated teeth, and feed impaction occurs. If untreated, or perhaps regardless of treatment, depending upon the situation, this may progress to periodontal disease, ***diastema***, pulpitis, and subsequent tooth death.

Retained deciduous teeth and impacted teeth

In the normal situation, as developing permanent teeth move toward the mouth, they put pressure on the roots of the deciduous teeth, gradually cutting off their nutrition and causing them to be ***exfoliated***.

Sometimes this doesn't happen correctly, and the deciduous teeth fail to shed. When they do, the deciduous tooth ("cap") becomes a retained tooth.

Retained teeth may cause overcrowding, leading to incorrect eruption of the permanent teeth, ***apical abscessation***, and crown elongations as discussed for supernumerary teeth, above. Even if the cap is not retained,

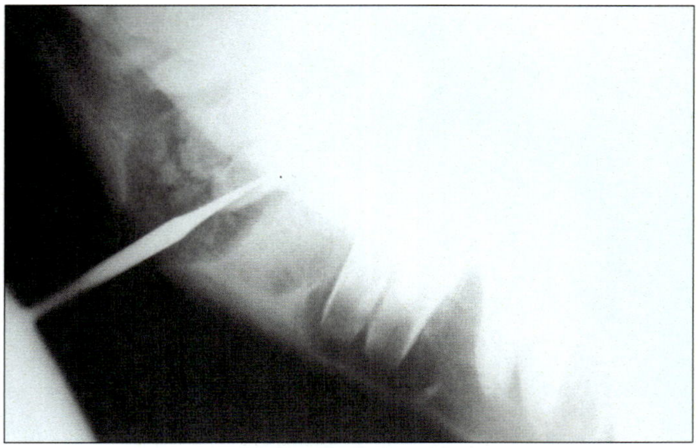

Radiograph of an apical infection with a mandibular draining tract in a five-year-old horse, likely due to anachoretic pulpitis. A large "fluffy looking" cementoma may be seen near the metal probe, which is shown in the draining tract exit. It was not fluffy, but gritty, calcified material at the end of the degraded apex of the tooth. The tooth and cementoma were extracted. Image credit Author.

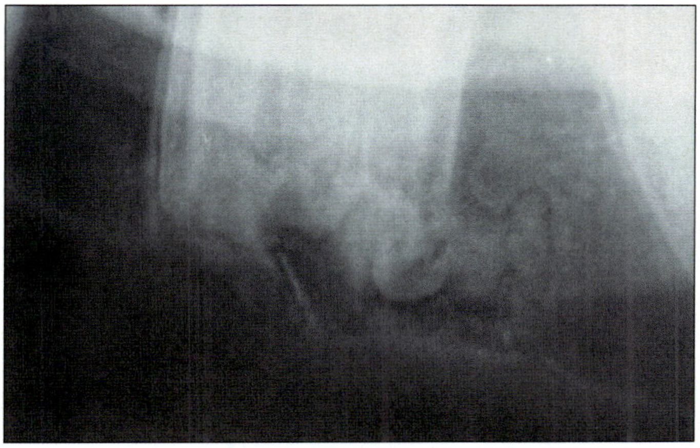

Abnormal apices of an impacted permanent tooth, likely caused by delayed exfoliation of a deciduous cheek tooth. Image credit Author.

some permanent cheek teeth (the '07s, '08s, and '11s) may not erupt properly because of entrapment from the limited space created by the eruption sequence, with these teeth having to fit in between or distal to already-erupted teeth.

Impacted deciduous caps or impacted permanent teeth may cause hard, bony swellings, or "eruption bumps" ***rostral*** to the facial crest and/or ventral to the mandible. Usually, the eruption bump is a temporary thing and resolves with the eruption of the permanent tooth. Impactions can, however, cause delayed eruption or ***lingual*** displacement of permanent teeth. However, if the line of eruption of a permanent tooth is blocked, or if the inflamed eruption cyst of the permanent tooth beneath it is invaded by bacteria from the bloodstream, the tooth may be in trouble. These situations may lead to a problem called anachoretic pulpitis, which may kill the tooth and result in draining tracts to the bottom of the mandible or out the side of the face. These require surgery.

If large tooth bumps are present, especially if they are not symmetrical or if the horse is exhibiting discomfort with its mouth, get your vet to check them. Radiographs may be indicated to determine the extent of the problem.

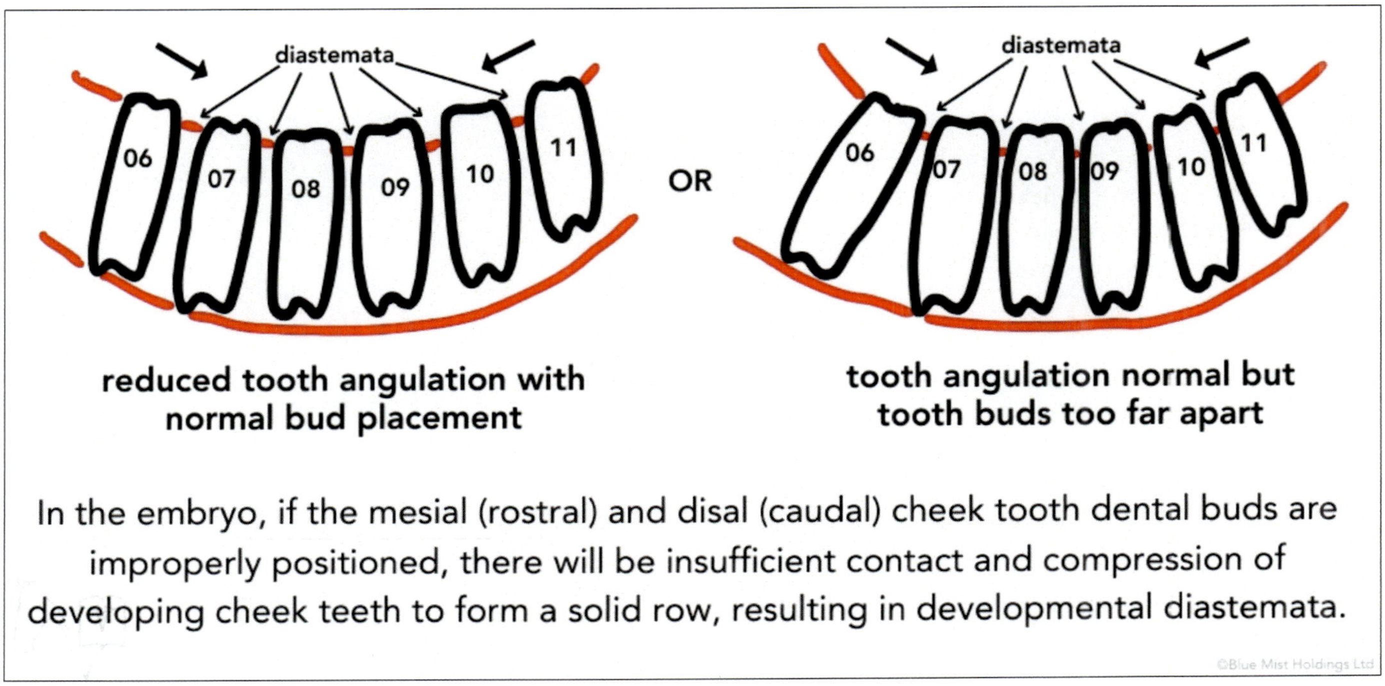

Two mechanisms for primary developmental diastemata in equids. Image credit Dr Padraic Dixon. Redrawn by Author.

What are developmental (primary) diastemata?

A ***diastema*** (pl. ***diastemata***) is a space between two adjacent teeth. Diastemata are classed as "open" or "closed". A closed diastema (also called valve diastema) is one which traps feed. An open one does not.

Developmental diastemata may occur as a result of either the developing ***tooth buds*** residing too far apart, or due to insufficient angulation of the teeth to tightly compress an arcade into one unit.

This latter is seen especially in the incisors and cheek teeth, which are meant to be tightly packed together. Diastemata tend to pack food and as such, they predispose the teeth involved in the diastema to developing periodontal disease.

Adult horses and geriatrics may also have "acquired diastemata". As teeth continue to erupt into old age, the occlusal surfaces and exposed crowns become smaller, which can lead to diastemata between the teeth. This will be discussed later in the chapter.

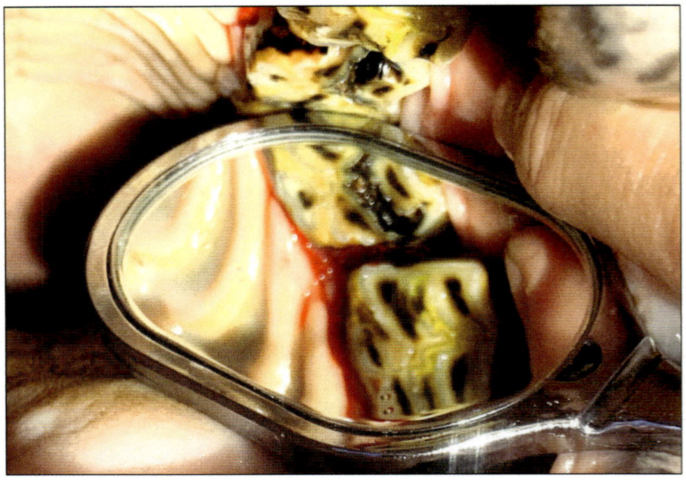

Cheek tooth diastema and infundibular caries. Image credit Author.

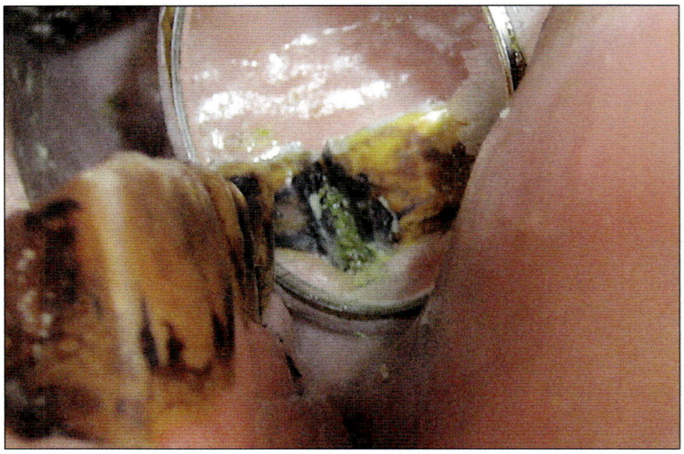

Feed-filled diastema in the 400 arcade. These are extremely painful and require sedation and perineural anesthesia (nerve blocks) to treat effectively. They should be treated as soon as possible. Image credit Author.

Retained root slivers

Root slivers which have been retained after incomplete exfoliation of deciduous caps may cause considerable discomfort due to resultant gingivitis and periodontal disease. Removal of these slivers may result in significant increase in their comfort level. Retained deciduous incisors can also be a source of trouble in young horses.

Remember that this occurs in young horses aged between one and six years of age, when most horses are beginning training and work. When deciduous teeth are loosening up, they are spiky and can be quite painful. These young horses often fuss with their mouth, rub their muzzles or faces on their buckets, stall doors, fences, etc. Good dental examinations are important for their health and happiness, starting at birth!

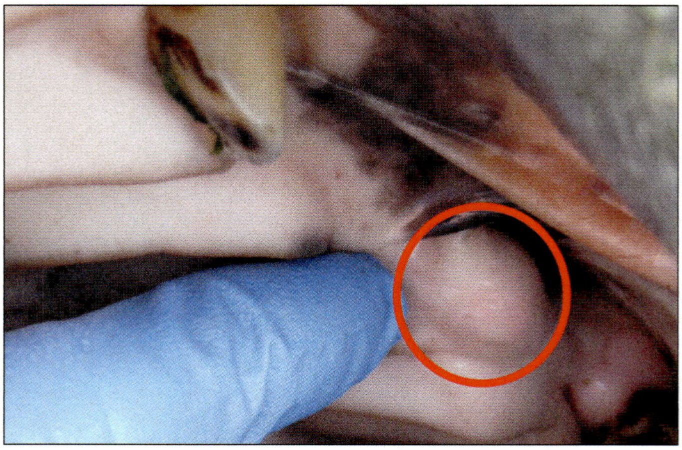

This unerupted 205 (wolf tooth) was pointed mesially and buccally. Every time the owner pulled on the left rein, the horse would throw its head, and sometimes rear. Its half-brother had the same issue on its 205. Both were extracted and the owner's left rein issues resolved. Unerupted wolf teeth are palpable with the fingers before placing a speculum. Image credit Author.

Unerupted canines and wolf teeth

Unerupted ***canines*** and ***wolf teeth*** are those which have erupted from the bone but are still covered with ***mucosa***.

Unerupted '04s (canine teeth) can cause subgingival pain and bit irritation, which may lead to head shaking or other bad habits. Unerupted canines may or may not cause pain issues in the *un*-bitted horse, but they are highly likely to in the bitted one. If they are painful when they are pressed upon, they should be surgically exposed by your veterinarian in a surgery called an operculectomy. In a bitted horse, it is vital to expose the unerupted tooth, as the bit can hit the sensitive mucosa over the sharp tip of a subgingival canine, causing pain. Unerupted '05s (wolf teeth) can cause pain for the same reasons and should be removed, as they are likely to cause pain upon contact with a bit. These unerupted teeth often lie parallel to the maxilla (or the mandible, if they are mandibular). I have found unerupted maxillary '05s in two half-brothers, which were directed mesially and buccally, causing severe bitting problems.

Tell me about Apical Infections, Pulpitis, Apical Abscessation, Peri-Apical Infections, and Tooth Root Infection!

PULP DISEASE IS extremely painful. Although the pulp may appear to be dead, the nerves are the last to die, and a tooth with pulp disease can cause excruciating pain for your horse. This disease can occur at any age, though the most likely causes of an apical infection tend to differ relative to the age of the horse.

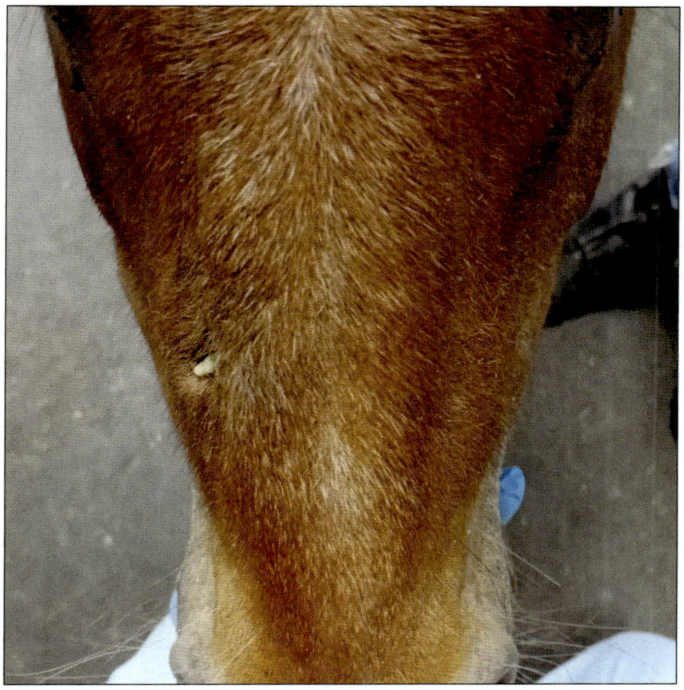

An apical abscess from one of the most mesial cheek teeth in the 100 arcade has caused a fistula to form from the apical infection through the bone of the maxilla to the outside. The yellow material is purulent exudate, or pus. Image credit Dr Elke Pollaris.

Inflammation of the pulp is termed "pulpitis". If pulpitis progresses and becomes contaminated with bacteria, it may become an apical infection, tooth root infection, apical abscessation or peri-apical infection. We tend to notice the result of pulpitis at the apex of the tooth, or the root, hence the use of "apical" in the names. This condition has many aspects, including the infection at the apical portion of the tooth, the infection and inflammation of the pulp, the hard, bony external swellings on the face or mandible over the apices of the teeth, discharging tracts either out the side of the face or beneath the mandible, and unilateral (one-sided) discharge from a nostril.

One of the common names for this condition, "tooth root infection" is not always technically correct, because for the first two years after a tooth has erupted into the mouth, the apical portions are not fully developed into roots, and so "tooth root infection" isn't appropriate at every stage of a horse's life, while "apical infection" *is*.

How would I know if my horse has an apical infection?

As we discussed in Chapter 1, How do I Know My Horse has Dental Disease?, historically, we have not been good at detecting dental disease, but that is changing as we learn to notice their subtle (or not so subtle) signs such as bitting problems, head shaking, difficulty eating or eating in an odd fashion, grumpiness, unwillingness to work, or by finding evidence of disease such as purulent discharge (pus) from under the mandible, from a single nostril, or out the side of your horse's face over the tooth apices. In extreme cases, you might see weight loss. Your thorough dental operator will see much more, which is detailed below under *Examination Findings*.

How do apical infections start?

- Anachoresis (through the bloodstream)
- Direct ***pulpar exposure***—traumatic pulp exposure
- Indirect pulpar exposure—traumatic near-pulp exposure
- Extension of periodontal disease
- Extension of infundibular caries
- Application of certain chemicals used in restoration of teeth

What the Heck is Anachoretic Pulpitis?

- In young horses (often 5-6 years old), pulpitis can occur subsequent to inflammation from:
- a normal eruption cyst
- a transient impaction during teething, or
- subsequent to trauma, such as a kick to the mandible from another horse.

Whatever the origin of this inflammation, bacteria from the bloodstream may invade the apical area (which is called "anachoresis") and set up an infection of the pulp. This is then called "anachoretic pulpitis" and tends to predominate in the mandibular '08s and the maxillary '07s and '09s.

These infections are termed apical infections. The above images show the case of a young horse who presented for a large swelling with a draining tract on the ventral mandible, or the bottom of her jaw. Transient swellings of the mandible or maxilla (tooth bumps) may occur as a result of normal eruption cysts and should recede over the next year and half or so unless there are restrictions to eruption of the permanent teeth. See Tooth Bumps later in this chapter.

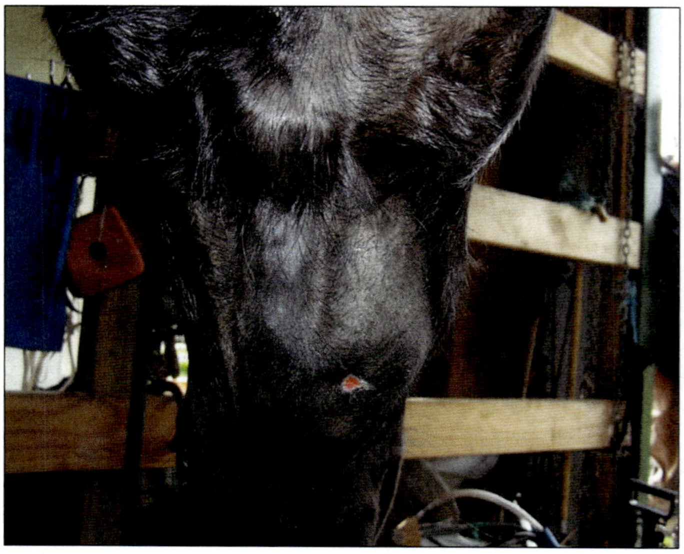

This five-year-old mare presented with a hard swelling on the bottom of her mandible, which was draining purulent material. Diagnosis: apical infection. Image credit Author.

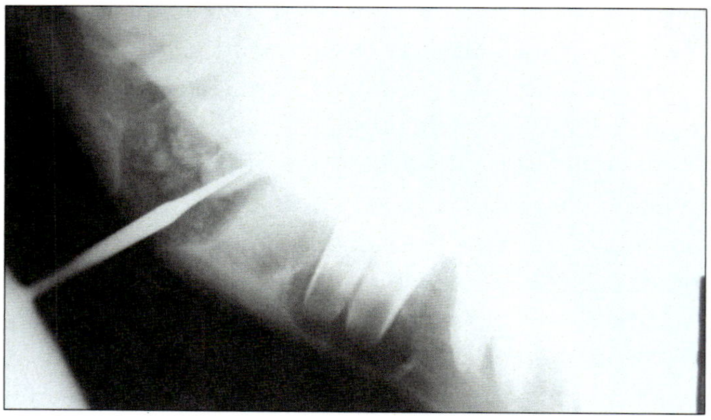

Radiograph of the above horse. A large "fluffy looking" cementoma may be seen near the metal probe, which has been placed into the exit of the draining tract. It was not fluffy, but gritty, calcified material at the end of the degrading apex of the tooth. This was extracted. Image credit Author.

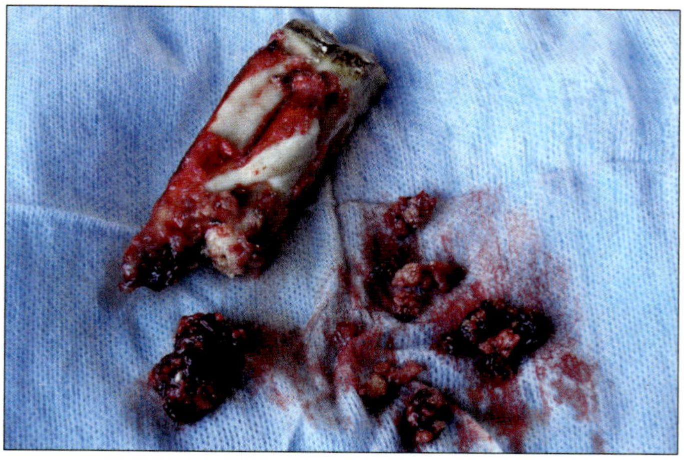

The tooth and cementoma and chunks of cementoma extracted from this horse, Image credit Author.

What is Direct Pulp Exposure, and How Does it Happen?

In horses of any age, a pulp may be directly exposed by traumatic injury to a tooth such as a tooth fracture, or by ***iatrogenic*** mistakes causing direct or indirect pulp exposure via overzealous odontoplasty (removing too much tooth and/or overheating the teeth), cutting teeth, or inadvertent pulp exposure during surgery. If any of these occur and a direct pulp exposure exists, a vital pulpotomy should be performed to try to save the life of the tooth. This needs to be done by an appropriately trained veterinarian within a few days, or bacteria can infect the pulp, causing a possibly irreversible pulpitis.

How about Indirect Pulp Exposure?

An indirectly exposed pulp, due to a near-pulp exposure, where the pulp is not exposed, but is within approximately three millimeters of the pulp, can have the same effect. Indirect pulp exposures may be treated by your dental veterinarian with multiple, cured, layers of appropriate treatment medications to attempt to prevent infection of the pulp by bacteria working their way down the tooth's ***dentinal tubules*** to the pulp.

Extension of Periodontal Disease

Pulpitis may result from extension of periodontal disease, with bacterial contamination from the mouth traveling down an unhealthy ***periodontal ligament*** and

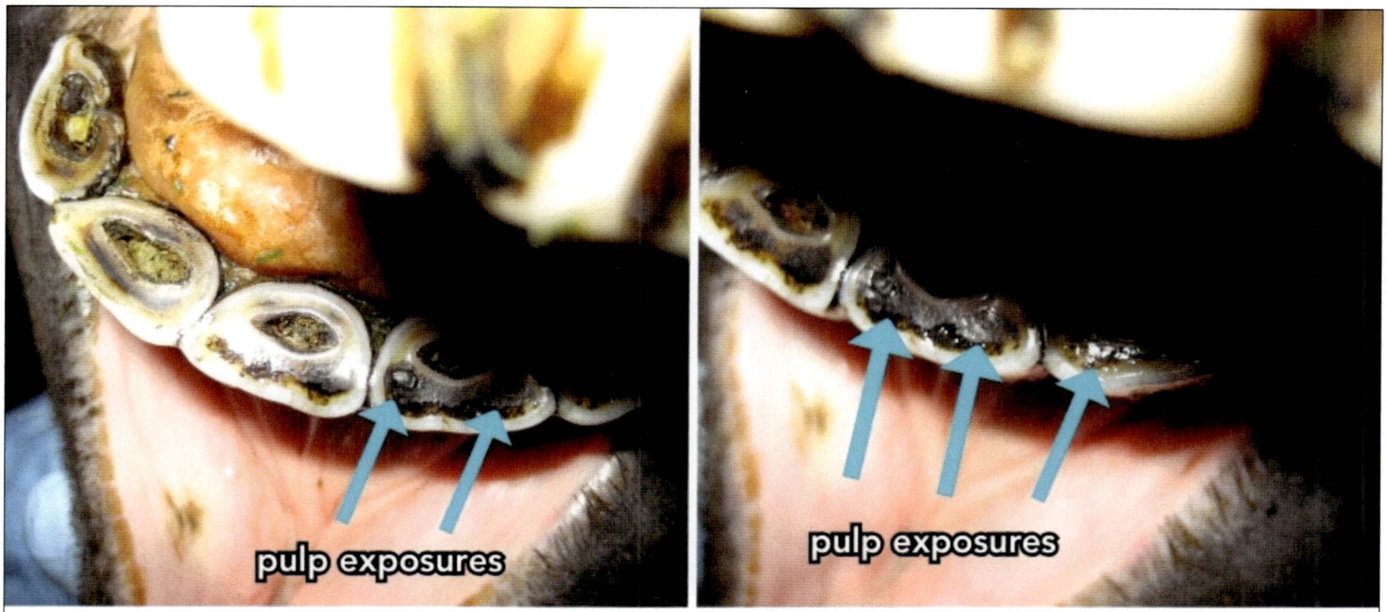

The incisors on this young horse were severely overheated and not cooled with water, causing pulpitis and severe pain. This horse was obsessively sucking on his knees (carpi).

This young horse was examined by Dr Elizabeth Thompson after he was found to be obsessively chewing on his carpi, or knees, due to the pain in his incisors. He sustained near pulp exposure in multiple teeth from power dentistry without water cooling. The arrows point to the shiny, wet pulp exposures between the open infundibula (normal for his age) and the labial border of the mandibular incisors. Image credit Author.

directly infecting the pulp at the apical end of the tooth. In older horses, pulpitis is more likely to occur due to extension of periodontal disease than to anachoretic pulpitis.

Extension of Infundibular Caries

If infundibular caries progresses through the end of the infundibular ***enamel*** and into the ***dentine or dentin***, a pulpitis may result, with subsequent damage as above. This type of pulpitis is more common in horses between eight and fourteen years of age and is primarily seen in distal maxillary cheek teeth.

Uh-oh, pulpitis and tooth death!

Regardless of how the inflammation of the pulp started, it is still termed "pulpitis". Pulps can attempt to protect themselves by filling the pulp chamber with reparative dentin. This is called formation of a "dentinal bridge", or a wall between the infected pulp and the rest of the tooth.

If the animal can fight the infection of the pulp and wall off the infection, there is hope for the tooth. If not, the pulp, and therefore the tooth, dies.

Signs of pulpitis on dental examination include discolored teeth, a black-colored pulp horn (vs. the brown normal pulp horn) on the occlusal surface, a black hole in a tooth (nonvital pulp exposure, pulp necrosis, necrotic dentin), sinusitis with purulent discharge from only one

This horse with pulpar exposure has formed a dentinal bridge:

a: abnormal (wide) pulp canal on occlusal side of dentinal bridge

b: dense dentinal bridge

c: normal (narrow) pulp canal on apical side of dentinal bridge

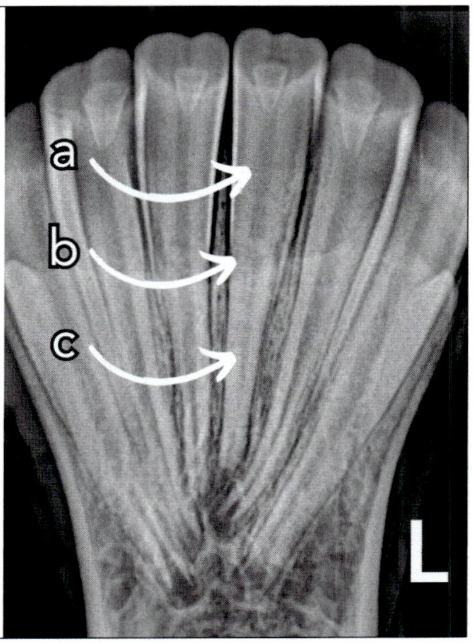

This horse had a pulpar exposure of his 301. Note the overly wide pulp at a) on the occlusal side of the radiodense dentinal bridge at b), which has formed to protect the normal pulp chamber at c), which is apical to the dentinal bridge. Image credit Dr Marieke van den Enden.

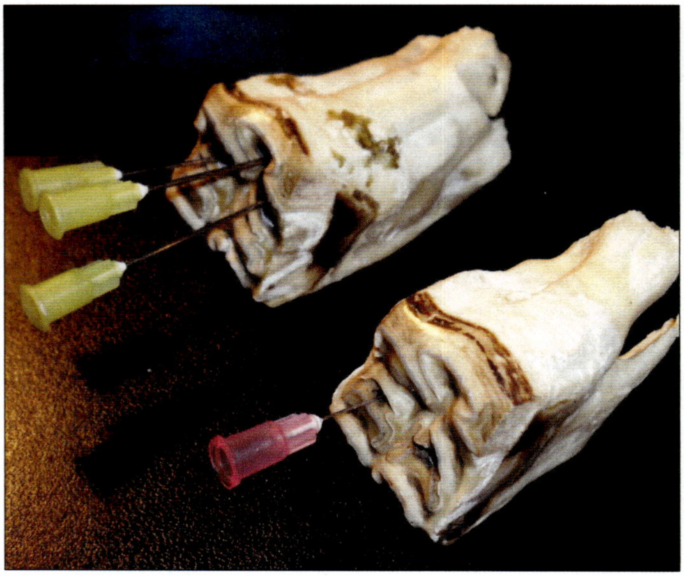

An extracted cheek tooth with nonvital pulp exposures from a mare with a unilateral, chronic sinus infection. A needle was not able to be inserted into the pulp horns for several months after extraction. Image credit Author.

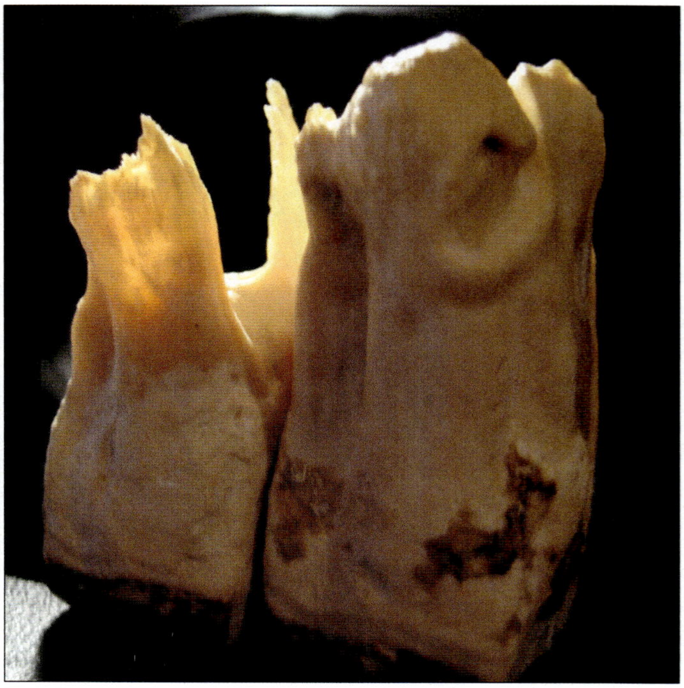

These are the apical (root) ends of two extracted cheek teeth. The thin, flaring root tips of the tooth on the left are relatively normal. The lumpy, thickened roots seen on the right-hand tooth, with the opening in the side of the tooth, are a result of pulpitis. This apical end was so dense, it appeared as a "cementoma" on radiographs, but it was in reality all one piece. Image credit Author.

nostril, draining tracts out the side of your horse's face or out the bottom of the mandible, or sadly, iatrogenic pulp exposure from someone performing dentistry. See Chapter 9, Iatrogenic Disease: What is Pulpar Exposure... Your dental veterinarian can check your horse and radiograph the skull and teeth to determine the condition of the pulp. Is it alive or not? Is it trying to repair itself? Repeat radiographs may be needed to assess the progression of the disease at three-to-six-month intervals.

Young horses are better able to counteract a pulpitis than an old horse. As mentioned in Chapter 3, Anatomy of the Mouth, young teeth possess a large, open pulp with a rich blood supply as well as many types of cells capable of helping to fight infection and repair damage (e.g. undifferentiated cells, immune cells, and odontoblasts). Their wide-open pulp is also helpful in moderating the increased pressure inside the tooth which may occur as a result of inflammation. All of this helps the tooth of a young horse fight pulp infection and survive a pulpar insult. If the tooth or teeth cannot survive this pulp insult, they will die.

As horses age, unfortunately, their pulp chambers narrow with each passing year. These older pulp chambers are thus smaller in diameter. They have fewer cell types to fight the infection, a much-diminished blood supply, and have a relatively poor ability to regulate the increased pressure from inflammation inside the tooth. All of these make it difficult for the older horse to fight pulpitis, which in these horses often results in tooth death.

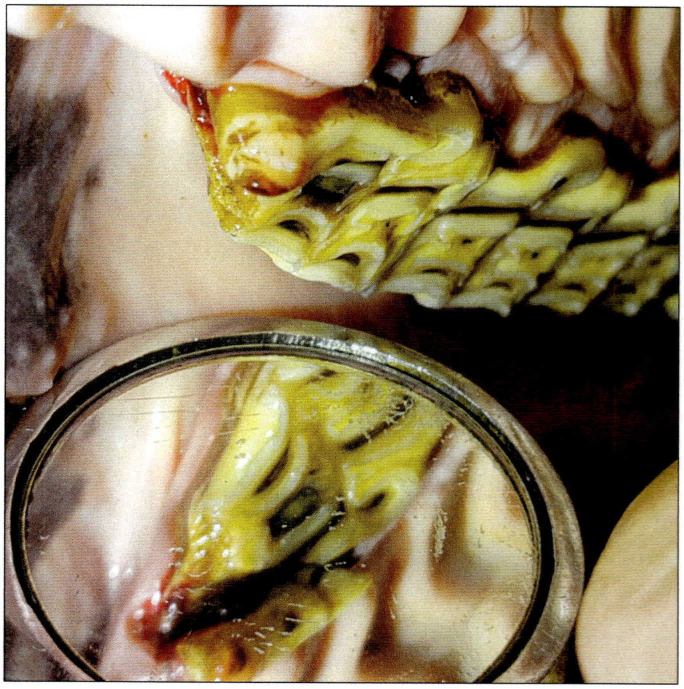

Fracture of palatal edge of 106, with pulpar exposure, evident with mirror. Image credit Cathie Heald Greenwell.

What can be done about pulpitis?

To relieve pain, a dead tooth must be extracted by your dental vet, or it may be treated endodontically by a specialist veterinary dentist if the specialist deems it an appropriate candidate for root canal or other endodontic therapy. See Chapter 15, Advanced Techniques to Help Your Horse: Endodontic Therapy in Equids.

Some teeth are more amenable to treatment by root canal therapy than others. In general equine veterinary dental practice, these are primarily incisors. Cheek tooth root canal therapy is a much more involved procedure and may be performed by specialist veterinary dentists on cheek teeth. Optimally, the veterinary specialist will utilize a CT or MRI, due to the extremely complex system of between five and seven interconnected pulp canals and cross-canals. A limited number of people around the world possess the expertise, experience, and equipment to successfully perform cheek tooth endodontics. It's not something your local equine vet will usually be set up or trained to do, and since it is dealing with live tissues, it is regarded as the practice of medicine in many locales.

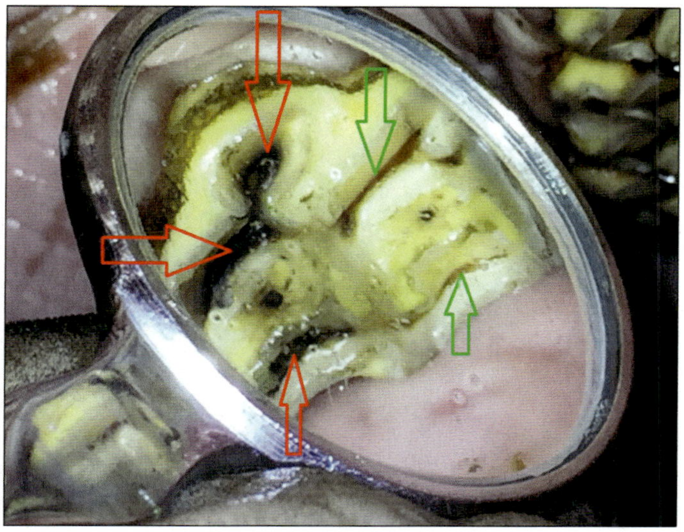

The red arrows at the blackened pulp areas indicate open pulps, or pulp exposures. The green arrows show normal brown pulps. This tooth was extracted. Image credit Dr Kirsten Jackson, Dental Vet.

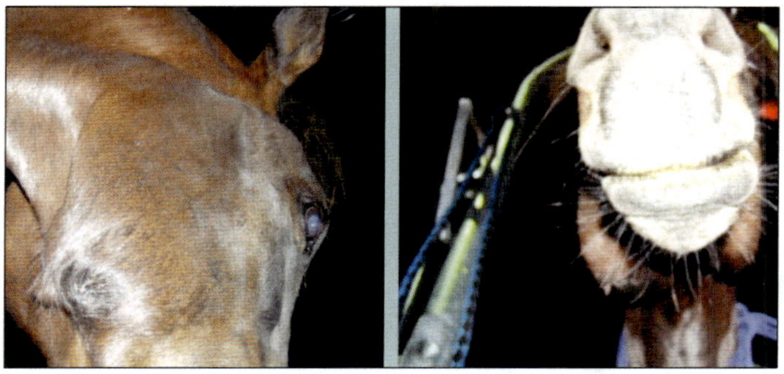

Comminuted fractures involving multiple mandibular cheek teeth in this stallion resulted in a draining tract exiting through his ventral mandible. Each tooth was fractured into many fragments. Image credit Author.

Examination findings

During a thorough examination, ideally, every pulp in every tooth may be scratched with a probe to check for open pulp cavities or roughness over the pulp cavity, evidence of possible nonvital pulp exposure. Unfortunately, one cannot always place a probe into a pulp canal, even if there truly *is* pulp exposure, as the dentin or feed material blocking it may be too dense. However, sometimes with time, the tightly packed rotted feed material filling the pulps will soften enough that the pulps may be probed.

Some clinical signs of apical infection include ***gingival*** recession, blackened pulps (instead of brown), ability to insert probe into pulp/s (although this isn't always possible even if apical infection is present, as mentioned above), and pain upon palpation or probing. If the apical infection is due to periodontal disease, there will often be deep periodontal pockets between the tooth and the gingiva, usually packed with putrid, rotting feed. Radiographs (X-rays) are used to diagnose the condition and detail exactly which tooth, or teeth are affected.

Advanced pulpitis or apical infection may be associated with a unilateral sinus infection which leaks purulent material from one nostril, or a draining tract with a purulent discharge. The location of the draining tract usually corresponds to the location of the tooth apex, unless the infection tracks mesially or distally to the tooth through the bone or soft tissue.

If the affected tooth is:

- a maxillary '06 or '07, a draining tract may exit out the side of the face in this area because these teeth reside in the maxilla itself.
- a maxillary '08-'11, a sinus infection (one sided, usually) may result, with a one-sided purulent nasal discharge, because the apices of these teeth reside in the rostral and ***caudal*** maxillary ***sinuses***. The discharge can be putrid (extremely foul-smelling) due to foul gas produced by the anaerobic bacteria causing the infection. Trust me, you do not want it all over you, but worse, the horse probably doesn't like it either.
- in the mandible, the draining tract will usually be on the ventral side (bottom) of the mandible.

Radiographic signs

While some radiographs of apical infections are obvious, some may be tricky to read. Your equine dental vet has been trained to properly radiograph, interpret, and diagnose dental conditions such as this. They will use all of this to make a plan and determine the next steps. If they are unsure, they will know where to send the radiographs for verification of their conclusions, or where to refer your horse if they don't feel comfortable with the necessary treatment and desire someone with more experience to perform further treatment.

If your horse has pulp disease, his options may include either root canal therapy or extraction of the tooth or teeth. See Chapter 16, Advanced Techniques to Help Your Horse: Endodontic Therapy in Equids. Many complications can occur if treatment is not started promptly, including pulp death, infection around the tooth, infection spreading to other parts of the body, and/or premature tooth loss. As previously discussed, the loss of a tooth in an equid, whether it is lost on its own or extracted, will have lifetime ramifications, including six-monthly odontoplasty throughout the horse's life. See Chapter 15, Veterinary Specific Procedures: Extraction Considerations.

What are Malocclusions?

HAVE YOU SEEN a horse chomp its food like a dog? It might look comical, but a horse only chomps in this way, with up-and-down motions of the mandible when it's unable to move its jaw horizontally with the equid power stroke as it should. A horse will only do this due to pain caused by dental pathology. How does this pathology occur? It has a lot to do with the horse's anatomy, so let's have a look. First off, malocclusions are a mismatch between the maxillary and mandibular teeth or between adjacent teeth, which cause a horse to have improper occlusion. This retards regular chewing and causes problems. There are many types of malocclusions which occur in the horse.

As we saw in the beginning of Chapter 3, Anatomy of the Mouth, we have bred horses for many things, but unfortunately, not for highly functional dentition. Historically, our breeding of equids has led to problems which we must solve if we can. Dental pathology results from many things, including disorders of wear, abnormal tooth placement, extra teeth, too few teeth, trauma, loss of teeth, and bone and tooth fractures. Most of these result in secondary focal crown elongations (overgrowths) and resultant pathology and pain.

As discussed earlier in this chapter in the section on Developmental Disorders Occurring at the Time of Eruption, if a tooth is unopposed for any reason, its previously opposed tooth isn't present to keep it in check at the appropriate length. Without an opposing tooth, the overgrowth of the existing tooth into the gap left behind will cause severe, painful problems with mastication. This will only get worse until effective treatment is provided to gradually reduce the crown elongations by careful, specific odontoplasty every two to three months to gradually reduce the tooth to the level of the rest of the teeth, then six-monthly odontoplasty for the remainder of the horse's life. See Chapter 15, Veterinary Specific Procedures: Ongoing Post-Extraction Care.

IMPORTANT: regarding the occlusion of the incisors and the cheek teeth, the incisors and the cheek teeth are not designed to be in contact at the same time, contrary to what some groups promote with "rebalancing". From a point where the incisors are ***in occlusion***, or in contact, the mandible moves sideways to bring the cheek teeth into contact with each other to grind their feedstuffs, which brings the cheek teeth "into occlusion", and causes the mandibular and maxillary incisors to separate from each other, effectively taking the incisors "OUT of occlusion". See Chapter 4, Examination of the Mouth.

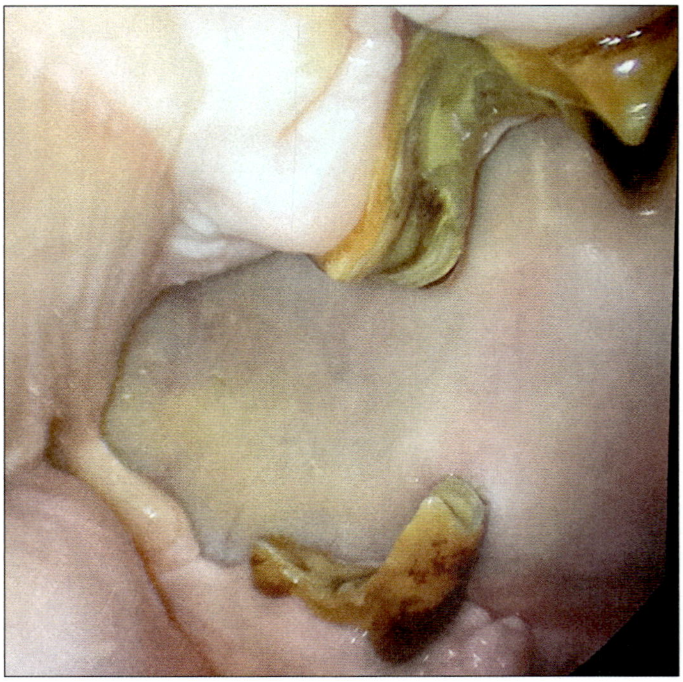

Oroscopic view of a severe wear disorder. Image credit Dr Elke Pollaris.

Cheek teeth malocclusions

Disorders of Wear

As we discussed in Chapter 3, Anatomy of the Mouth, equids are anisognathic, with the maxillary cheek teeth set wider than those of the mandible. This creates a situation where, in grinding their feed with a horizontal power stroke, the ***palatal*** edges of the maxillary teeth and the buccal edges of the mandibular teeth are ground off the most.

This allows the buccal edges of the maxillary cheek tooth crowns and the lingual edges of the mandibular cheek tooth crowns to elongate and become sharp, resulting in ***sharp enamel points*** (SEPs). The SEPs of the mandibular cheek teeth can cause mucosal ulcers by cutting into the tongue and the opposing maxillary gingiva if the crown elongations are extremely long, while the buccal maxillary sharp points may lacerate the buccal mucosa, especially when the mouth is open. This is made worse when the SEPs are under the cheek pieces of halters and bridles. If these elongations are long enough to become ***hooks***, they can cut into the opposing gingiva and bone if the opposite tooth is absent and cause severe ulceration and even ***osteomyelitis*** (bone infection).

The space between the maxillary cheek teeth and the buccal mucosa is very narrow at rest, but when the mouth is opened, the cheeks press tightly onto the teeth and against any SEPs. This may create painful buccal ulceration

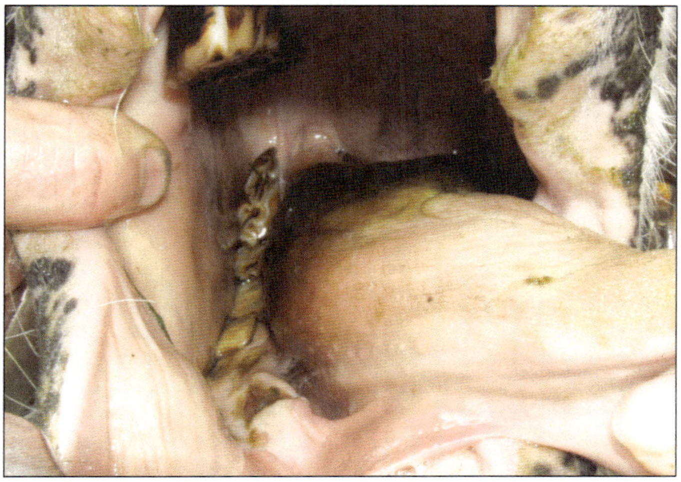

Result of above 106/ 206 crown over-eruptions or overgrowths: bilateral ulcers in the opposing mandible. Image credit Author.

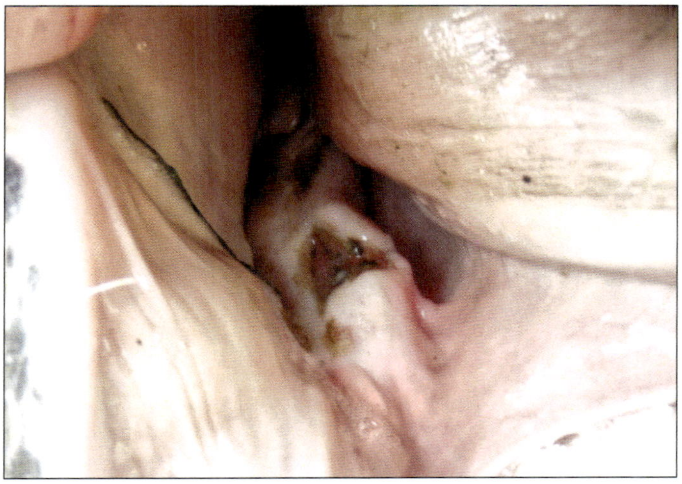

Ulceration of mucosa of mandible opposite the above cheek tooth overgrowth. Scarring of tongue also evident. Image credit Author.

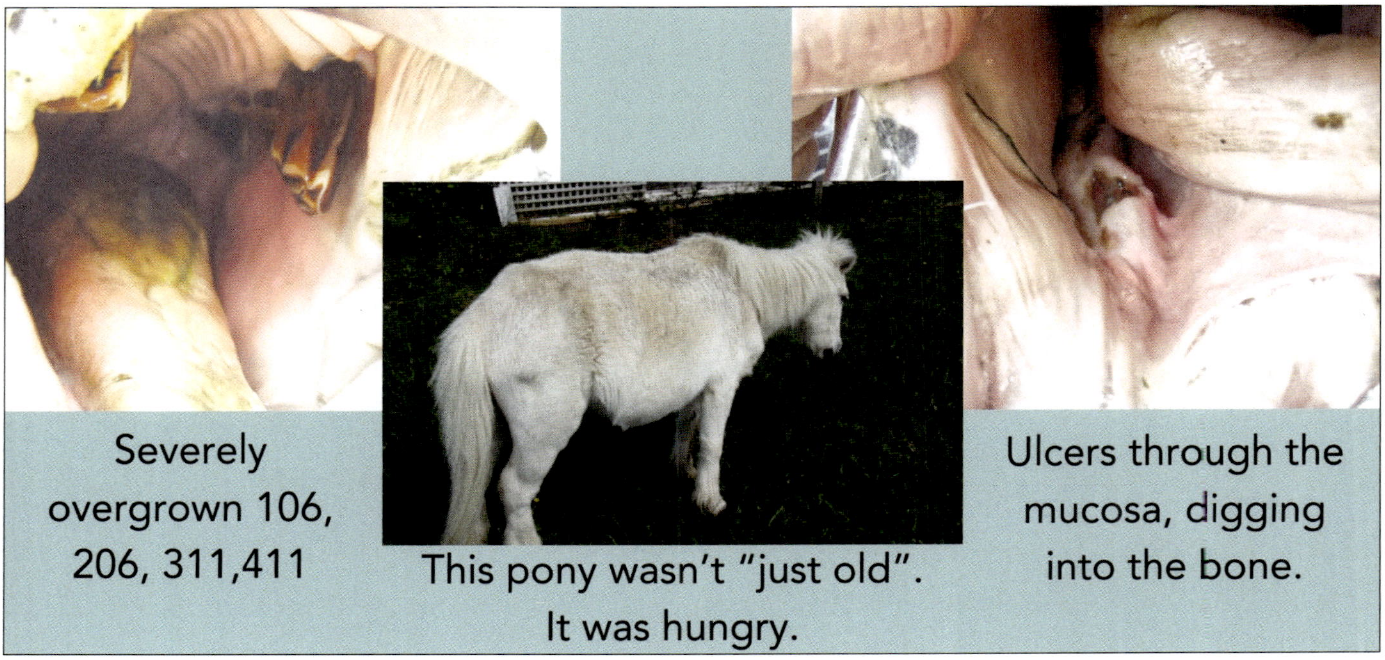

Poor condition due to extreme overgrowth into opposing jaw, tooth loss, and neglect. Image credit Author.

(***lacerations***) in the cheek mucosa. This pain may cause the horse to chew abnormally. In turn, this leads to uneven wear patterns and crown elongations, called malocclusion. Malocclusion leads to feed entrapment and stagnation adjacent to the affected teeth, with bacterial overgrowth and resultant acid formation by the bacterial replication. All of these result in damage to ***oral*** and dental tissues and promote conditions like periodontal disease and many of the other dental diseases to be discussed later in this chapter. Regular odontoplasty helps prevent development of many malocclusions by removal of sharp points and overgrowths. It helps repair damage which has occurred over time by dental neglect. This may take some time and several rounds of treatment.

Crown Elongations (Overgrowths)

Crown elongations are wear disorders which result when a tooth or a portion of a tooth over-erupts past the plane of the rest of the adjoining occlusal surfaces.

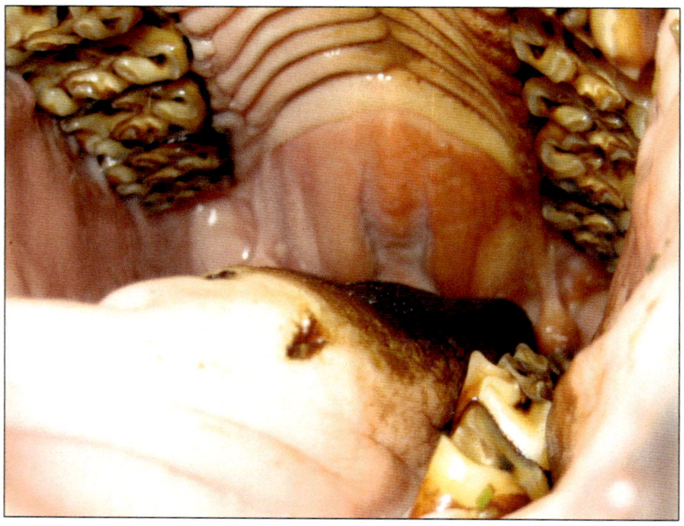

Lingual SEPs have lacerated this horse's tongue, while smaller buccal lacerations have occurred as a result of buccal SEPs of the maxillary cheek teeth. Image credit Author.

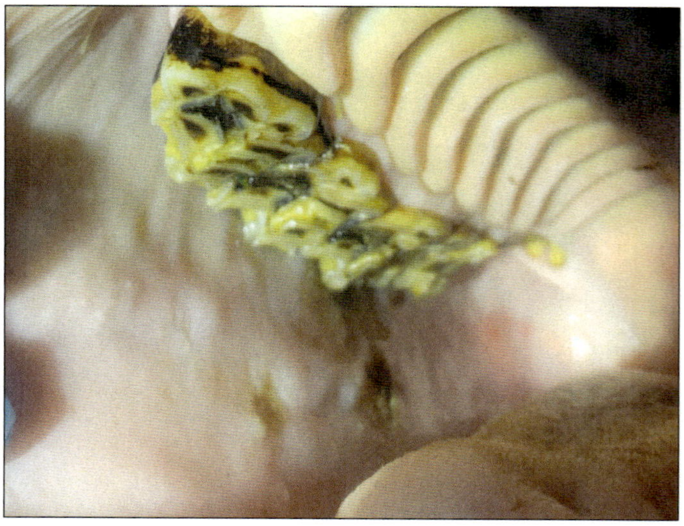

Sharp enamel points (SEPs) of cheek teeth and resultant buccal ulceration. Image credit Cathie Heald Greenwell.

Elongations occur whenever ***hypsodont*** teeth are not evenly opposed by teeth in the opposite arcade. They are involved in all of the below malocclusions, or "bad" "occlusions/meeting of teeth".

What are Sharp Enamel Points (SEPs)?

SEPs are common crown elongations of the buccal, palatal, and/or lingual edges of the cheek teeth, but are most commonly found on the upper buccal edges of the maxillary cheek teeth and the lingual edges of the mandibular cheek teeth. While they can cause buccal lacerations if they become overly long, in their moderate state they probably have a function in improving mastication.

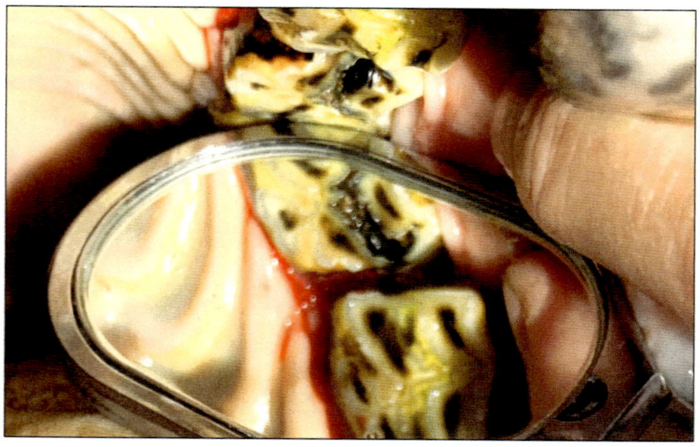

Cheek tooth diastema and infundibular caries. Image credit Author.

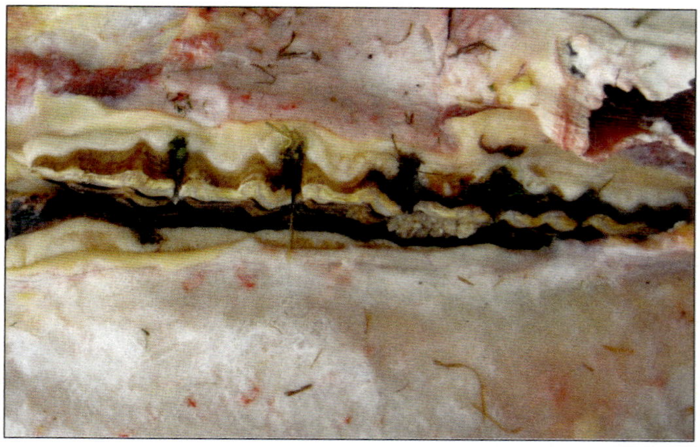

Diastemata existed between every cheek tooth in this horse cadaver, which likely had PPID, or Cushing's Disease, which caused immunosuppression. Image credit Author.

SEPs form as a result of the anisognathia of the mouth and the chewing cycle. See Chapter 3, Anatomy of the Mouth: Anisognathism... Your horse's feed will influence how quickly they form, with highly abrasive high silicate grasses, hard grains, grit, and sand causing more rapid ***attrition*** than soft grasses or softer feeds.

What are Diastema/Diastemata?

A cheek tooth diastema (Pl. diastemata) is an abnormal increase in the interdental space, or the space between cheek teeth, which may or may not have food impactions in these spaces. Portions of opposing teeth may erupt unchecked into the diastema and further widen the diastema by focal crown elongations or overgrowths.

Diastemata may be of "open" or "valve" (closed at the occlusal surface, hard to keep clean!) types and may occur in only one interdental space or may affect multiple interdental spaces. Immunosuppressed equids, such as those with PPID or Cushing's Disease may have multiple diastemata, as these patients have difficulty fighting infections. See the image on the previous page.

Hooks?

Hooks are a wear disorder comprising pointed elongations of the mesial or distal edges of the cheek teeth at the ends of the mandibular and maxillary arcades, usually the upper '06s and the lower '11s.

These elongations can be pressed against the cheeks and lips by the bit and cheekpieces of a bridle or halter, often

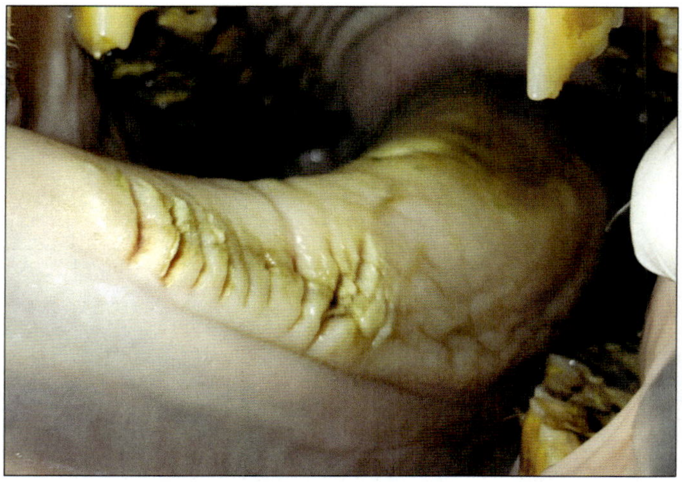

106 and 206 hooks will have caused problems for his horse for quite some time. Severe tongue lacerations from sharp 206 hook and sharp enamel points. Image credit Dr Kirsten Jackson, Dental Vet.

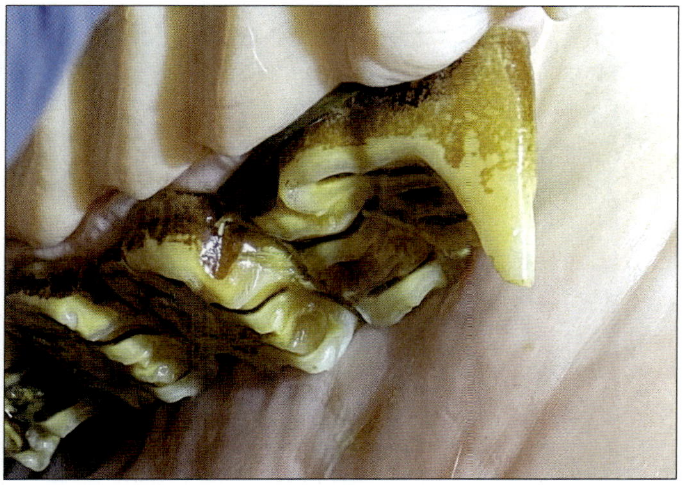

This is a mesial 206 hook and 207 and 208 ETRs. It will likely not be able to be fully reduced in one go, as the pulp will be close to the occlusal surface in this unopposed tooth. Image credit Dr Elke Pollaris.

resulting in pain and bitting problems. If unchecked, hooks continue to erupt and may protrude into the opposing jaw, causing extreme pain to the horse.

Hooks may restrict the normal ***mesiodistal movement*** of the mandible, which is essential to a horse's comfort and ability to work and eat properly. See Chapter 4, Examination of the Mouth: What Makes a Dental Exam Thorough?.

Feeding horses from the ground or in a bin near the ground, rather than from a high hay net or rack, can help prevent occurrence or recurrence of hooks after their gradual removal by repeated odontoplasty at 60-90-day intervals after pulps have had time to retreat, and the color-coding on the occlusal surfaces of the teeth has returned (secondary occlusal dentine has stained from feed pigments again).

Horses with incisor overbites or overjets (parrot mouth, ***brachygnathism***) are predisposed to acquiring upper '06 hooks and lower '11 hooks. Horses with incisor underbites (sow mouth, ***prognathism***) tend to get lower

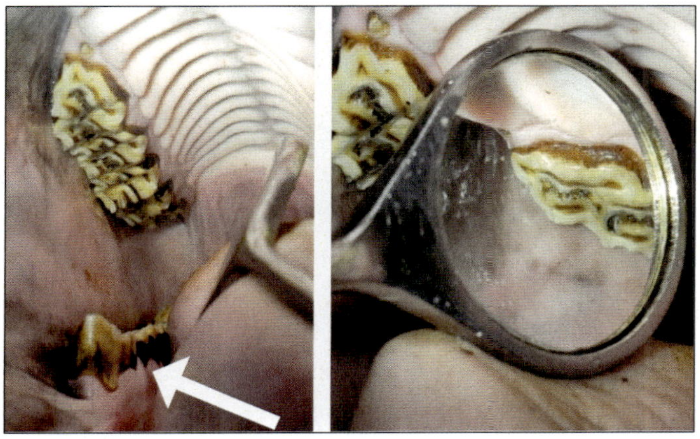

The 406 ramp is shown to the left (white arrow), while its wear effect upon the 106 can be seen in the right-hand image. Images credit Cathie Heald Greenwell.

'06 hooks and upper '11 hooks. These hooks must be addressed in these horses to keep them from living in severe discomfort.

What are Ramps?

Ramps are a wear disorder with a gradual lengthening elongation of the crown of a cheek tooth (see the lower image on the far left). The opposing tooth has a corresponding shortening of its crown. These tend to be of a more gradual slope than a hook.

Cupped Teeth

A stage of tooth wear where the crown is exposed past the infundibulum, but there is still exposed crown above the gingiva.

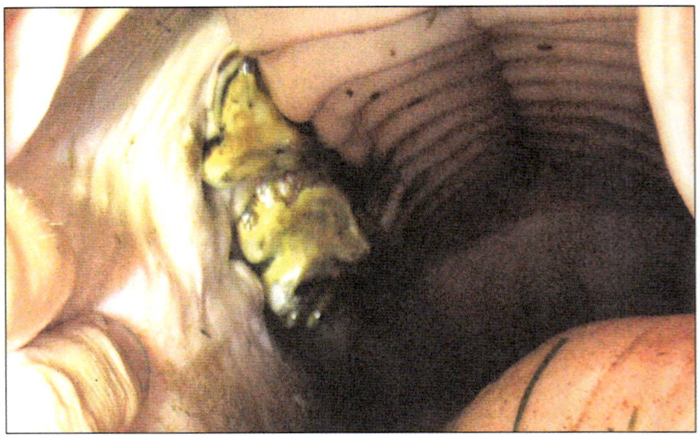

Cupped teeth in an aged horse. The loss of the majority of white enamel, leaves mostly yellow, smooth dentin. Hence the historical term "smooth-mouthed (old) horse". Image credit Author.

Expired Teeth

The wear stage past cupped, where the whole occlusal surface of the tooth is worn down to the level of the gingiva, and the roots are still connected to each other by a thin crown.

Expired with retained tooth root

The final stage of tooth wear where the tooth is worn to the gingiva, but the remains of the roots are no longer connected by the crown.

Excessive transverse ridges (ETRs)

ETRs are a wear disorder with ridges on the occlusal surfaces which run perpendicular to the cheek teeth arcades. Some ridging is normal, but ETRs are deeper and higher on the opposing side than they should be. When the mouth is closed, they restrict rostral movement of the lower jaw, causing discomfort to the horse. In the author's opinion, take for example, a dressage horse with ETRs wearing a tight cavesson or noseband. When it attempts to lower its head and work, its jaw cannot lower or drop, causing discomfort to the horse. Try it with your dressage horse with ETRs and see. When they become pronounced and elongated, as the teeth do not line up perfectly, I have seen the long portions begin to drive into gaps between the opposing cheek teeth and creating or worsening diastemata.

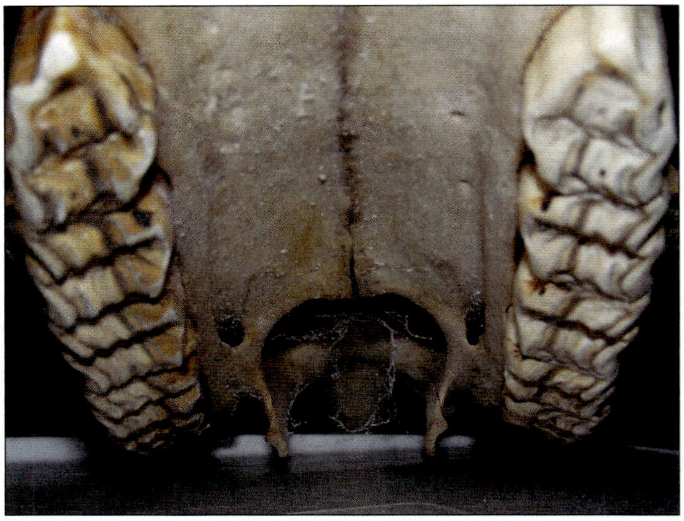

Excessive Transverse Ridges, or ETRs are evident on this skull. Image credit Author.

Waves

Waves are a wear disorder with elongation of two or more sequential teeth in an arcade, with opposing teeth shortened. This displays an undulating, wave-like appearance.

Steps

Steps are a wear disorder which usually includes individual teeth, giving an abrupt change in arcade height. One or more teeth may be involved.

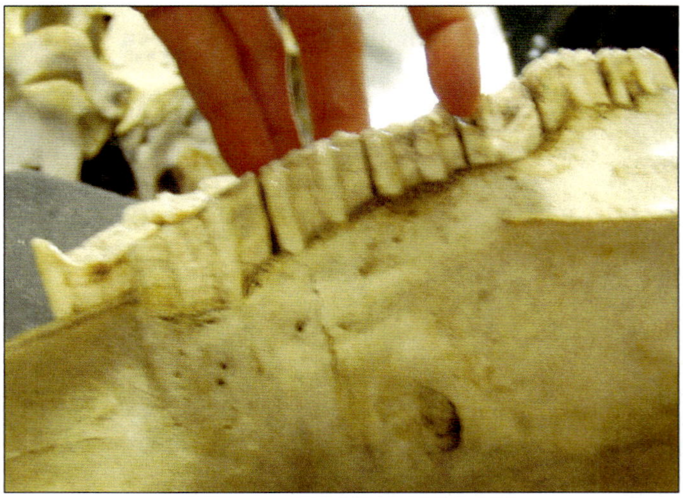

This horse has a wave and a hook. Image credit Author.

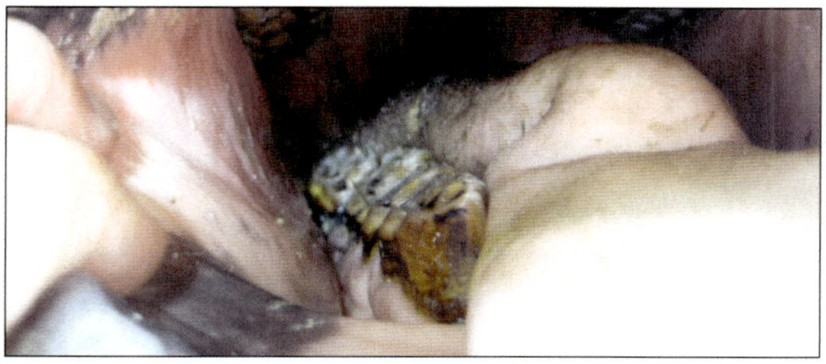

Aged horse with shear mouth and widespread periodontal disease. Image credit Author.

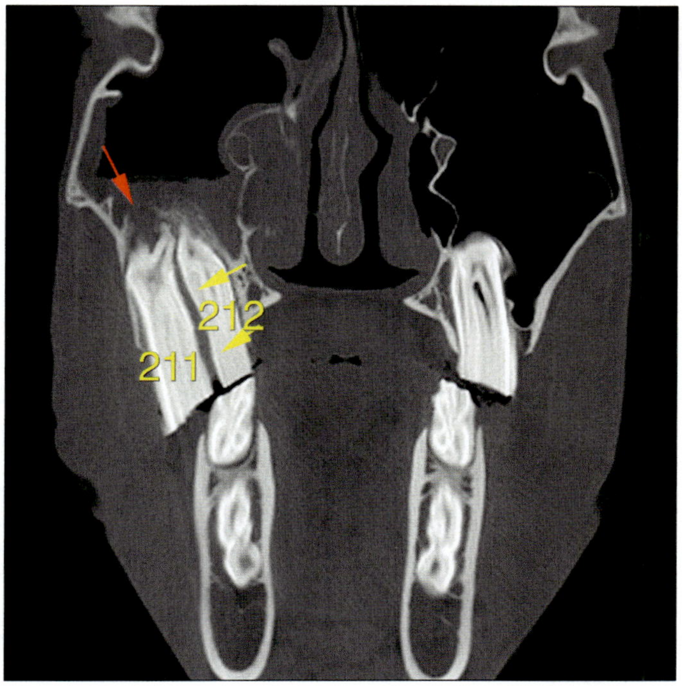

This CT image clearly shows a 212 which has erupted palatal to the 211. As you will remember from the Anatomy chapter, there should only be six teeth in the arcade, finishing with the 211, this horse therefore has a supernumerary tooth. One can also contemplate the space between the 211-212 that has ultimately led to sinusitis due to ascending food accumulation and infection in the space towards the sinus. Image credit Dr Denis Verwilghen.

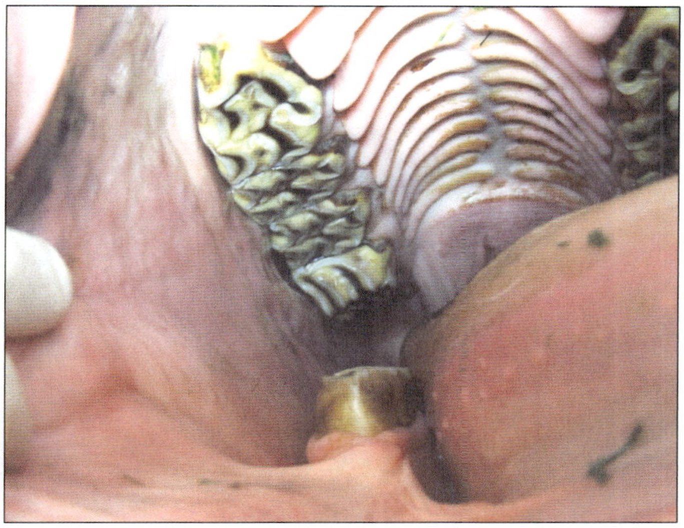

An abrupt crown elongation called a step. This is a severe problem for the tooth or lack of tooth in the opposing arcade. Image credit Author.

Shear mouth

Shear mouth is a wear disorder where the occlusal angulation is steeper than normal, usually 45 degrees to the normal occlusal plane. It usually occurs in response to a painful condition causing a horse to chew abnormally and is rarely the primary pathological issue, therefore the source of the problem should be found and corrected rather than only attempting to correct the sheared occlusal surfaces.

Supernumerary teeth

Supernumerary teeth have been covered before, but here are a few more examples. Supernumerary teeth are extra teeth in an arcade, consisting of more than the normal six teeth per cheek tooth arcade, or incisor arcade. They tend to have irregular shapes and cause overcrowding, and can erupt in any configuration. These

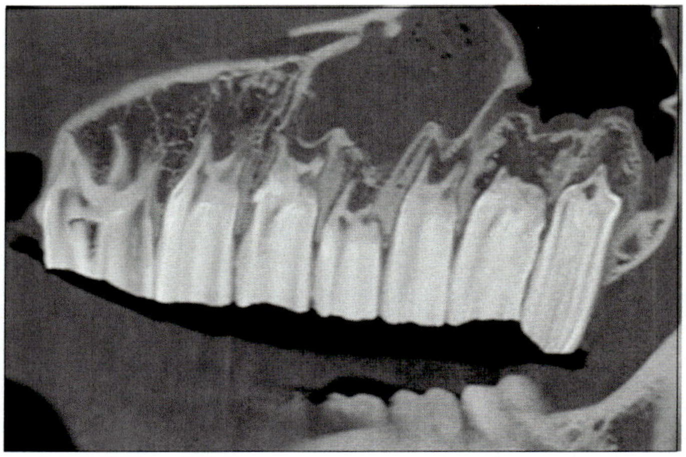

CT image showing seven maxillary cheek teeth. Note the length of the seventh tooth (the '12). What might happen if this supernumerary tooth was ignored and never filed? Image credit Dr Tracy Tinsley.

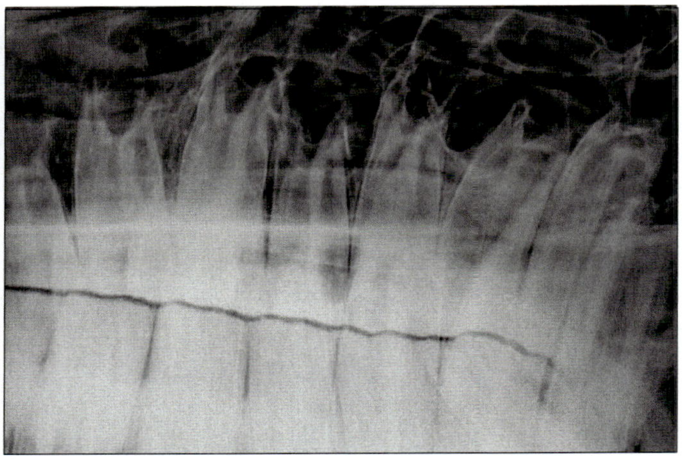

There should be six teeth in each cheek tooth arcade. How many do you see in this maxillary arcade? Image credit Dr Denis Verwilghen.

cause problems because they are not usually opposed by corresponding teeth in the opposite arcade, causing tooth overgrowths in the opposing arcade.

Rotated teeth

Rotated cheek teeth can cause lifelong problems, including formation of diastemata and buccal or lingual mucosal ulcers due to lack of proper apposition of teeth in the opposing arcade.

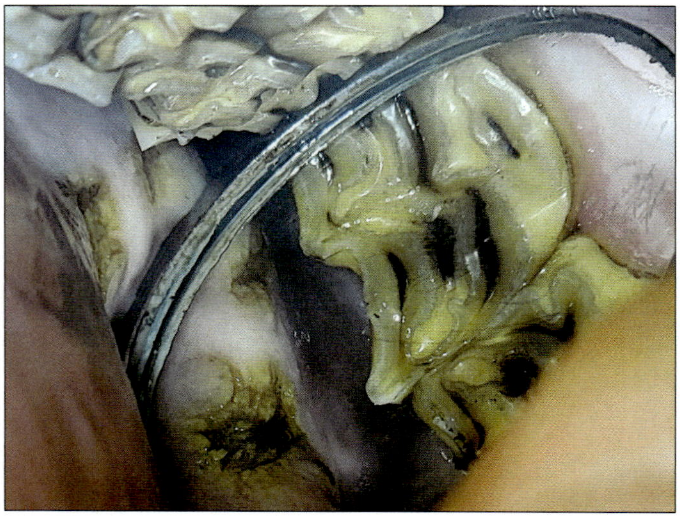

Rotated 110 which has created severe buccal ulceration. Image credit Cathie Heald Greenwell.

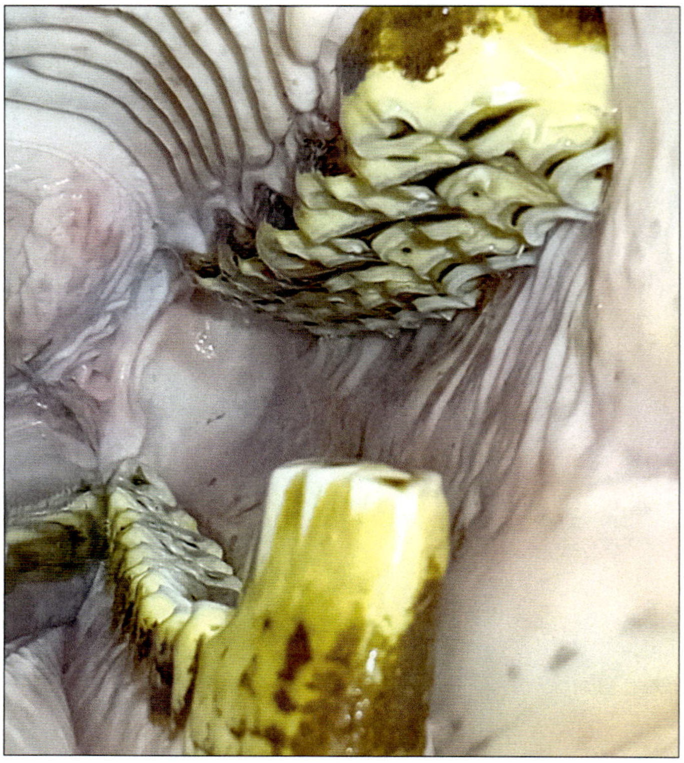

This horse is missing its 206 and there is an extremely long 306 crown eruption creating serious problems. Image credit Dr Elke Pollaris.

Missing teeth

Missing teeth are absent teeth or functionally absent teeth such as dead or broken teeth.

These cause problems because they are not usually opposed by corresponding teeth in the opposite arcade, causing tooth overgrowths in the opposing arcade.

Developmental diastemata

Developmental diastemata (plural of diastema) may originate from 1- inadequate mesiodistal angulation of the mesial and distal cheek teeth during foal development, or 2- from tooth dental buds which have normal angulation, but develop too far apart, both of which cause an imbalance between the size of the cheek teeth and of the supporting bones. See image above.

Developmental diastemata are common in miniatures, which possess small supporting bones for the size of their relatively overlarge teeth. These cause overcrowding and lead to impaction of the cheek teeth, especially the '08s, which are the last teeth to erupt into the arcade. If the teeth can erupt into the mouth at all, they may be displaced from the normal position.

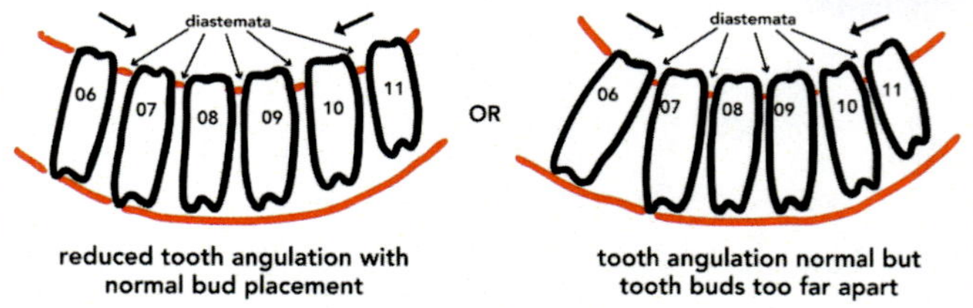

In the embryo, if the mesial (rostral) and disal (caudal) cheek tooth dental buds are improperly positioned, there will be insufficient contact and compression of developing cheek teeth to form a solid row, resulting in developmental diastemata.

Two mechanisms for developmental diastemata in equids. Image credit Dr Padraic Dixon. Redrawn by the Author.

Incisor malocclusions

While some incisor malocclusions are due to problems with the incisors themselves, most of these occur because of malocclusion or pain distally in the cheek tooth arcades. The majority of minor incisor malocclusions will correct themselves when any pathology in the rest of the mouth is appropriately treated, especially via reduction of cheek tooth crown elongations.

If the incisors do not make full contact, however, as seen in severe cases of brachygnathism or prognathism, there will be significant consequences. A newborn foal's "bite", or incisor occlusion, should be checked on its neonatal vet check, as any corrective procedures must be attempted as early in life as possible for the best chance of correction.

Some may be corrected with early orthodontics, while others may require surgery, and some may not be reparable at all.

Brachygnathism ("short jaw"/mandible)

Also known as parrot mouth, overbite, and overjet, brachygnathism is a congenital deformity in which the mandible is short, leaving the maxillary incisors further rostral than the mandibular ones. It is important that this is checked with the head in a neutral position. There are two different conditions of brachygnathism:

- overjet: with a maxillary overjet, the maxillary incisors protrude further rostrally than the mandibular incisors.
- overbite: with a maxillary overbite, the portion of the maxilla containing the incisors curves downwards, (and the portion of the mandible containing the incisors curves upward, as in the figure to the right.

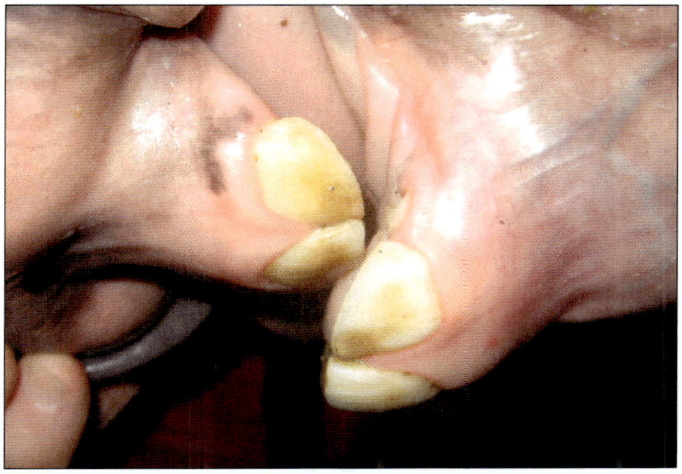

A yearling with a severe brachygnathia, with an overjet of 25mm and am overbite of 15 mm. Image credit Author.

This young horse had a severe overbite. The maxilla was curving ventrally (downward), and the mandible was curving dorsally (upward). This was only noted by the owners when the imported horse was over a year old.

Prognathism ("protruding jaw"/mandible)

Also known as underbite, sow mouth, or monkey mouth, prognathism is a congenital deformity in which the mandibular incisors are further rostral than the maxillary incisors. This is the opposite of brachygnathism. Often prognathism is accompanied by hooks on the mesial edges of the mandibular '06s and the distal edges of the maxillary '11.

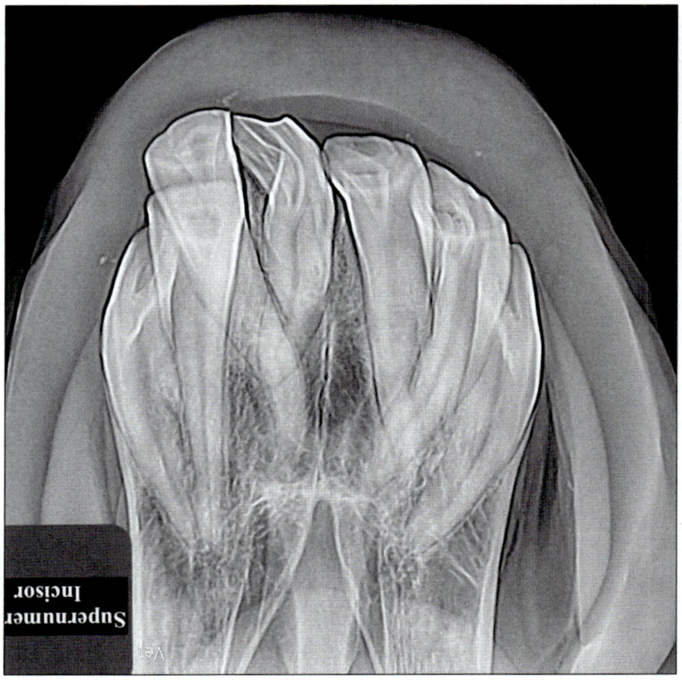

This supernumerary incisor has forced the rest of the incisors in the arcade out of place. Image credit Dr Tracy Tinsley.

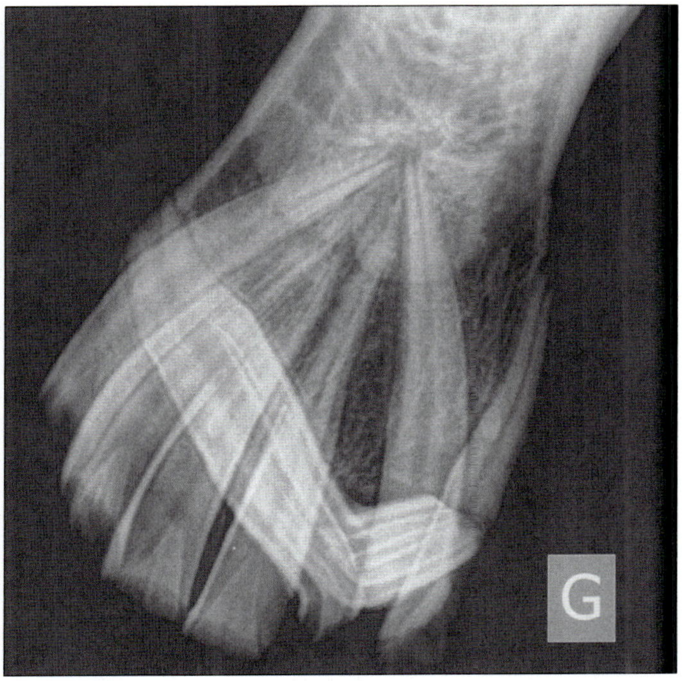

This supernumerary tooth has caused incisor displacement. Without X-ray it would not have been possible to identify the orientation of this tooth. Following X-ray, it was decided not to attempt extraction as this would have disrupted the entire incisor arcade. Image credit Dr Denis Verwilghen.

Incisor Diastema

An incisor diastema (Pl. diastemata) is a gap between incisors, often packed tightly with feed. Portions of opposing teeth may erupt unchecked into the diastema and further widen it. Developmental diastemata are common in equids with EOTRH. It is also common in miniatures and small ponies, which possess small tooth-supporting bones (the mandible and maxilla) for the size of their relatively overlarge teeth and developmental abnormalities which cause overcrowding. These problems lead to impaction and wear disorders. See Chapter 12, Special Equids: Miniature Horses. Certain incisors (often the '03s) may erupt in a reverse or otherwise abnormal direction, which causes wear disorders and allows feed impaction with subsequent painful periodontal disease. If the most significantly affected displaced teeth are not extracted, progression of the periodontal disease may result in tooth death and more pain.

Crown elongations (Overgrowths)

Teeth which have erupted (part or all of the teeth) past the level of the rest of the teeth in an arcade.

Retained deciduous incisors

Deciduous incisors which have not been exfoliated as they should have. They can block the proper eruption pathway of the permanent incisors and cause them to erupt in the wrong place, which is usually palatally or lingually.

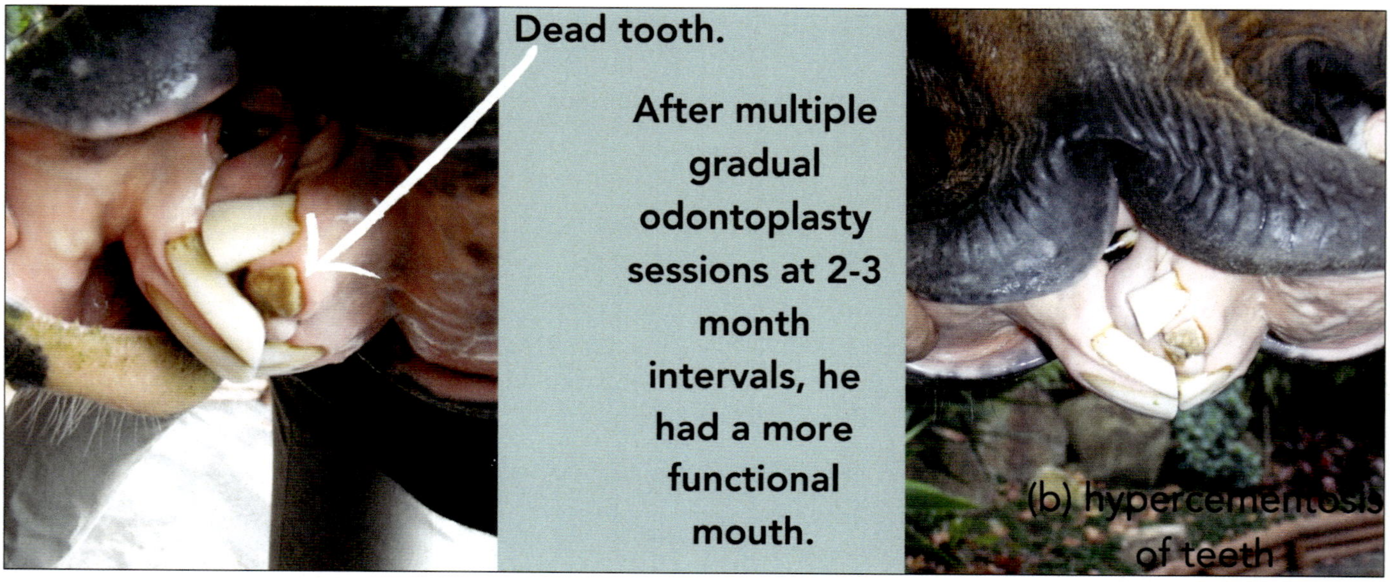

Trauma and a dead 102 contributed to this malocclusion with severely overgrown teeth impinging onto the opposing gingiva. Image credit Greg Miller-Hard.

Supernumerary incisors

Extra teeth in the arcades. These cause problems because they are not usually opposed by corresponding teeth in the opposite arcade, causing crown elongations in the opposing arcade. If they are occlusally opposed, they may be left in place, but this is rare.

Haplodont supernumerary incisors are cone-shaped incisors (may appear cylindrical) which aren't opposed. They can cause problems by occupying space where incisors should lie and allowing crown elongations in the opposing arcade, so extraction is recommended. Six-monthly odontoplasty is required post-extraction while shifting of the other incisors to fill the gap occurs. Correct occlusion may or may not be attained.

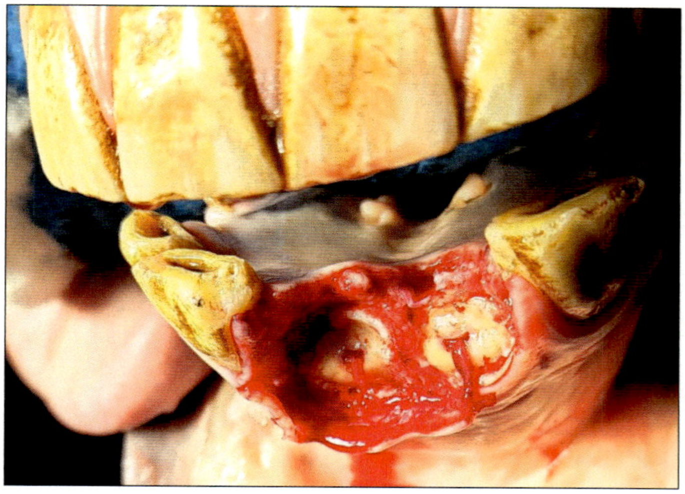

The 301 and 401 incisors have fractured near the gumline. Note the red pulps exiting the center of these two teeth. This horse will be in serious pain and is in need of vital pulpotomy as soon as possible. Image credit Dr Elke Pollaris.

Missing teeth

As with supernumerary teeth, these cause problems, first, because the missing teeth don't usually have missing teeth in the opposite arcade, hence allowing crown elongations in the opposing arcade, and second, because they could experience dental drift of the teeth adjacent to the missing tooth. In situations of hypodontia (see above), dental drift of the adjacent teeth into the site of a missing tooth is absent or reduced when compared to the amount of drift which occurs following an extraction.

Fractured teeth

Fractured teeth often leave a gap into which the opposing teeth can erupt. Fractured teeth are painful if the fracture line enters or is near the pulp. If caught within the first few days, restoration may be possible, and the tooth saved. The horse at the top right will be in serious pain due to the pulps hanging out of its fractured teeth.

Irregularly shaped (e.g. tubular, or connate) incisors

Like extra or absent teeth, these tubular, or "connate" teeth don't match up with the opposing teeth, resulting in crown elongation of the opposing teeth.

Hooks

Hooks are pointed overgrowths of the '03s on the distal edges, usually seen in the upper incisors.

Dorsal curvature (frown)

An incisor malocclusion where the upper '02s and '03s are overly long while the lower '01s are overlong.

Ventral curvature (smile)

An incisor malocclusion where the lower '02s and '03s are overly long, as are the upper '01s.

Slant or diagonal mouth

A wear disorder where the occlusion angle of the incisors varies from the horizontal, usually due to wry nose or a cheek teeth disorder (e.g. when pain causes the horse to chew with only the non-painful side of its mouth).

The slant shown to the right is unlikely to be due primarily to the incisors themselves. This is a hint to look elsewhere in the mouth for the real problem, such as a fractured tooth, diastema, etc. Changing the slant is not usually the answer, and the primary problem needs to be found and corrected.

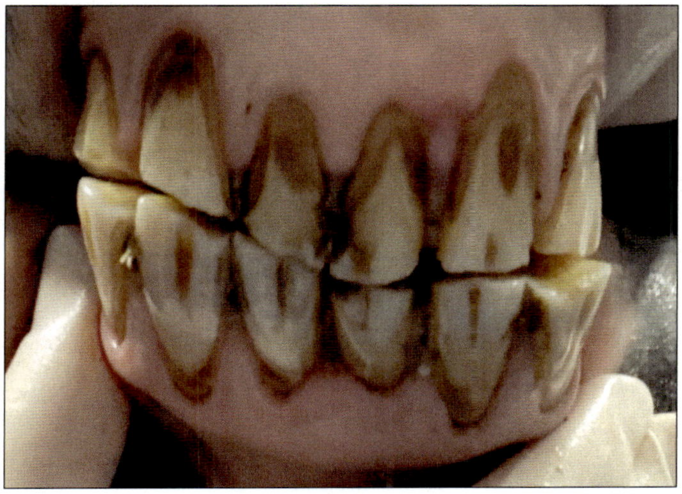

This horse shows a diagonal or slant incisor bite. Image credit Dr Elke Pollaris.

Over-long incisors

Sometimes seen in horses which are always stabled and do not graze grass outside, but not nearly as common as some believe.

Rotated incisors

Rotated incisors can cause lifelong problems, including formation of diastemata and buccal (cheek) or lingual (tongue) mucosal ulcers due to lack of proper apposition of teeth in the opposing arcade.

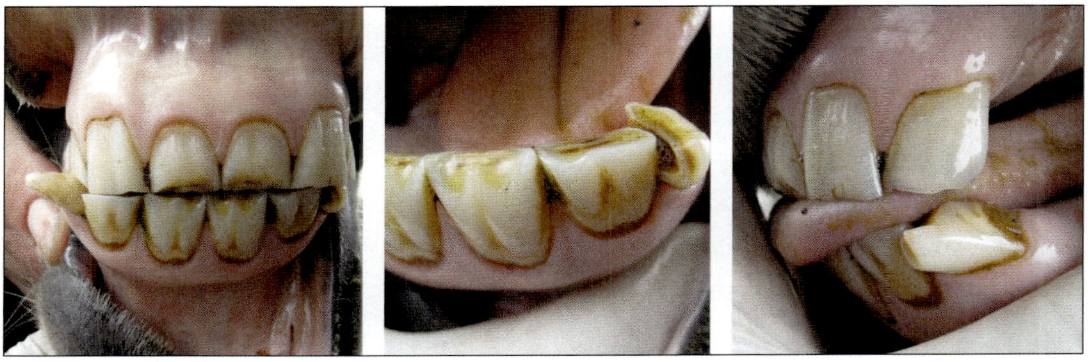

This miniature's ectopic maxillary corner incisors are rotated and have painful pulp exposures and periodontal disease. Image credit Author.

What the Heck are Infundibular and Peripheral Caries?

CARIES (PLURAL AND singular are both "caries") is a form of dental decay, or demineralization (the minerals are drawn out) of the tooth structure caused by either:

- malformation of the tooth during development (called infundibular hypoplasia or secondary caries), or
- environmental causes such as sweet or acidic feeds or water (called ***peripheral caries***).

This demineralization occurs either from the mouth bacteria metabolizing sweet feeds in the diet to produce acid, or directly from acidic feed or water. If the fluid around the teeth stays acidic for a prolonged period, then the teeth begin to demineralize. Once the minerals are gone from that part of the tooth, the connective tissue is no longer protected and is abraded away, and that part of the tooth is lost.

The two main forms of caries in horses are peripheral and infundibular. They are classified by the structures invaded and destroyed by the caries process, starting from the most external (Grade 1) and going deeper into the tooth structure (Grade 5), using the modified Honma classification system. PC refers to peripheral caries and IC to infundibular caries.

The two main forms of caries in horses are peripheral and infundibular. They are classified by the structures invaded and destroyed by the caries process, starting from the most external (Grade 1) and going deeper into the tooth structure

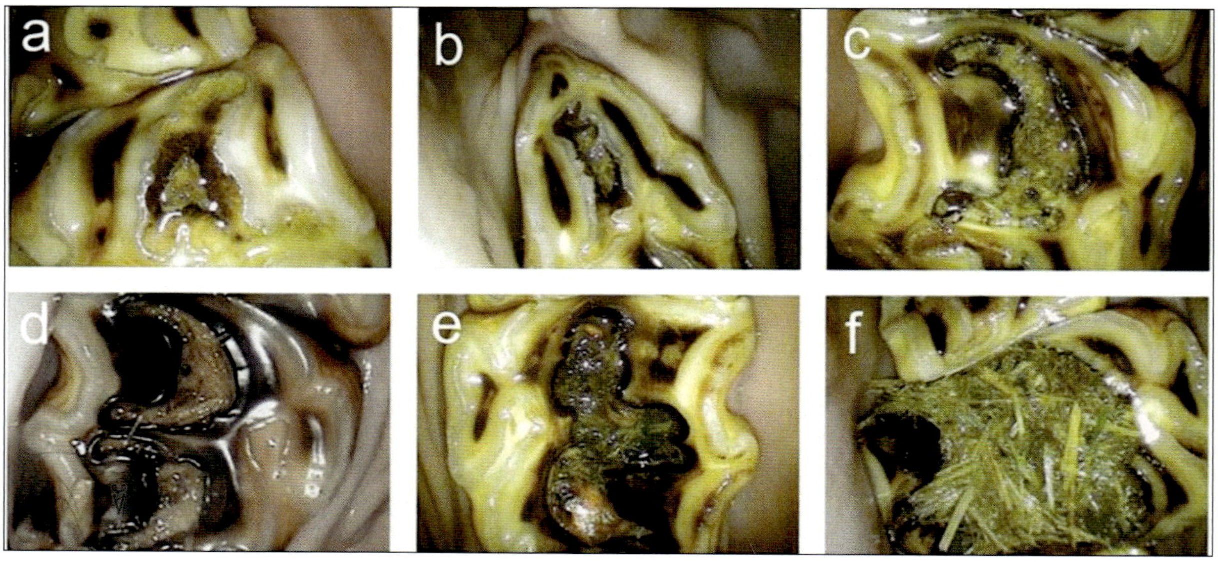

Examples of cheek teeth with occlusal infundibular caries classified using the modified Honma classification system. (a) Grade 1: caries of infundibular cementum only, (b) Grade 2: caries of cementum and enamel, (c) Grade 3: caries of cementum, enamel, and dentine, (d) Grade 3+: grade 3 mesial and distal infundibular caries, (e) Grade 4: as grade 3 but coalescence of mesial and distal infundibular caries, (f) Grade 5: advanced caries; pathological structural loss, fracture. Image credit Dr Pearce C. (2020). Image originally published in Pearce C. Recent developments in equine dentistry. New Zealand Veterinary Journal 68, 178-86, 2020. ©NZVA

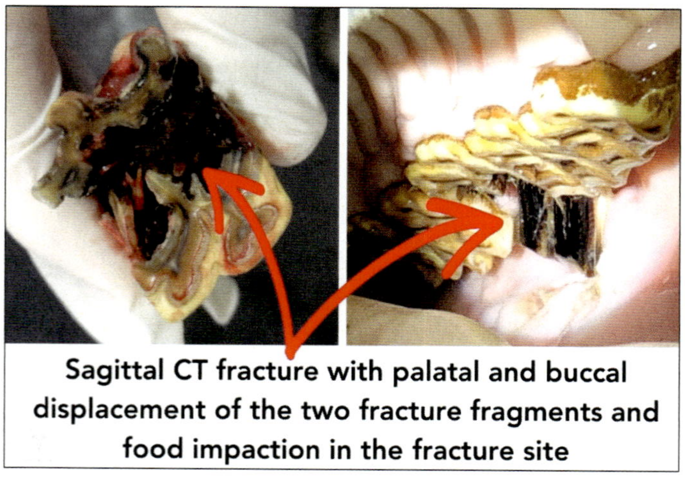

An example of infundibular caries as a cause of sagittal fracture in this horse. Image credit Dr Kirsten Jackson, Dental Vet.

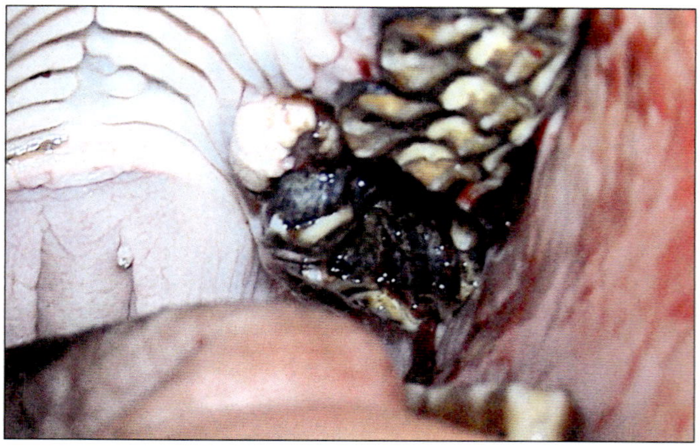

A 16-year-old horse in full work, this was found on oral exam for routine dentistry. Unfortunately, this is not uncommon. Shown is a sagittal fracture of 209 subsequent to advanced, Grade 5 infundibular caries. Image credit Author.

(Grade 5), using the modified Honma classification system. PC refers to peripheral caries and IC to infundibular caries.

- Grade 1 - PC and IC: caries of cementum (caries occurs at only a mildly acidic pH of 6.7). PC: this is further divided into:
  - Grade 1.1 - PC: caries have superficial pitting and small cemental caries lesions.
  - Grade 1.2 - PC: caries have larger areas of cemental caries exposing enamel.
- Grade 2 - PC and IC: caries of cementum and enamel (*enamel* is affected at pH of 5.5).
- Grade 3 - PC and IC: caries of cementum, enamel, and dentine (*dentine* is affected at pH of 6.2) In IC there is a Grade 3+:
  - Grade 3+ - IC: Grade 3 affecting both the mesial and distal (rostral and caudal) infundibula.
- Grade 4 - PC: Loss of structural integrity of tooth with possible secondary dental fracture or pulp exposure. IC: As Grade 3 with coalescence (joining) of mesial and distal (rostral and caudal) infundibula.
- Grade 5 - IC: Advanced caries with secondary tooth fracture (most commonly a mid-sagittal fracture), pulp exposure, and/or apical infection.

We get particularly concerned at Grade 3 and above because if it is affecting the dentin, it is destroying the protective layer overlying the pulp cavities. If this infection enters the pulp, it can kill the tooth.

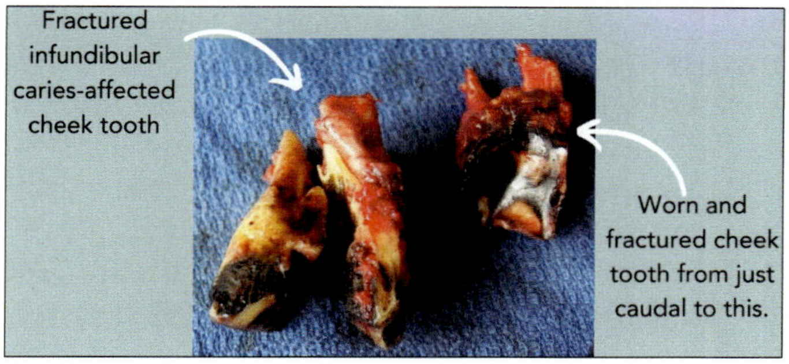

The 209 and 210 extracted from above horse. This must have been a painful issue for many years, from the pathology evidenced by the teeth. The left-hand tooth had extensive infundibular caries and had split from the palatal to the buccal side. The right-hand tooth had been worn away by the distal portion of the fractured tooth. It may have had caries, but there was little left to tell. Image credit Author.

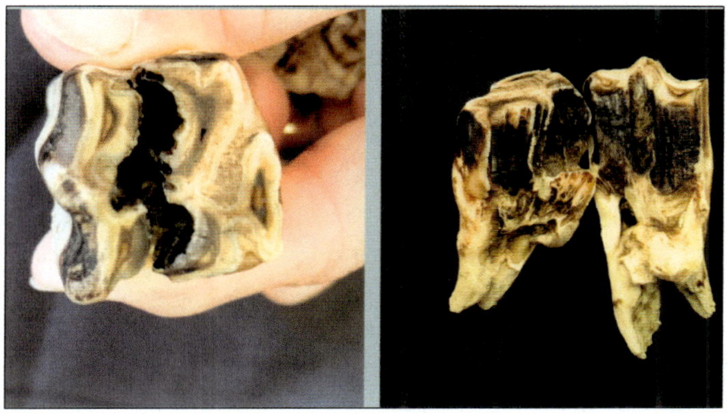

Close up, cleaned detail of the 209 from above. Held together on the left and opened on the right. Image credit Author.

Infundibular caries

Infundibular caries is the most common form of caries.

One study found them to be present in up to 100% of horses aged over 12 years. Another study found the prevalence of occlusal infundibular caries to increase significantly with age, from 23% at 3-5 years of age through to 69% at over 20 years of age. They affect the maxillary cheek teeth. They won't be found in mandibular cheek teeth because the mandibular cheek teeth have no infundibula.

Caries are graded as mentioned above. Following is a visual grading chart for infundibular caries:

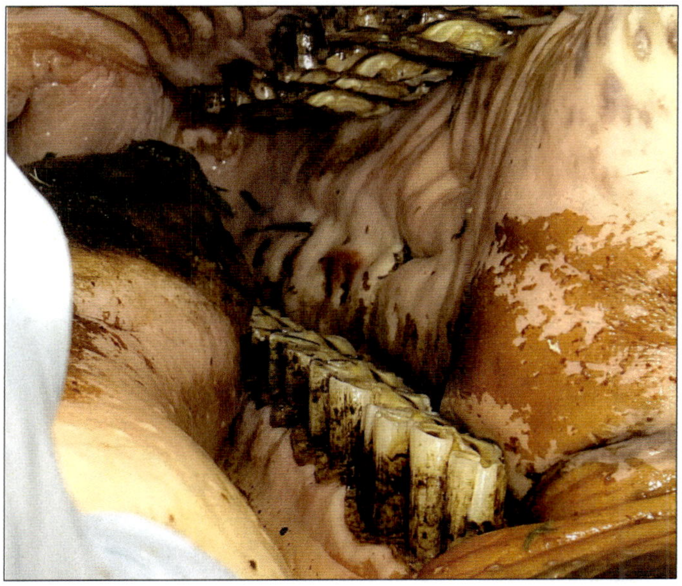

Extensive Grade 1.2 peripheral caries have removed all of the cementum from these teeth. The horse was routinely fed on a diet of very acidic corn silage. Image credit Dr Elke Pollaris.

How do infundibular caries develop?

As discussed earlier in this chapter under Central Infundibular Cemental Hypoplasia, developmental cemental hypoplasia predisposes horses to infundibular caries as their teeth undergo attrition with age (as they get worn down with age). The more the teeth are worn toward the apex, the more common are areas of cemental hypoplasia, due to faulty incomplete filling of the infundibula during tooth development. The filling of the infundibulum with cementum occurs from the occlusal surface toward the apex, which leaves more gaps in the cementum (hypoplasia) toward the apex, gaps which can be then become impacted with feed and invaded by bacteria as that part of the tooth is exposed by wear over time, and so caries takes hold.

What's the big problem with infundibular caries?

For one, if they are extensive, they can destabilize the affected tooth, or teeth, and sagittal fractures may result.

When a horse has advanced caries of both infundibula and the tooth in between them coalesces (joins together), the tooth can fracture along the line of both infundibula. This is called a sagittal fracture.

What makes infundibular caries worse? How can prevent my horse from getting infundibular caries? If he does get it, can I do anything to help him get over the disease?

Monitoring your horse's diet to reduce sweet or acidic feeds and water, as well as maintaining regular dental examinations and ***odontoplasty*** as needed, will probably make a big difference. Treating any diastemata feed impaction on a regular basis will likely help to slow progression of the disease. If warranted, many dental veterinarians can perform restorations ('fillings'), where the impacted feed material is thoroughly evacuated (cleaned out) and disinfected, and then the area of hypoplasia is filled with dental material to try to eliminate feed impaction and stop the progression of decay inside the tooth. The 'fillings' just wear down with the teeth.

Peripheral caries

Caries affecting primarily the outer layers of the teeth are termed peripheral caries and are largely diet and/or environment related. They preferentially affect the teeth toward the back of the mouth, with the most commonly affected areas being the buccal aspect of the mandibular and the palatal aspect of the maxillary cheek teeth. In peripheral caries cases, the ***peripheral cementum*** is lost, and the caries can progress to affect the enamel and dentin as well. Recent research has been progressing our understanding of this painful condition. There are several articles in Bibliography and Further Reading, if you wish to study this topic in more depth.

In a normal tooth, the cementum provides strength to the tooth and protects the harder, but more brittle enamel. It also creates the rectangular shape of the mandibular cheek teeth. If the cementum is lost, the gaps which arise between

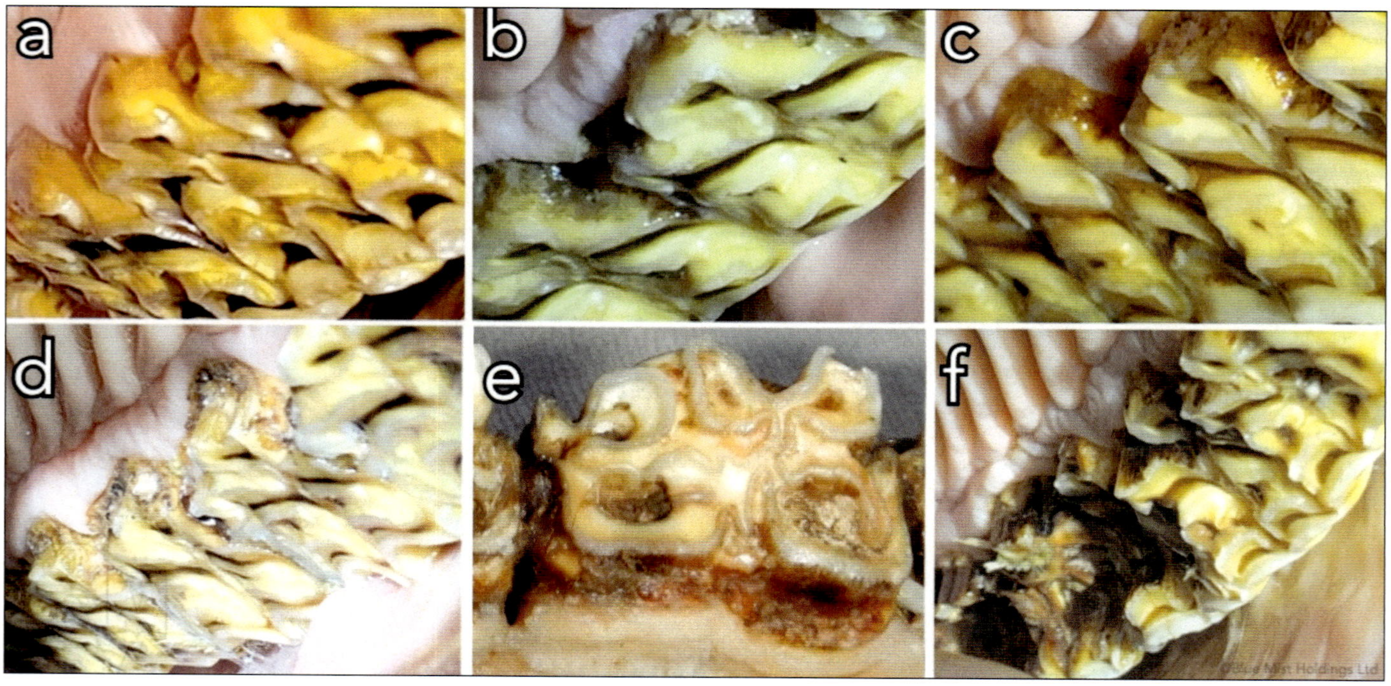

Classification of peripheral caries in equine cheek teeth using the modified Honma classification system (Dacre 2005). (a) Grade 0: No peripheral caries. Some discoloration may be present, but no pitting. (b) Grade 1.1: Only cementum is affected by caries. Caries have superficial pitting or partial loss of cementum. (c) Grade 1.2: Almost total loss of peripheral cementum with some exposed enamel. More severe cases have total cementum loss in some areas. (d) Grade 2: Cementum and underlying enamel are both affected. Enamel is completely exposed and discolored. (e) Grade 3: Cementum, enamel and dentine are affected. (f) Grade 4: Loss of integrity of the tooth with possible secondary dental fracture or pulp exposure. Individual images credit Dr Kirsten Jackson, Dental Vet, graphic credit Author.

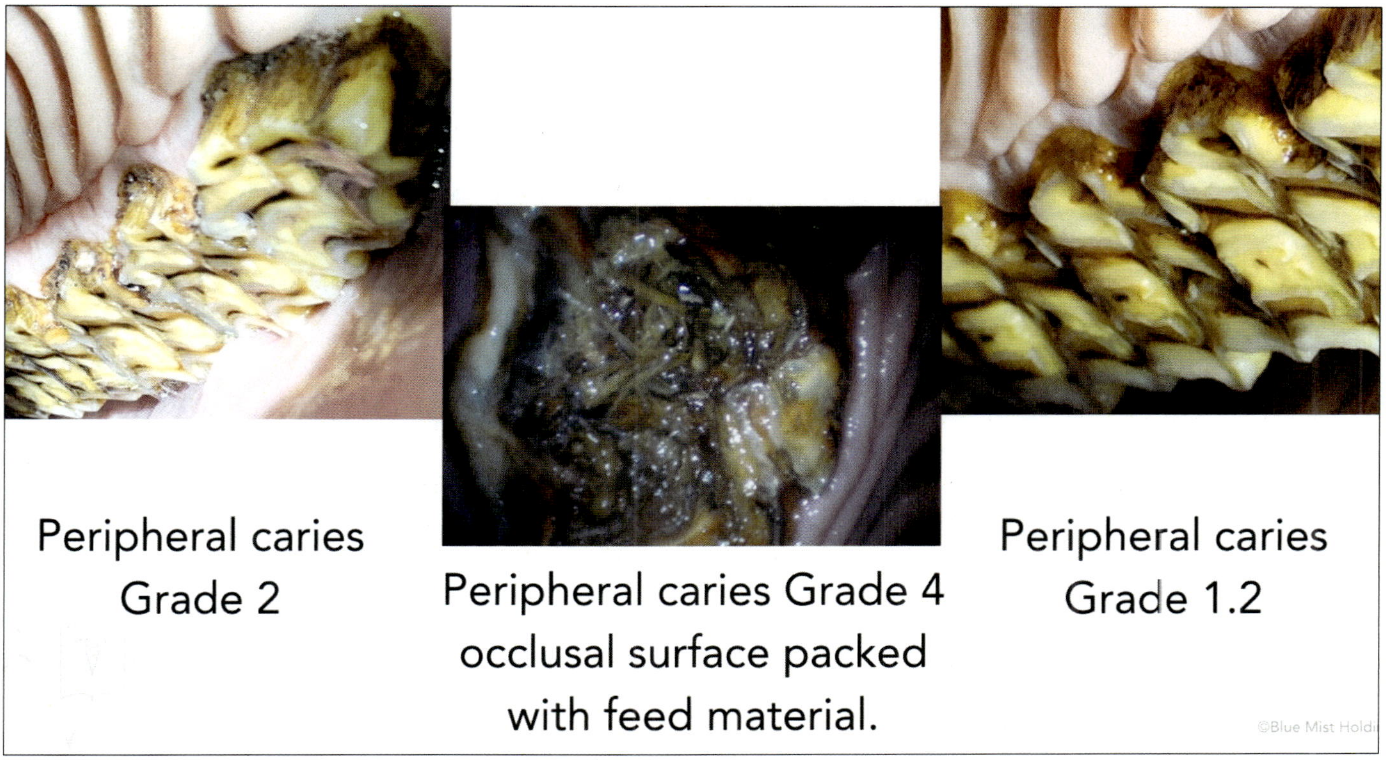

A client's horse fed honey daily for a year developed severe peripheral caries of Grade 2, and appeared much like the horse on the left, with affected cementum and the adjacent enamel. The central image shows the occlusal surface of a grade 4 horse, with feed material packed into the caries sites. The right image at grade 1.2 exhibits almost complete loss of peripheral cementum and the enamel is exposed in some areas. Original image credit Dr Kirsten Jackson, Dental Vet, graphic credit Author..

the teeth allow feed entrapment and periodontal disease can then develop. Peripheral caries, in advanced stages, weakens the tooth by causing loss of the cementum, which allows increased wear and may lead to tooth fracture.

In severe cases, there is almost no tooth material left inside the mouth (though the ***reserve crowns*** and roots are still present) and caries can kill the tooth if the infection enters the pulp cavities. Affected horses are also very prone to periodontal disease as feed becomes trapped in the gaps between the teeth caused by the lost dental material. The sole good thing about this condition is that only the ***clinical crown*** (portion of the tooth already erupted into the mouth) is affected, and the tooth below the gumline is normal. Since a horse's teeth exhibit ***prolonged eruption***, if the cause can be removed and the healthy tooth below the gum replaces the damaged tooth by eruption, the affected teeth can recover. The normally large flow of saliva and the frequent chewing motions in a horse's mouth are protective against caries, but with modern feeds, or a problem with saliva delivery, the chewing and saliva alone cannot compete. Horses with a damaged parotid salivary gland duct on only one side have been found to have severe caries on the ipsilateral (same side) of the mouth, giving us an idea how important that full flow of saliva really is. See papers in Bibliography and Further Reading.

How Do Peripheral Caries Develop?

Have you seen how calcium-containing items are demineralized in the presence of an acid? Try this sometime: Put a whole uncooked egg (still in its shell) in vinegar (which is weak acetic acid) and leave it overnight. What happens? This will prove to you how quickly an acid solution can pull the calcium out of a relatively hard object. It does the same thing to teeth, unfortunately.

Frequent feeding of easily fermentable carbohydrates like sweet feeds and sugars increase acid production in the mouth and encourage demineralization. Plaque, a biofilm which sticks to the tooth and contains bacteria, plays a part here as well. The acid-forming bacteria gain some protection from hiding in the biofilm while they make even more acid and decrease the pH of the biofilm, creating perfect conditions for acid-caused demineralization, or caries, to occur.

What Makes Peripheral Caries Worse?

New research indicates the most significant causative factor in peripheral caries is dietary sugars or acidity. The researchers found these components to be associated with peripheral caries formation:

- Specific types of hay which are high in soluble carbohydrates. E.g. cereal hays such as oaten hay

- Feeds which promote acid formation. E.g. sweet feeds, concentrate feeds
- Drinking water of low pH (acidic). E.g. In Australia, from rainwater, or dam water
- Lack of access to grazing
- Concurrent dental or periodontal disease, especially cheek teeth diastemata with interdental feed accumulation and gingival recession
- Breed. E.g. Thoroughbreds are more likely to get the disease than Warmbloods and Western breeds in Australia

Can I do Anything to Help My Horse with Peripheral Caries?

The researchers found that reversal of the condition may be possible when the inciting cause/s are identified and corrected, and the reserve crown is allowed time to replace the damaged clinical crown. Since the changes in the teeth only occurred above the gumline, dietary change to reduce acidity may result in the eruption of normal teeth as they continue to emerge.

Their recommendations for treatment and prevention of peripheral caries include:

- Avoid feeding fermented forage or cereal hays (in particular, oaten hay)
- Feed meadow/grass hay if supplementing pasture
- Provide horses only neutral or slightly alkaline pH drinking water (pH 7-8). E.g. using ground water (bore/well) water rather than rainwater, or dam water, although should still pH test the water as some bore water can be acidic.
- Provide year-round grazing
- Correct dental and periodontal disease

Again, take heart, peripheral caries is one of the few dental conditions we can treat by simple changes to equine management.

What is Pituitary Pars Intermedia Dysfunction—PPID?

THE ENDOCRINE DISEASE Pituitary Pars Intermedia Dysfunction (PPID), also known as Cushing's Syndrome, or

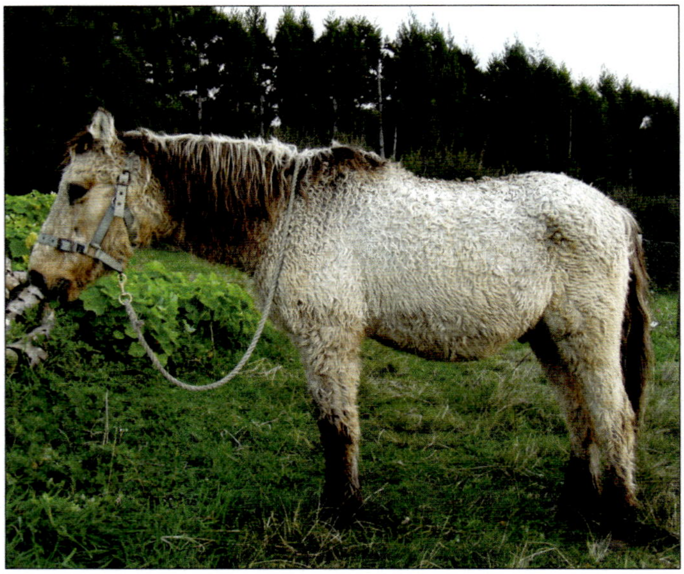

An equid with advanced PPID often appears as this one, with an extremely long haircoat, pendulous abdomen, and chronic laminitis. The associated immune system dysfunction can cause problems with healing and result in severe dental disease. Image credit Author.

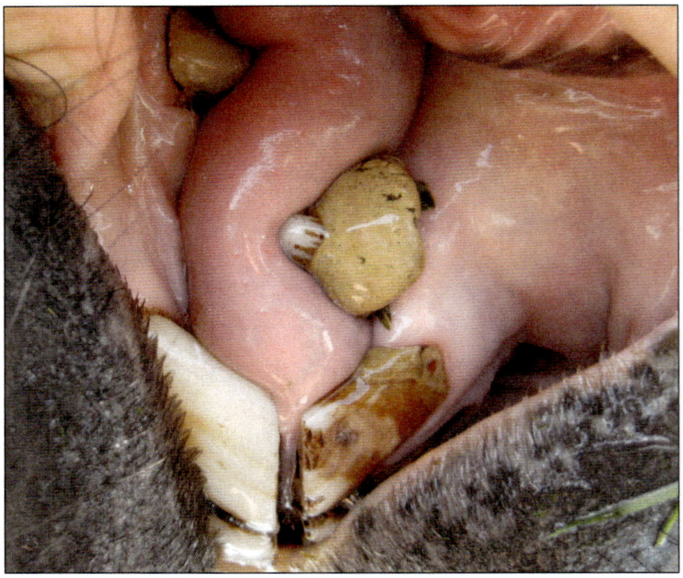

Severe calculus accumulation on canine 304. An equid with advanced PPID often looks like this, with an extremely long haircoat, pendulous abdomen, and chronic laminitis. The associated immune system dysfunction can cause problems with healing and result in severe dental disease. Image credit Author.

Cushing's Disease, causes high levels of the horse's own steroids to be released into their bloodstream. These steroids cause immunosuppression, which prevents wounds from healing properly and decreases the horse's ability to fight infections, in addition to causing other conditions such as laminitis.

It is most common in older horses, and many aged horses with widespread diastemata, non-healing wounds, or periodontal disease may suffer from this condition. It is wise to test older patients for adrenal function (PPID) before you get too far with extensive dental treatment. If the horse is positive for PPID, it may benefit by treating first for the PPID, and when immune function is restored, the dental treatment is more likely to have a positive outcome.

Do Horses get Calculus (aka Tartar)?

HORSES TEND TO accumulate ***calculus*** on the canines, the ***interproximal spaces*** of the cheek teeth, and the gingival margins of the incisors, all places which don't get a lot of "brushing" from the feeds horses eat, especially grass and hay. Calculus is only rarely found in other locations in the equid mouth.

Calculus forms when the dental plaque on the tooth surface mineralizes. The calculus is bad enough, but unfortunately, it covers up pathology. It is important for your dental operator to ensure they remove all attached calculus from every tooth and examine the tooth and tissue beneath. There will often be local gingivitis and caries of the tooth (especially the canine) beneath the calculus. Human curved scalers are perfect for cleaning up equid calculus.

It is a good idea to carefully observe equids with these calculus-affected canines and incisors for evidence of Equine Odontoclastic Tooth Resorption and Hypercementosis (***EOTRH***). Calculus is commonly found on canines and incisors affected by EOTRH and can hide this disease's erosive or proliferative tooth lesions. See Chapter 7, EOTRH.

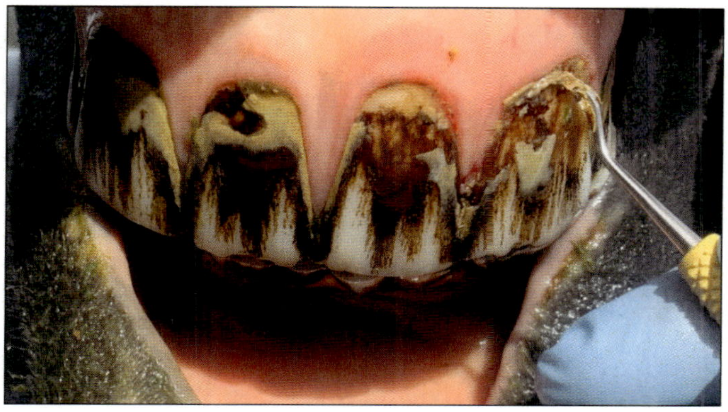

Incisor calculus being removed by Dr Thompson with a scaler. Image credit Author.

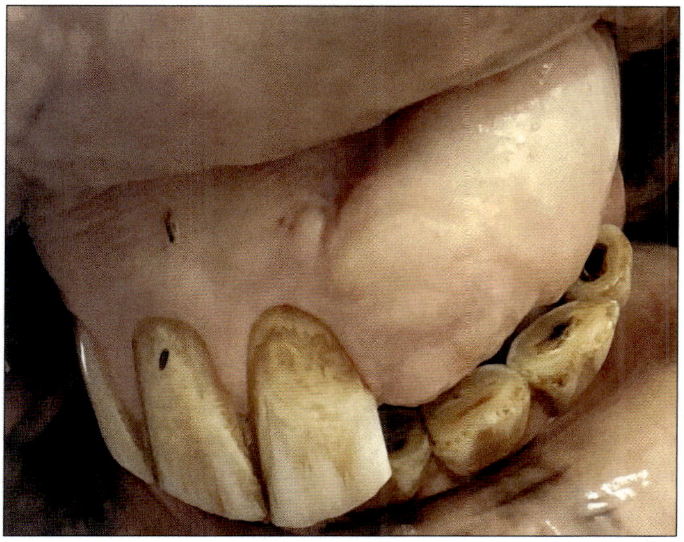

A large mass which displaced the 200 arcade incisors. Image credit Dr Elke Pollaris.

Masses, Tumors, Lumps & Bumps!

TO TAKE THE fear out of this chapter, the term "tumor" simply means an abnormally localized tissue growth.

The types of cells in a tumor define whether it is benign, pre-malignant, or malignant:

- **Benign**, or not containing cancerous cells. These may be locally invasive but won't spread elsewhere.
- **Pre-malignant**, or containing certain abnormal cells which have the potential to become cancerous, or
- **Malignant**, or containing cancerous cells. Normal cells stop replicating when they come into contact with the cells beside them, but malignant or cancerous cells have lost their contact inhibition, meaning that they keep replicating and result in a cancerous mass, or neoplasia, and may spread further in the body.

We will start with some of the more common and innocuous benign lumps and bumps before moving on to the malignant ones.

As we move through the tumor types, remember that these are the typical presentations of these tumors, but they didn't always read the book. You'll have to trust your veterinarian on this!

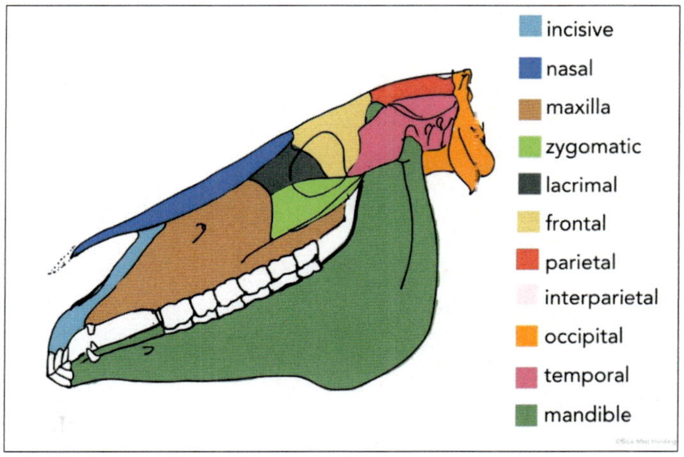

The lines where two bones join are called the "sutures". Note especially the suture between the nasal (dark blue) and frontal(gold) bones while looking at the injury in the figure below. Image credit Author.

Non-malignant facial swellings

Suture Periostitis, ***exostosis***, ***separation*** or ***suturitis***: Usually a one-sided or bilateral firm, non-painful swellings near the suture (joining) line between the nasal and frontal bones of the skull. See Chapter 3,

Some of these deeper tissues which may be involved include the naso-lacrimal or lacrimal-maxillary sutures. Periostitis of these sutures can cause chronic epiphora, or tearing. Bone sequestra may also form, which may result in chronic draining tracts until the condition is surgically repaired. Less severe cases usually resolve by themselves over time, but if they persist, radiographs and in tricky cases, CT, should assist with the diagnosis and treatment.

Eruption Cysts (Pseudocysts, as no cyst lining exists): Also called 3- and 4-year-old bumps, or "tooth bumps", are the normal, enlarged areas of soft tissue at the apex of developing permanent cheek teeth.

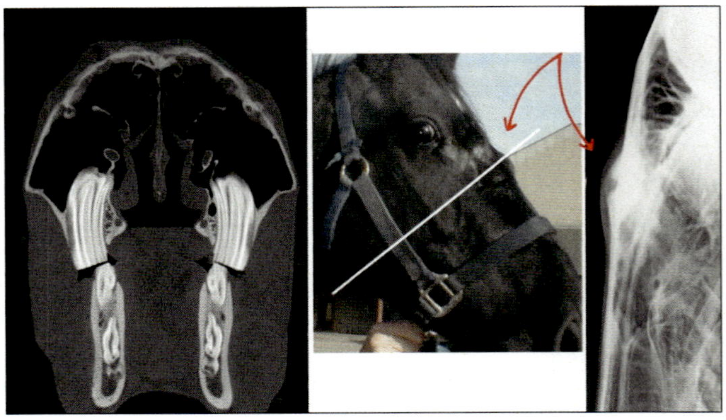

Suture Exostosis: Image on left is the Computed Tomographic (CT) image in a transverse (cross) section of a horse's skull. The top of the image shows clear reaction (roughening) of the naso-frontal suture line with some gas. The central image is the horse with its firm swellings over the front-maxillary region. The white line is approximately where the CT section was located. On the right is a radiograph showing suture exostosis. These cases are most likely related to trauma or infection of the suture line. Unmarked image credits Dr Denis Verwilghen, graphics credit Author.

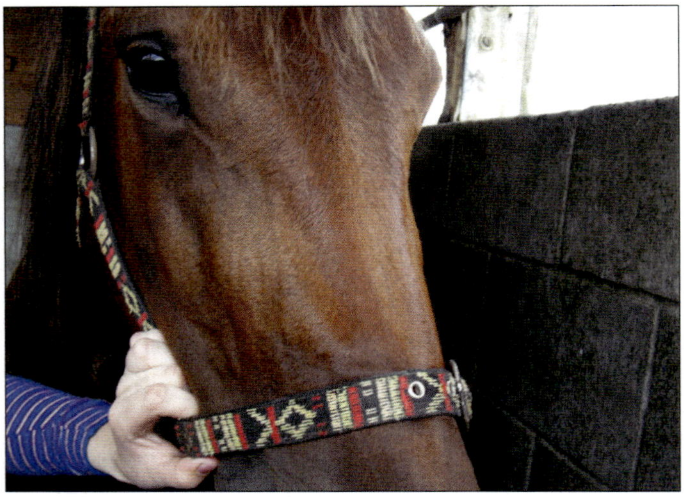

Image of a five-year-old mare with eruption cysts, commonly known as "tooth bumps". The mouth should be checked for retained deciduous, so that the impediment to eruption is resolved before damage occurs to the permanent tooth apices. Image credit Author.

If there is an impediment to eruption which is not resolved, such as overcrowding of the '07s or '08s or a retained deciduous cap, there may be bony swelling of the maxilla or mandible over the pseudocyst, and in extreme cases, it may result in an apical infection with or without draining tracts. See Chapter 6, Developmental and Acquired Conditions, Malocclusions.

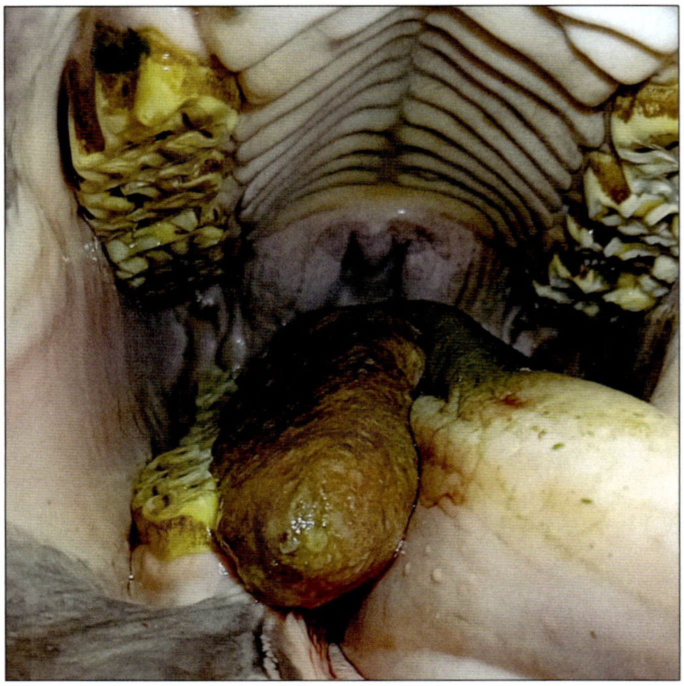

A large mass beside the tongue. Unfortunately, the diagnosis by histological examination of the tissue was not 100% conclusive. Image credit Dr Elke Pollaris.

Potentially more serious tumors

Tumors are characterized by their origin and their behavior, or how they grow. They can be:

- Malignant (cancerous)
- Benign (non-cancerous)
- Invasive (invade locally by infiltrating the tissues adjacent to them)
- Proliferative (creating bulges of tissue)

- Ulcerative (destructive, or eroding the surface and forming open ulcers)

Tumors of the head and face are quite rare and difficult to diagnose for the following reasons:

- They are usually not recognized until they are quite far progressed even for the most observant owner, as they tend to be out of sight.
- Since they have been there for so long, they tend to have significant infection or granulation already, which changes their appearance, both grossly (to the naked eye) and histologically (under a microscope).
- Grossly, they can be similar to other benign and malignant conditions and require histological examination of the tissue.
- Even if one has histological samples, their appearance on slides is not necessarily consistent with the type of tumor they truly are.
- The rarity of these tumors, combined with the variation in their appearance and classification under the microscope make it difficult for the pathologist viewing the slides to give definitive diagnoses, especially because they see them so rarely.

What does this all mean?

Their rarity, meaning lack of comparative studies to use in diagnosis, combined with often-delayed detection make it difficult to give a prognosis (expected outcome) in many of these cases, whether or not the tumors are treated. You will need your veterinarian and a good pathology lab to try to solve these cases.

What will I see?

There may be no obvious signs, or you may see oral bleeding, an abnormal mass on the head or inside the mouth, weight loss, or difficulty eating or chewing. You may also note changes in other adjacent organs such as the respiratory tract (nasal discharge) or nervous system (your horse may self-injure from rubbing itself, sometimes all the way through the skin because nerve damage from the mass has caused a loss or alteration of sensation to that area of skin—sometimes itchiness.)

Call your veterinarian right away!

They may:

- Perform a thorough physical examination to evaluate the nature and extent of the lesion and to see if any gross lesions (lumps or erosions) are palpable anywhere and check the larger lymph nodes for evidence of metastases (masses due to the spreading of the cells of a tumor).
- Take note of the structures included in the area affected by the tumor, or area of infection around it.
- Biopsy (take a tissue sample) for submission to a veterinary diagnostic lab. As these are weird tumors, it may be helpful to discuss the case with the pathologists first.
- Perform bloodwork. While bloodwork may only rarely show which specific tumors are present, it can reveal patterns which may help in the diagnosis, although tumors of the head and neck rarely affect distant organ systems.
- Use diagnostic equipment. Depending upon the structures involved, your vet may also take radiographs and/or use endoscopy, oroscopy, sinoscopy, ultrasound, CT, MRI, or nuclear scintigraphy.

Types of oral tumors

There are two main types of oral tumors:

1. Tumors of dental origin, which include
    - Odontogenic tumors (tumors of tooth tissue origin)
    - Osteogenic tumors (tumors of bone origin)
    - Soft tissue tumors (tumors of soft tissue)
2. Tumors of non-oral tissues in the oral cavity, which are rare.

Odontogenic Tumors

These are rare in all species. The most common or significant ones are:

Ameloblastoma: Usually found in the mandible in older horse and occasionally in young foals. They usually appear as a swelling of the affected side of the jaw. Due to their usually late detection and expansive nature, the prognosis is usually guarded (a poor prognosis).

Cementoma: usually found in the apical region of a developing tooth. Cementomas are accumulations of excessive amounts of cementum into a large lump of hard tissue at the apex of the tooth. They result from dental impaction, tooth fracture, periodontal disease, and supernumerary teeth. Secondary changes like infection make this hard to differentiate from a standard apical infection. Extraction of the tooth affected by the cementoma is curative of the condition, but these teeth may be difficult to extract. The good news is that this is a benign tumor and, as said before, extraction cures the condition.

Complex/Compound Odontomas: Appear outwardly as firm, painful swellings between the eyes and the top of the nostrils (over the roots of the maxillary cheek teeth) in very young or very old horses. The prognosis is reasonable, with surgical treatment, though it may require several surgeries to resolve the odontoma.

Cysts and Pseudocysts

Temporal teratoma, radicular cysts, and bone cysts.

Osteogenic Tumors

Osteoma: Benign, dense bony proliferation usually occurring on the mandible. The etiology is unknown, but may be due to trauma, infection, or of embryological origin. It occurs at all ages and is slow growing. Surgical excision is curable if no damage occurs to adjacent structures. Does not metastasize.

Osteosarcoma: Very rare in horses, but usually seen as a hot, painful swelling on the mandible. This is highly malignant. Radiation therapy is often only hope of success. If it is slow growing, may be okay for a while, but prognosis is guarded.

Tumors of Soft Tissue

Squamous Cell Carcinoma (SCC): Malignant tumor of soft tissue which may occur in the mouth, around the eyes or nose, or on/in other skin. It is destructive, ulcerative, and spreads widely into the local tissue, though metastasis is rare. You may smell a foul odor from your horse's mouth. Treatment options include surgical excision for small lesions (but high recurrence), irradiation or injection/application of anti-cancer drugs. Since it is locally invasive but slow to metastasize, survival for some time may be expected. However, if it has advanced to the point where the horse doesn't want to eat, has loosening teeth, has facial distortion, or breathing obstruction, the prognosis is poor.

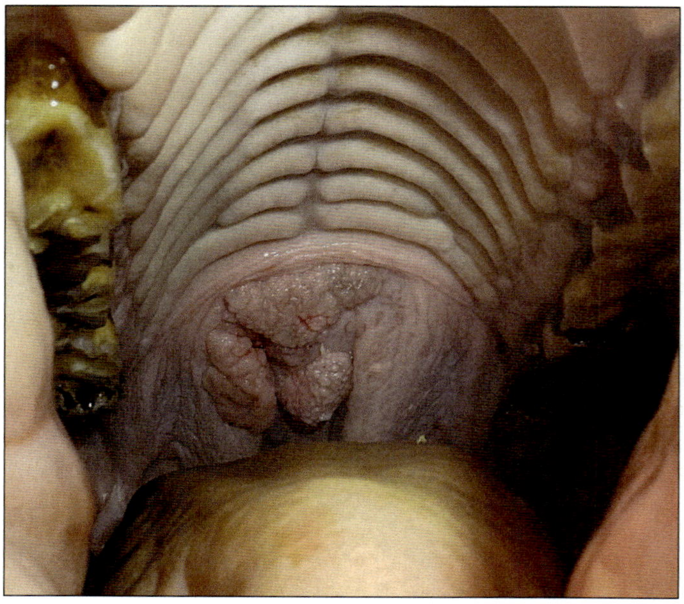

Squamous cell carcinoma of the soft palate. Image credit Dr Elke Pollaris.

Melanoma: Solitary round dark masses, tending to be found on the lips (and perineal area) of horses, especially grays. They tend to be benign, but some are aggressive. Biopsy gives a firm diagnosis and an idea of how fast they are growing, and if they are metastasizing. Prognosis is usually favorable, but occasionally they are aggressive and cause secondary effects.

Myxomatous Tumors of the Jaw: A rare, very destructive yet proliferative, tumor of maxilla with secondary nasal or sinus occlusion, loose teeth, and alveolar bone infection. Wide tumor margins usually make surgical excision difficult to impossible. This group of tumors is unpredictable. Some are slow growing while others are very aggressive.

Oral Hemangiosarcoma: A malignant solid tumor of older horses. More than one lesion doesn't necessarily mean it's metastatic. Excision is difficult but may be effective.

Salivary Adenocarcinoma: An uncommon tumor of the parotid or mandibular salivary glands in horses between seven and eighteen years old. Usually only see enlargement of gland on one side of horse, which is uncomfortable, but not painful to touch. Excision is possible, but normally it's not diagnosed before it spreads. Many of these tumors metastasize to the lungs.

Tumor-like lesions of soft tissue

Abscess: Abscesses can occur anywhere, due to infection, which may contain a foreign body (like a grass awn or a piece of stick or metal). Your vet will help you with this.

Sarcoid: This poorly understood mass may show up as nodules (lumps), ulcerations, or verrucae (spiky protrusions jammed together) in the commissures of the mouth, cheeks, and skin around the mouth or elsewhere on the body. If you're going to treat them, it is best to treat early with your vet's choice of treatment. If they are flat and out of the way they are best left alone, as they become reactive when you annoy them. Prognosis is guarded if they are in a bad location due to tack, harness, or movement, or if they don't respond to therapy.

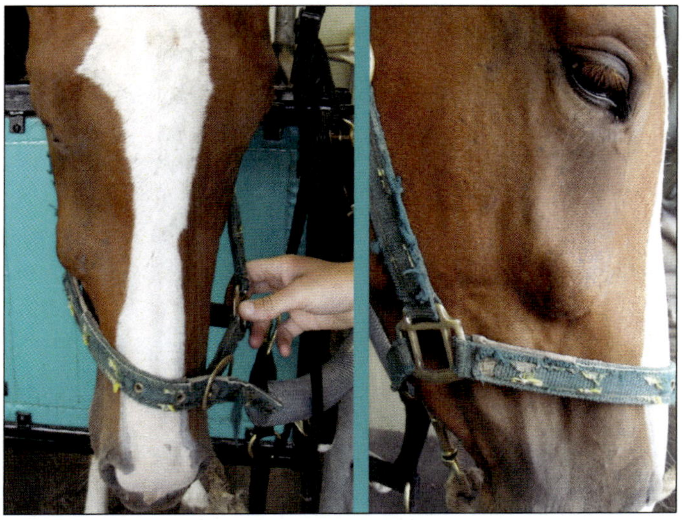

Ossifying fibroma in a young horse. Image credit Author.

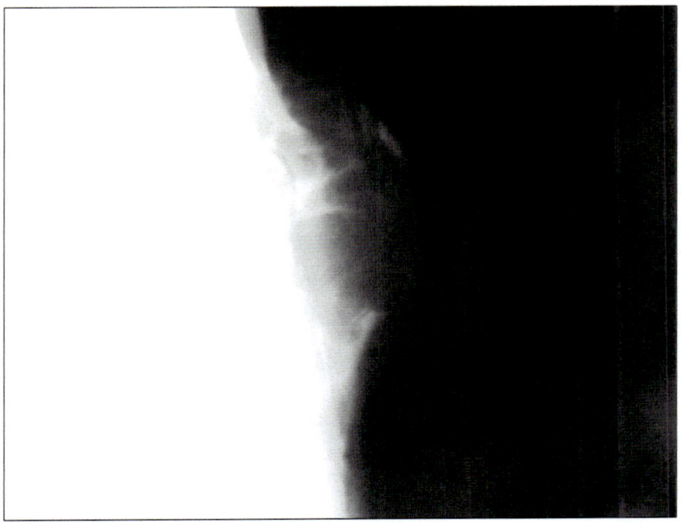

Radiograph of the above horse with ossifying fibroma. Image credit Author.

Oral Papilloma: Usually seen in young horses, though it also occurs in immunosuppressed older horses (e.g. PPID). May appear as multiple or single discrete or coalesced, verrucose, gray-pink papules on the ***mucosa*** of the mouth, which usually don't ulcerate. They usually resolve spontaneously, but can be treated with surgery for individual lesions, autologous vaccines, or topical therapy. Ask your vet!

Epulis: A benign thickening of the gingiva at the gingival/tooth margins, usually secondary to long-term inflammation, such as from calculus accumulation. Removal of the cause (removal of the calculus or damaged dental/ soft tissue) is usually curative.

Ossifying Fibroma: Normally seen in equids less than one year old, this usually shows up as a firm mass on one side of the rostral mandible. It may cause a gross distortion of the lips and associated teeth. Excision is usually curative as long as all of abnormal tissue is removed, but regrowth is common. Irradiation after excision is best. See images on the following page.

Gingival hyperplasia: proliferation of the gingival mucosa due to irritation from pasture and forage, chemicals, or infection under the gingiva (such as with EOTRH). The primary cause must be found and eliminated. It mimics several other more severe tumors.

Abnormalities of Jaw and Teeth Resembling Neoplasms

Bone Cysts: Bony swellings of the jaw consisting of cystic lesions which may affect chewing. Odontogenic bone cysts are noninflammatory, while radicular bone cysts occur adjacent to tooth roots and are reactive and associated with inflammatory disease. Removal of the cyst and its lining may be curative. If associated with apical infection, that must be addressed as well.

Epidermal Inclusion Cyst: A cyst formed between the skin and the mucosal lining of the nostrils which contains a viscous, keratin containing substance inside a cyst lining. It is not neoplastic and is curable by surgical removal of the cyst, especially the entire cyst lining.

Fibrous Dysplasia: A non-neoplastic smooth bone deformity with a loss of bone structure which is replaced with a form of fibrous-bony matrix.

Sialolith: A concretion of calcium and other minerals within the salivary duct or gland, often around a nidus of infection such as a grass seed or hay splinter.

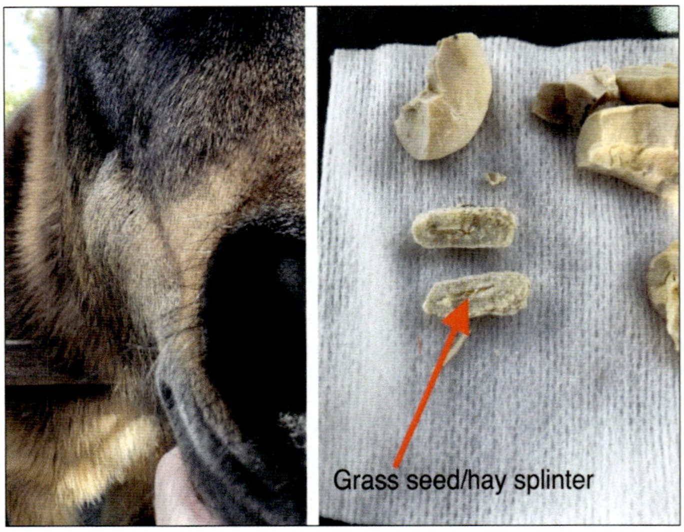

This sialolith had formed in a salivary duct around a grass seed and was broken up by the time it was removed. Individual image credit Dr Kirsten Jackson, Dental Vet, graphic credit Dr Elizabeth Thompson.

Non-Oral Origin Tumors Affecting the Mouth and Jaws

Lymphosarcoma: Lymphosarcoma appears in the mouth as poorly defined nodules in or below the ***mucosal*** surface which may or may not ulcerate. If it affects tonsil tissues, lymphosarcoma may affect swallowing. Anemia, lethargy, or weight loss may indicate systemic involvement.

Pituitary Adenoma (PPID)

As previously discussed, PPID causes secondary disease due to immunosuppression, usually in older horses. The secondary signs of PPID: oral ulceration, non-healing wounds or incisions, anemia, extensive periodontal disease, early shedding of teeth, sinusitis and/or oronasal fistulae. Discovery of any of these pathologies may be the first indication your horse should be checked for PPID. If possible, treat your horse if positive for PPID before further dental or other surgical work.

CHAPTER SEVEN

EOTRH: WHAT THE HECK DOES THAT STAND FOR?

WHILE WE DON'T yet know what causes the excruciating condition called EOTRH, or equine odontoclastic tooth resorption and hypercementosis, we do know it's a painful, progressive condition seen in equids which primarily affects the canine and incisor teeth. While horses over fifteen years are at higher risk of the disease, moderate to severe radiographic (X-ray) changes in the canines and incisors may be seen in horses from around eleven to thirteen years old. This underdiagnosed and frequently misdiagnosed condition existed in the past but has only been named and studied in the past few decades.

Tell Me More About EOTRH

While EOTRH is more common in canines and incisors, it has recently been reported in ***cheek teeth***. A thorough dental exam can hint at a diagnosis of EOTRH by showing many of the clinical signs, but the diagnosis can only be made by dental radiographs, or better said, EOTRH is a "radiographic diagnosis". Dental radiographs also help your ***veterinarian*** make a prognosis (what is likely to happen and when) and suggest an appropriate treatment plan. Histopathology (lab analysis of abnormal ***tissues***) may be indicated to differentiate this from other similar-looking diseases. It is vital that you, as the owner, are aware of this disease, because the ***clinical crown*** (the part of the tooth you can see) and the ***gingiva*** (gums) around the affected teeth may not appear diseased until it is significantly advanced under the gums. It can be hard to be told X-rays are needed when you can't see a problem yourself. And hard to accept that a condition so painful can only be seen on X-rays! Luckily, horses with complete or multiple incisor extractions have been shown to have a favorable prognosis. EOTRH is a reason why every dental exam should be a veterinary dental exam.

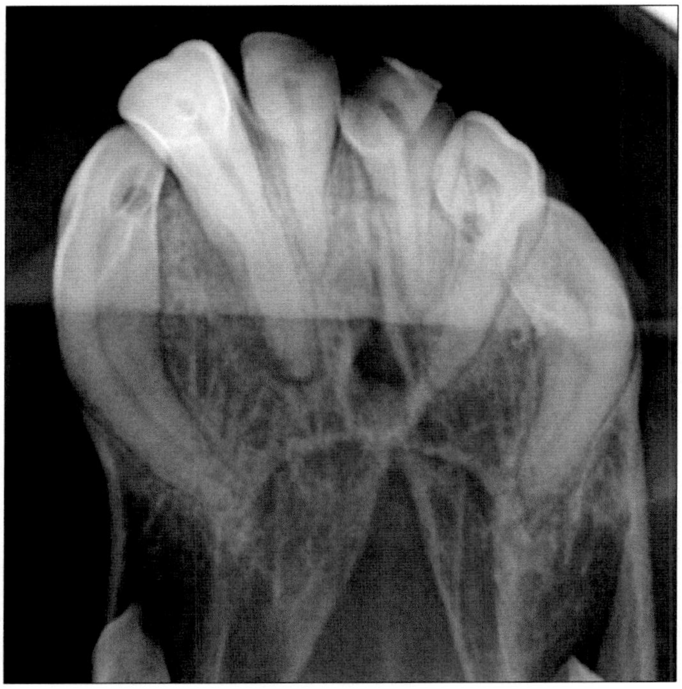

This patient stopped head shaking after extraction of his affected incisors. Image credit Author.

Owners of horses with EOTRH rarely recognize their horse is showing ***oral*** pain until the disease is diagnosed by their veterinarian, though they do mention wide-ranging signs. Their horses may be asymptomatic (showing no signs) or have a wide variety of clinical signs: pain, ***quidding***, behavioral changes, difficulty chewing, halitosis (bad breath), drooling, increasing unwillingness to be haltered or bridled, head shaking, increasing irritability, increasing refusal to bite whole carrots with their incisors (the "carrot test"), periods of poor appetite, and only in advanced cases, weight loss. Owners often attribute subtle, progressive changes in their horse's temperament or attitude to "old age", but after extraction of all affected teeth, owners usually notice signs of improvement. These older, stoic horses may not show obvious signs of pain as we understand it, which unfortunately allows the disease to progress until the damage and pain is so severe, they begin to lose weight due to reluctance to graze. Some horses with EOTRH-caused pain in their incisors are head shakers. The horse on the right stopped head shaking after extraction of his affected incisors.

So, what is EOTRH, really?

EOTRH is a disease of equid teeth which usually begins at around 15 years of age. It causes the inside and the outside of the teeth themselves to be resorbed (dissolved and assimilated into the body), combined with excessive hypercementosis (over-deposition of ***cementum***) and ***periodontal*** disease around the EOTRH-affected teeth. Basically, the disease turns the canine teeth, and then the incisors, into Swiss cheese. Lumpy, gritty Swiss cheese. Not ideal, and extremely painful for the horse.

Since the disease begins in the ***reserve crown*** (the part of the tooth inside the ***alveolus***, where you cannot see), EOTRH is often not picked up until periodontal disease associated with the disease becomes severe.

The disease usually starts with the canine teeth, then progresses from the '03s (the corner incisor) toward the '01s (the central incisors). As mentioned before, EOTRH has been reported in cheek teeth. Whether the relative scarcity of EOTRH in cheek teeth is due to true scarcity or whether it is not being detected remains to be seen. Watch this space.

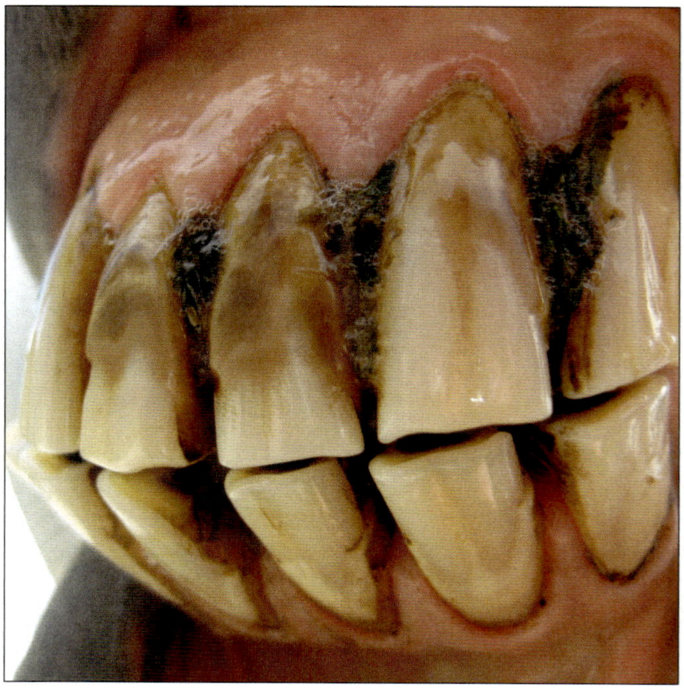

Severe signs of periodontal disease with diastemata and feed impaction. This horse was confirmed to have EOTRH by radiographic diagnosis. Image credit Author.

What causes EOTRH?

Unfortunately, we don't know what causes EOTRH, so we cannot make changes to prevent it yet. Recent histopathologic studies have revealed much about the microscopic changes in the teeth, but we still don't know exactly what causes this disease. A recent veterinary report hypothesized that the hypercementosis portion of the disease is a reparative, rather than a pathologic process, but although veterinarians around the world have been studying this condition for years, we have more work to do to solve this problem.

What, as an owner, can I do?

THE CARROT TEST!

You can monitor likely pain levels by offering whole carrots to your horses on a regular basis, holding them tightly in your hand and letting them bite it off with their incisors. When the pain from their incisors is significant, they tend to stop biting it and try to take it away from you and chew it with their cheek teeth. Since we don't know what causes it, we cannot prevent it, but we *can* look for it in your horses. We can perform thorough clinical exams every year at least, looking for any visible signs of the disease, and begin to monitor for radiographic signs of the disease in your horse's canines (if they have them) and their incisors by taking X-rays, starting when your horse is around thirteen years of age, or earlier if you see any of the signs in the figure below:

Possible sign of dental pain	Defined
quidding	dropping wads of hay into the paddock or feed bowl
attitude changes	behavioral changes such as increased grumpiness or irritability
abnormal mastication	difficulty chewing, or chewing strangely
halitosis	bad breath
hypersalivation	drooling
head shaking	shaking head when free or when bitted
inappetance	loss of appetite
fussy about bridling	unwillingness to be haltered or bridled
weight loss	loss of body weight, usually only seen with severe dental problems
positive "carrot test"	unwillingness to bite a carrot in half with its INCISORS. Horse will often suck the carrot in and grind it with its cheek teeth. This is a positive test.

Signs you may see in your horse with incisor pain. Image credit Author.

How is EOTRH diagnosed?

The outward clinical signs of early EOTRH are subtle and your vet will need to do a proper examination with at minimum: sedation, a full mouth speculum, light, water flushing, a mirror or oroscope, and radiographs. Your EOTRH-affected horse may seem to wake up when the speculum is placed into their mouth or when the mouth is opened. This may mean incisor pain. Any ***calculus*** or feed accumulation on or between the teeth can hide areas of tooth resorption, so they must be removed, and the underlying structures checked. You may see areas of discolored tooth, or an area of resorption, which may be surrounded by dark pink, bubbly granulation tissue. As the disease becomes more severe, horses may have difficulty eating, and their lymph nodes may enlarge. However, EOTRH requires radiographs for a definitive diagnosis.

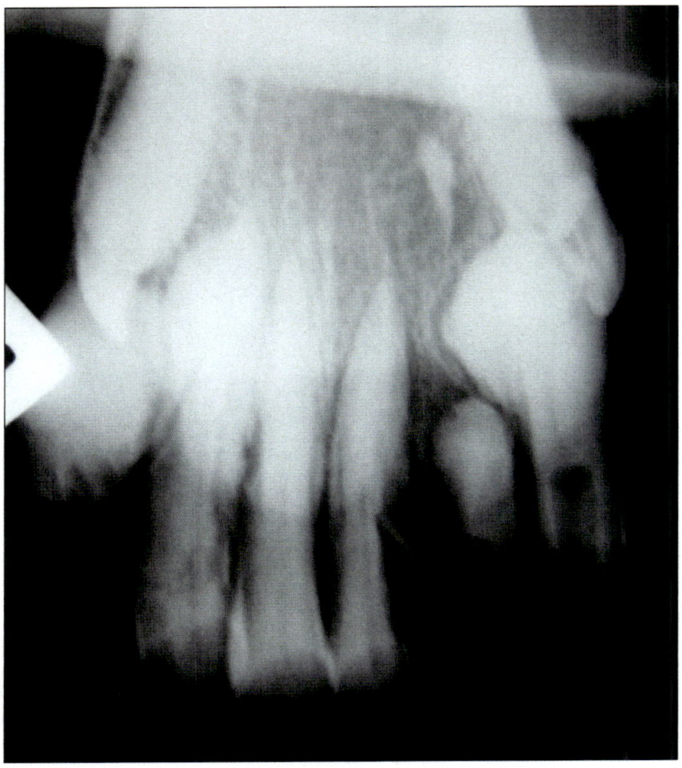

Radiographs are required for a definitive diagnosis of EOTRH, and to determine how best to approach therapy. Image credit Author.

What does EOTRH look like in affected incisor and canine teeth?

In your horse's mouth, EOTRH-affected canines and incisors may show several signs. The disease usually begins in the canines and progresses ***mesially***, toward the ***midline***.

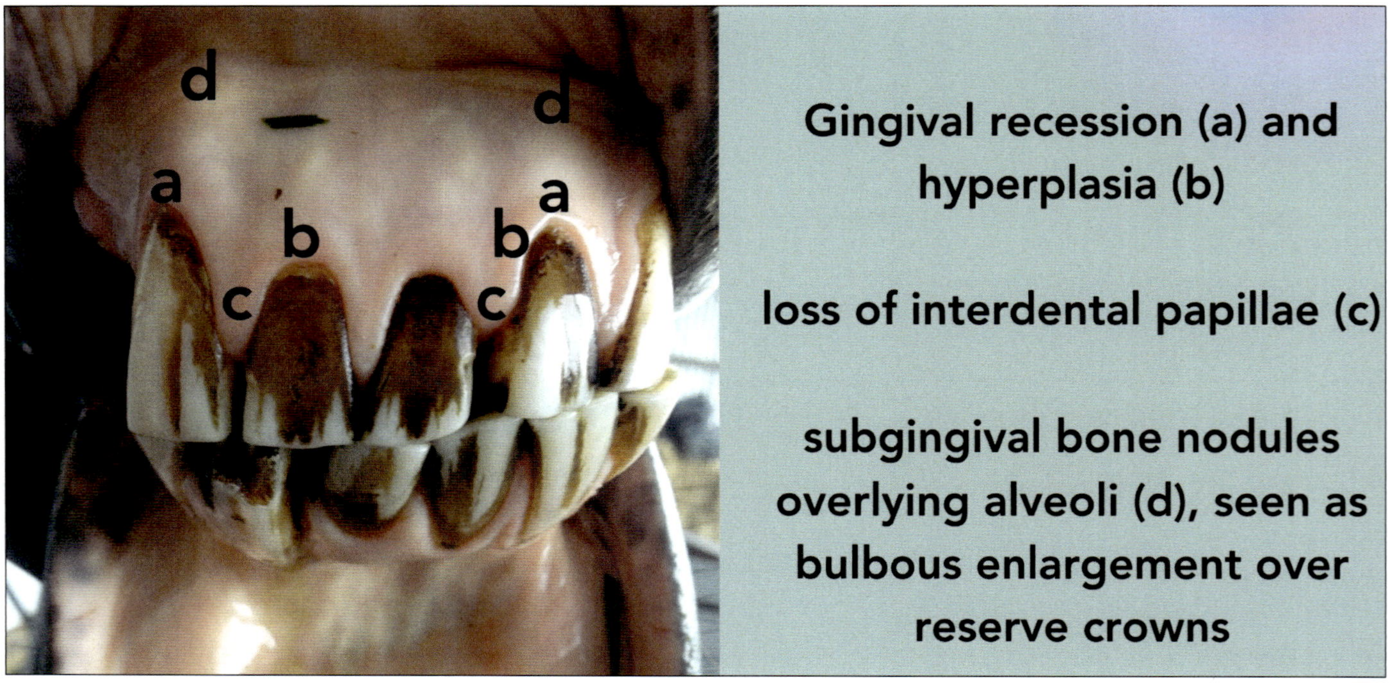

Some EOTRH clinical signs labelled on image. Unlabeled mage credit Dr Marieke van den Enden, graphic credit Author.

Letters in parenthesis below refer to the above image. Your vet may note:

- pain on tooth manipulation or probing.
- either gingival recession (shrinking away) (a) and/or hyperplasia (bulging) (b) where the gingiva meets the teeth.
- loss of the interdental papilla (c), which appears as receding gingiva, where it should rise up between the teeth.
- prominent reserve crowns (d), appear as hill-like swelling or lumpiness of the unerupted portions of the incisors beneath the gingiva due to hypercementosis.
- severe inflammation of the gingiva (gingivitis, or inflamed, red gums), periodontal disease.
- draining tracts (gingival fistulae), which appear as small red dots, often purulent, over the reserve crowns.
- bulbous enlargement of teeth, seen just above in the draining tract image.
- pulp exposure or pulp horn defects, seen as holes in the tooth over the pulps
- tooth fracture due to weakening of the tooth from resorptive disease.
- tooth mobility (loose tooth).
- tooth loss.

If any of these signs are present, especially in your middle-aged or older equid, it may be time to talk with your veterinarian about radiographing its mouth. X-rays will show you the ***pathology*** behind the signs listed above!

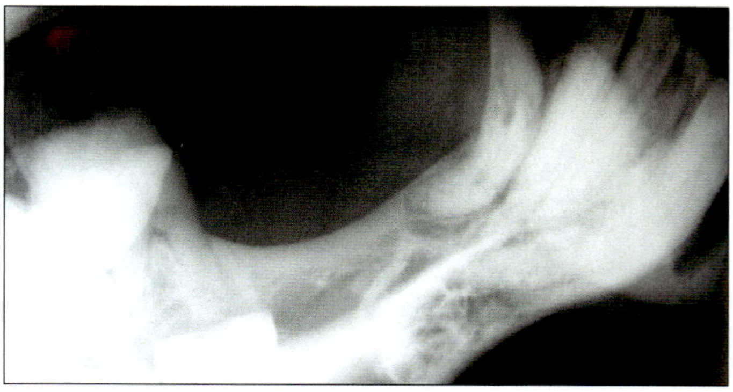

The canines on this horse were extremely painful when they were touched or gently wriggled. Image credit Author.

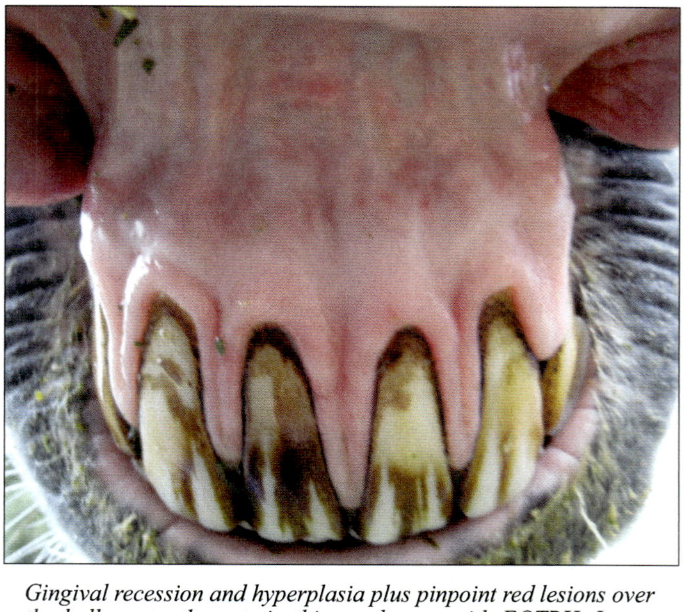

Gingival recession and hyperplasia plus pinpoint red lesions over the bulbous tooth roots in this aged mare with EOTRH. Image credit Author.

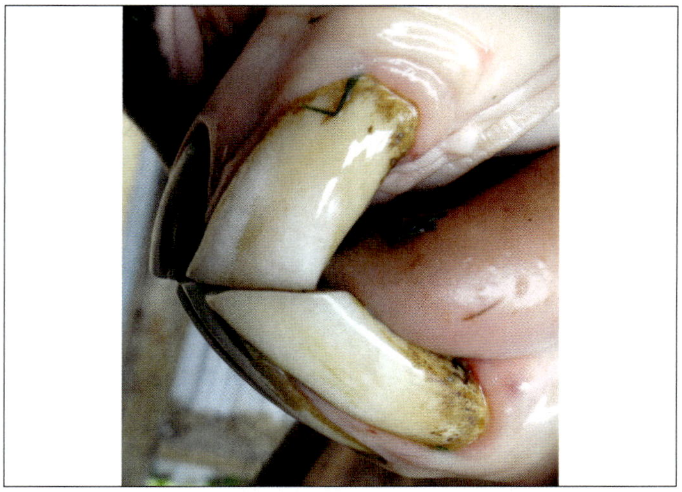

Gingival recession and inflammation. Image credit Dr Marieke van den Enden.

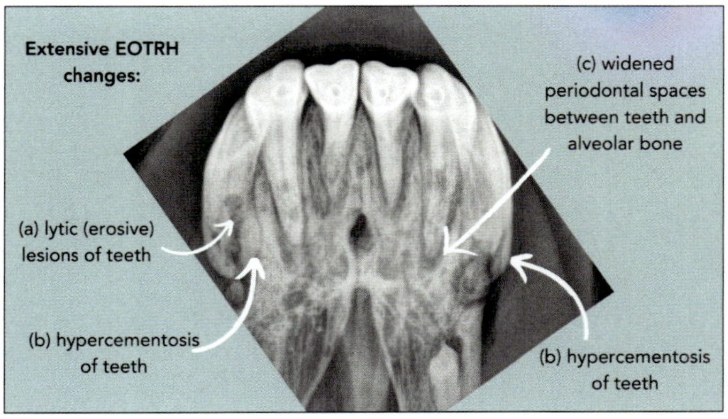

Combined resorption and hypercementosis. Image credit (unmarked image) to Marieke van den Enden, graphic credit Author.

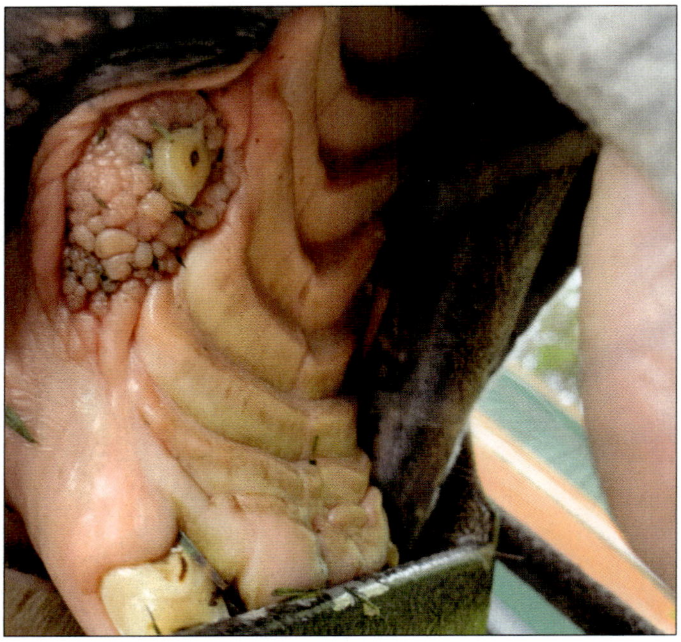

EOTRH horse exhibiting longstanding severe periodontal disease with gingival hyperplasia around this 204. This horse resented even a padded speculum. Image credit Author.

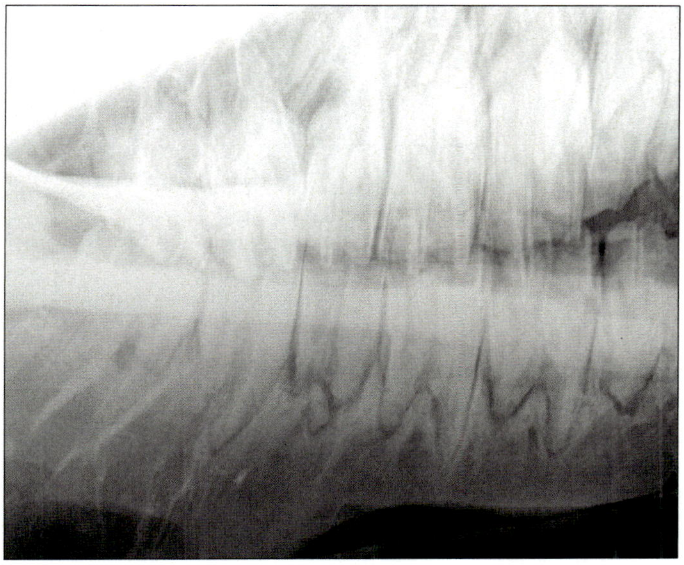

EOTRH patient with severe periodontal disease throughout mouth. He was likely a PPID sufferer, which could explain the extreme degree of changes on radiographs. Image credit Author.

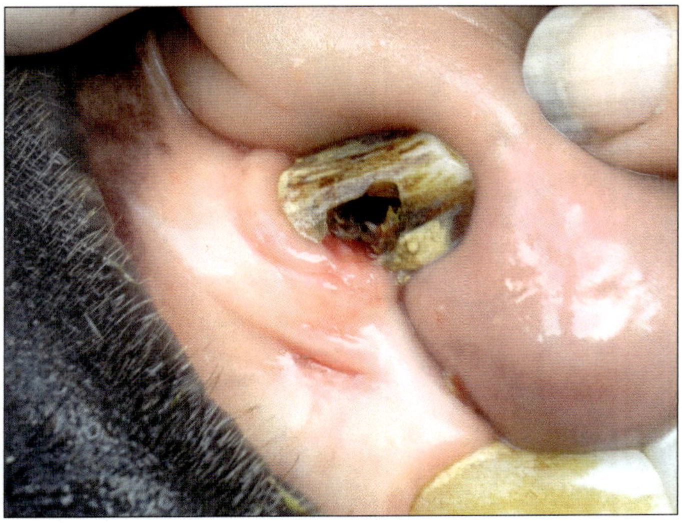

Periodontal disease around affected canine 404. Image credit Dr Marieke van den Enden.

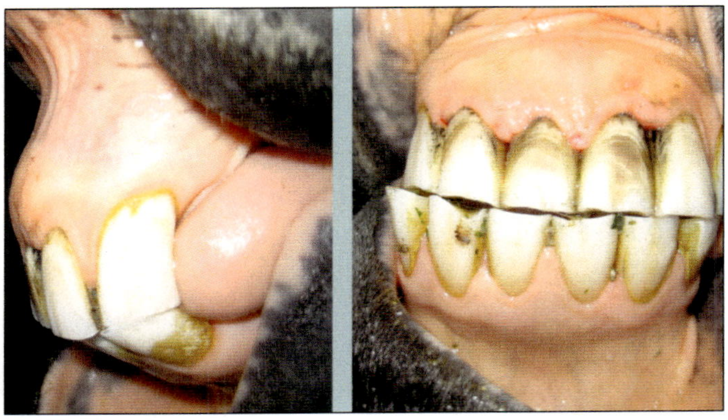

Mare with EOTRH displaying gingival recession and hyperplasia and bulbous enlargement over reserve crowns. Image credit Author.

How does EOTRH appear in affected cheek teeth?

Clinical signs of EOTRH in cheek teeth may also include areas of gingivitis, periodontal disease, tooth fractures, hypercementosis, draining tracts, pulp horn defects, tooth fracture, or mobility.

EOTRH in cheek teeth has been rarely reported, but it may be underdiagnosed because we haven't really been looking. Examination of each ***cheek tooth*** and the surrounding gingiva using an intraoral mirror or oral endoscopy may indicate radiographs are needed to assess your horse for this disease.

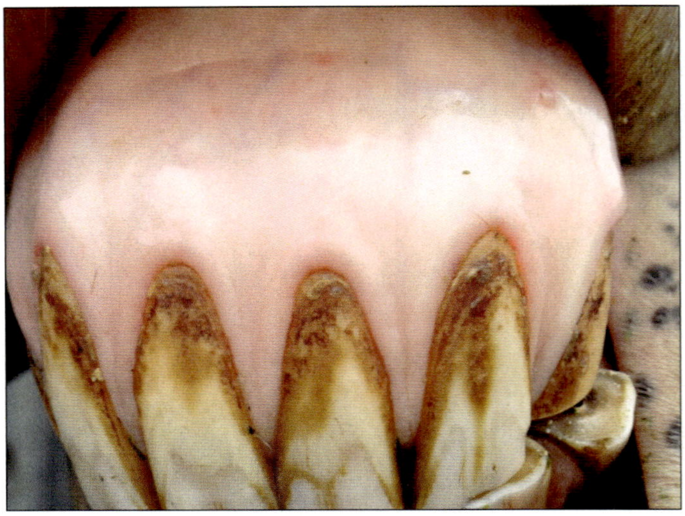

EOTRH-affected tooth. Image credit Dr Marieke van den Enden.

Is EOTRH the reason my horse resents a speculum or a bit?

Many horses affected with EOTRH show a significant pain reaction during oral examination with an incisor-contacting speculum, even under deep analgesic sedation. This may be seen as the horse "waking up early" and throwing its head around with the speculum in place. These horses will often not tolerate a speculum touching their incisors, even just seven or eight minutes into their sedation or after repeated re-doses with sedation and analgesics. This occurs whether the speculum is open or closed, and with metal or plastic bite plates. The reaction is worse when the speculum is opened. Repeated doses of heavy analgesics have allowed me three to six minutes of working time per re-dose, after waiting for each dose to take effect before opening or replacing and opening the speculum.

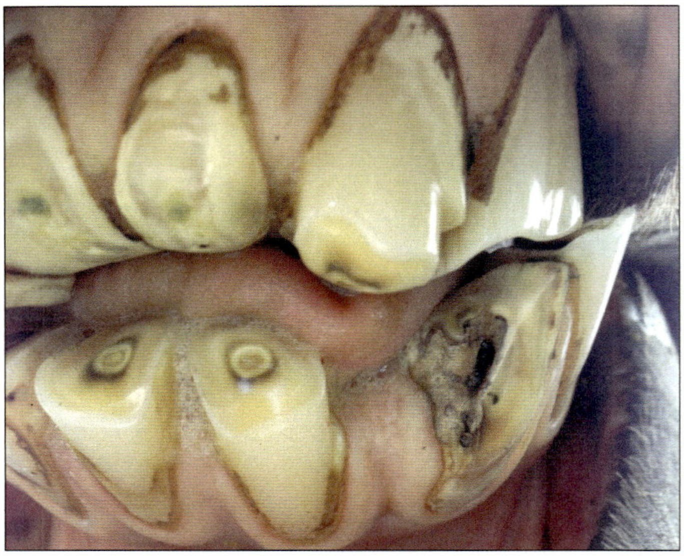

Pulpar exposure and pathologic fracture of incisors. Photo credit Dr Marieke van den Enden.

So, why do we need X-rays?

X-rays are required to assess the subgingival (beneath the gums) portion of the teeth and the ***mandible*** or ***maxilla***. This lets your vet determine the extent of the damage and which teeth are affected. Even cases with mild clinical signs (what you can see from looking at the horse) can have advanced radiographic changes and significant pain. The radiographic signs help us determine the stage of the disease and tells us which teeth need to be extracted now and which may wait until future radiographic and oral exams tell us it's time for extraction.

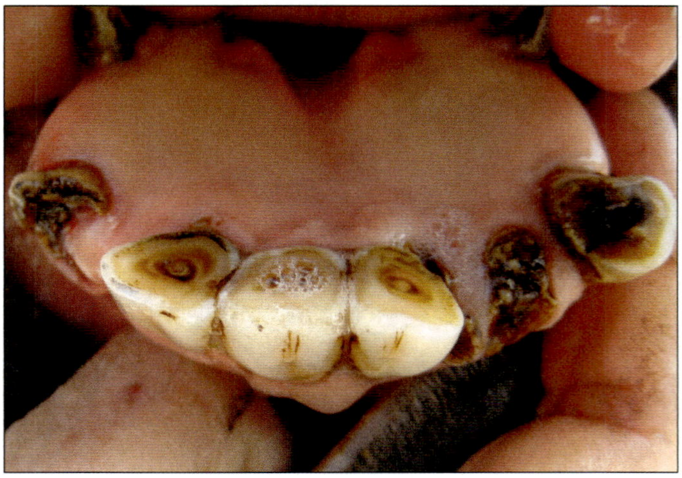

Is this EOTRH or just trauma causing these incisors to have fractured off? Image credit Author.

It's important to follow up these horses with repeat assessments, at least yearly, to ensure your horse's quality of life. These radiographs may be taken in the field with a well-sedated horse (preferably in ***stocks***) and portable radiography equipment. A dental halter or head stand helps for the incisor views, and a small table covered by a foam cushion for the horse to sink its nose into improves the quality of radiographs by stopping movement of both the X-ray receiver and the horse. Multiple radiographs taken at different angles, including obliques, must be taken to clearly visualize pathology in all of the teeth.

What are you looking for on the radiographs?

Radiographic changes on the incisors and canines include erosive resorptive lesions of the cementum and ***enamel*** layers of the reserve crowns, root, and/or surrounding alveolar bone, which over time progresses through to ***dentin***. As the disease progresses, we see hypercementosis of the reserve crown and/ or roots, widening of the ***periodontal ligament***, ***erosion*** or thickening of the alveolar bone near the apex (the root end) of the tooth, expansion of alveolar bone, dental fractures, tooth displacement, or tooth loss. Radiographic signs in EOTRH-affected cheek teeth are similar to those of affected incisors and canines.

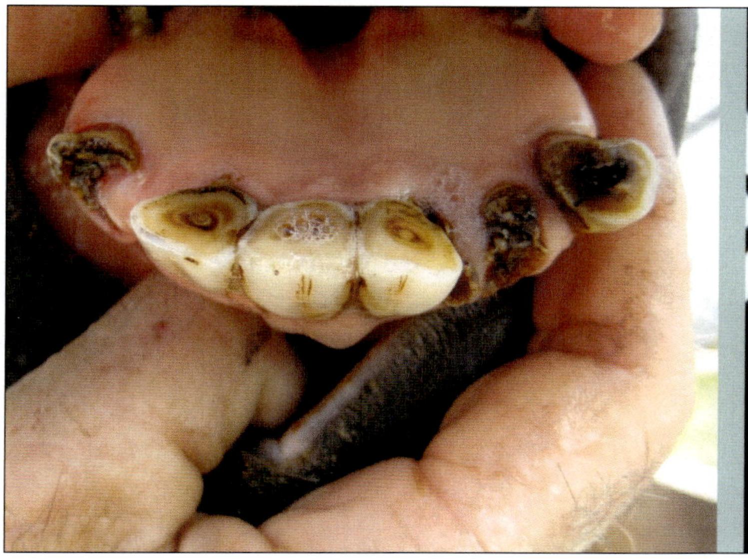

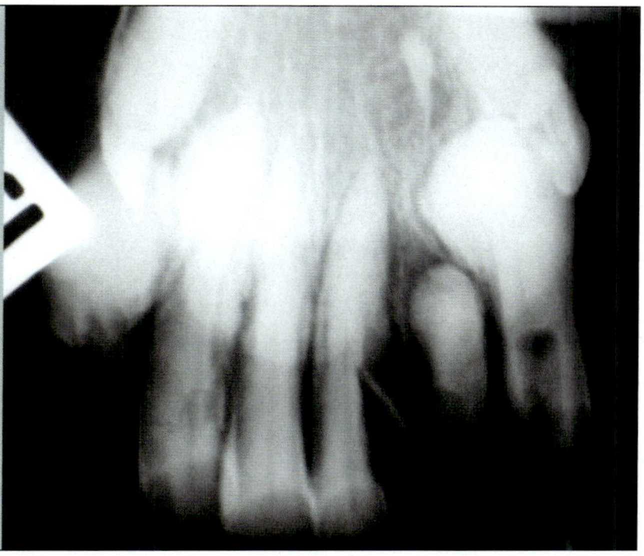

The incisors again from the horse above... it looks even worse on radiographs and confirms his diagnosis of EOTRH. This has likely caused this horse pain for a long time. Image credit Author.

The syndrome is said to have three main manifestations, which is why radiographs from individual patients with EOTRH differ so vastly. These are:

- Predominantly tooth resorption.
- Predominantly hypercementosis.
- Combined resorption and hypercementosis.

The proper names of the radiographic changes of EOTRH?

Some or all these changes may be seen in radiographs of equids suffering from EOTRH:

- lytic resorptive lesions of reserve crown/root/alveolar bone
- lysis of dentin underlying resorptive lesions
- hypercementotic reserve crown and roots
- periodontal ligament widening
- periapical alveolar bone lysis
- alveolar bone expansion
- periapical bone sclerosis
- dental fractures
- tooth displacement, avulsion, and loss.

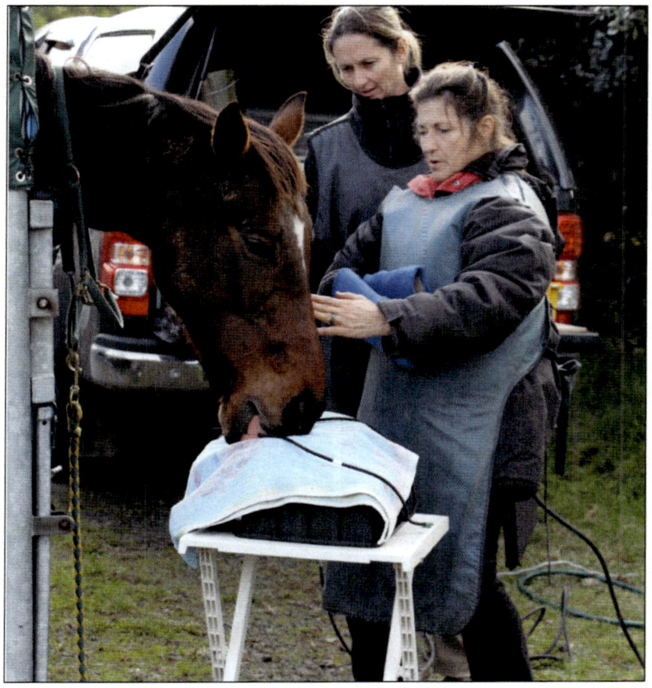

Dr Orla Roan and the Author show an effective setup for taking cheek teeth radiographs. A dental halter or headstand and aluminum speculum bite plates are useful for taking incisor views. Image credit Matthew Mole.

What do I really need to know if my horse has EOTRH?

You need to know the only currently proven treatment of moderate to severe EOTRH is extraction of affected teeth. The prognosis is good for horses with multiple-tooth or full mouth extractions. Choosing not to extract painful EOTRH-affected horses is detrimental to the health and welfare of the horse. Regardless of the type of disease noted in a patient, progression of the disease results in increased mobility and often fracture of teeth. Incisors and canines, from one to multiple, may be extracted with sedated standing surgery with local ***perineural anesthesia*** (nerve blocks) in stocks. Tetanus coverage, antibiotics, and analgesics will likely be needed at the discretion of your veterinarian, as will be discussed in Chapter 15, Veterinary Specific Procedures: Extraction Considerations. Horses respond ***Diastemata*** were covered in Chapter 6, Developmental and Acquired Conditions to extraction of these teeth and are usually able to eat effectively and happily the day after surgery, using their lips to pull grass and graze. A soft diet for several weeks is recommended. Most horses bounce back soon after surgery and temperament problems and other issues which may have been noted before the surgery tend to improve dramatically. Riding with a bit may be resumed after post-op examination reveals proper healing, usually three to four weeks after extraction.

As I've said, we still don't know what causes the disease, so prevention is a challenge, but gold standard of care should be regular screening radiographs of incisors and cheek teeth of horses over the age of fifteen years to evaluate for resorptive lesions to identify subtle, yet significant, signs of EOTRH before it can progress to the truly painful state of moderate to severe disease. Let's aim to keep horses pain-free in their golden years!

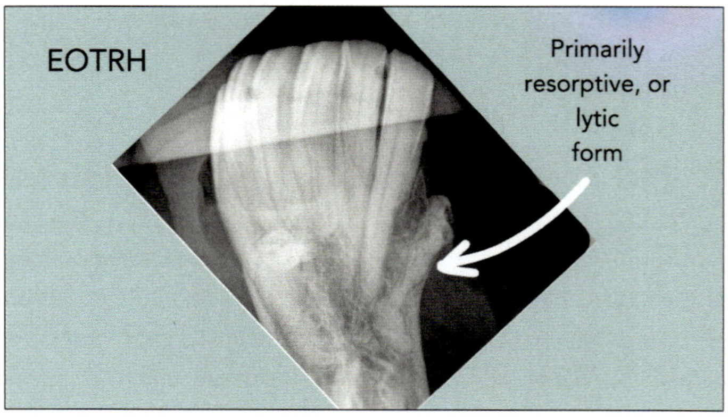

Primarily lytic, resorptive lesions in this canine. Image credit (unmarked image) to Dr Glenn Beeman, graphic credit Author.

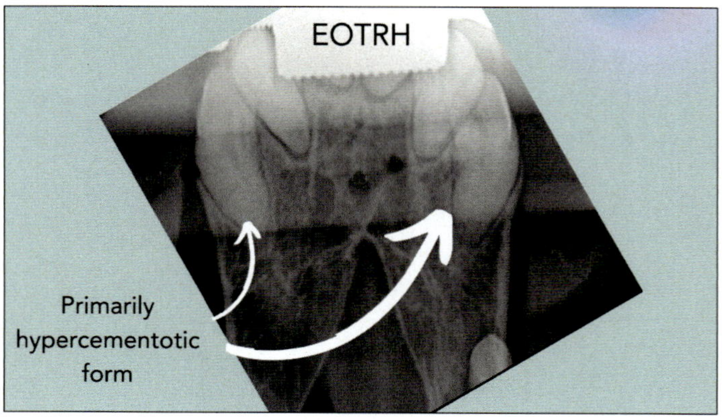

Primarily hypercementotic lesions in these incisors. Image credit Author.

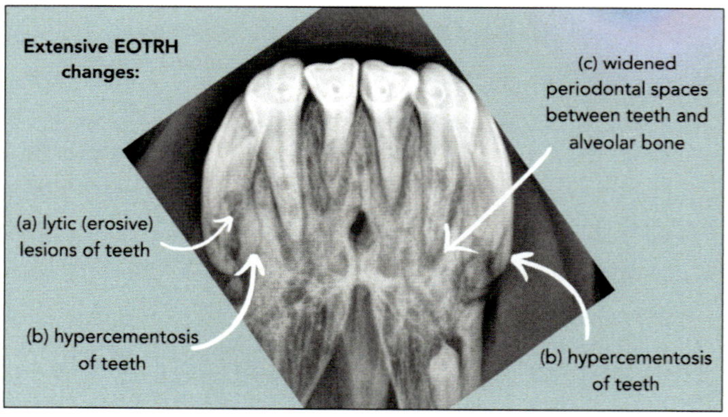

Combined resorption and hypercementosis. Image credit (unmarked image) to Marieke van den Enden, graphic credit Author.

What About Alternative Treatments and Rebalancing?

WITH RESPECT TO EOTRH, some people are claiming that osteopathy, diet, "rebalancing the mouth", etc. can stop progression of the disease. I am more "alternative" than most vets out there, having achieved my IVAS Veterinary Acupuncture certification in 1992 and trained in other modalities since then, but please do not make your horse suffer for any longer than it need to. By the time your horse has been diagnosed with EOTRH, it has likely already progressed to a constantly painful state and it needs veterinary care and probably extraction now, or in the near future. Repeat radiographs will let you monitor which teeth need extracting, and when. Sure, decreasing your horse's stress, supplementing to improve the general health of the horse, etc. may help keep inflammation down, but when your horse's teeth are like a block of gritty Swiss Cheese, filled with abscesses draining purulent material (pus) either into the periodontal space or out through the gingiva, I'd bet he would appreciate some help to make his life less of a hell—and leaving the seriously-affected teeth in place is not going to help his pain levels.

CHAPTER EIGHT

WHAT ARE SECONDARY FORMS OF DENTAL DISEASE?

SECONDARY DENTAL DISEASE is one which occurs secondary to (as a result of) another disease or pathological condition.

How do Equids Get Mucosal Ulceration?

THE SOFT ***TISSUES*** of the mouth may become ulcerated due to many causes. See Chapter 3, Anatomy of the Mouth. The most common dental causes include: ***abrasions*** or ***lacerations*** inside the cheeks and on the tongue result from ***crown elongations*** and ***sharp enamel points*** cutting into the cheeks or tongue when your horse is eating, or anytime it opens its mouth. Other causes include infectious (viral, bacterial, fungal, or parasitic) and non-infectious (nutritional, immune-related, organ failure, or neoplastic) disease.

Dental-related ***mucosal*** ulcers may also be caused by other ***oral*** problems such as loose teeth, displaced teeth, fractured teeth, or loose caps. Most of these ulcers will heal within a matter of days following effective ***odontoplasty*** to remove the sharp enamel points or extraction of the offending tooth or teeth. Other causes of mucosal ulceration such as infections of the ***alveolus*** or ***gingiva*** require treatment of the infection before they can heal.

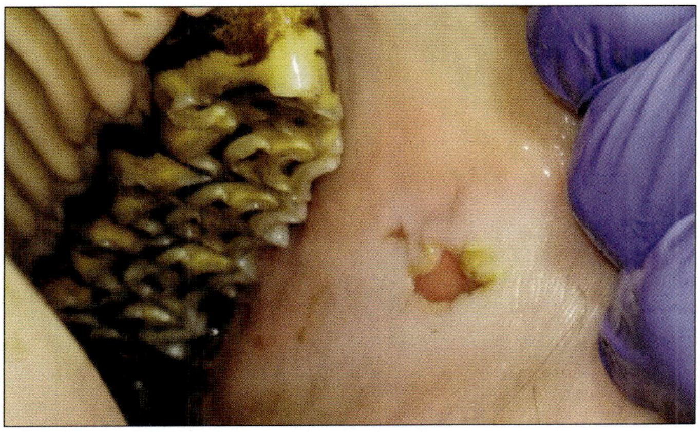

Buccal ulceration adjacent to sharp enamel points of cheek teeth. Image credit Cathie Heald Greenwell.

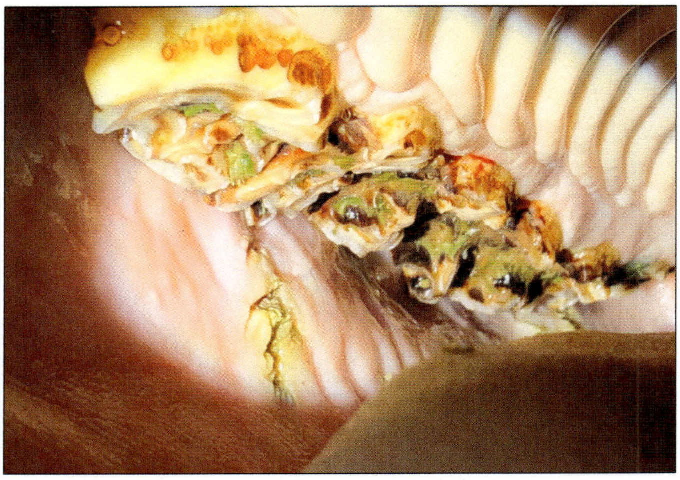

This horse with peripheral caries has extremely sharp enamel points which have caused severe buccal ulceration. Image credit Dr Kirsten Jackson, Dental Vet.

Buccal mucosal ulcers may also form due to trauma, such as a horse sustaining a kick on the face from another horse or colliding with a heavy, solid object. The adjacent buccal mucosa and/or lips may be lacerated from either the source of the injury, from the sharp edges of a tooth inside the mouth, or both. The mandible or ***maxilla*** may also sustain fractures.

The tongue or the mucosa over the ***bars of the mouth*** may become ulcerated by a horse playing with something sharp or holding something like a wire or thin cable in their mouth and then pulling back. They can also fracture their mandible or maxilla this way.

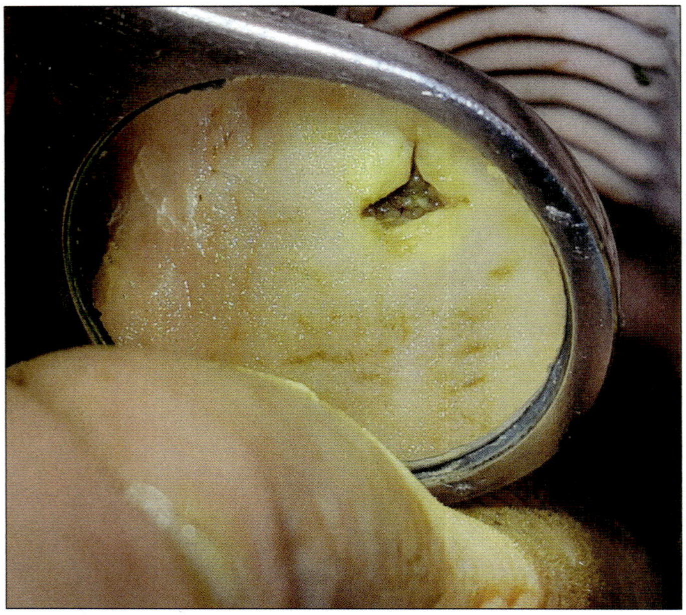

Aged, healing tongue ulceration. Image credit Cathie Heald Greenwell.

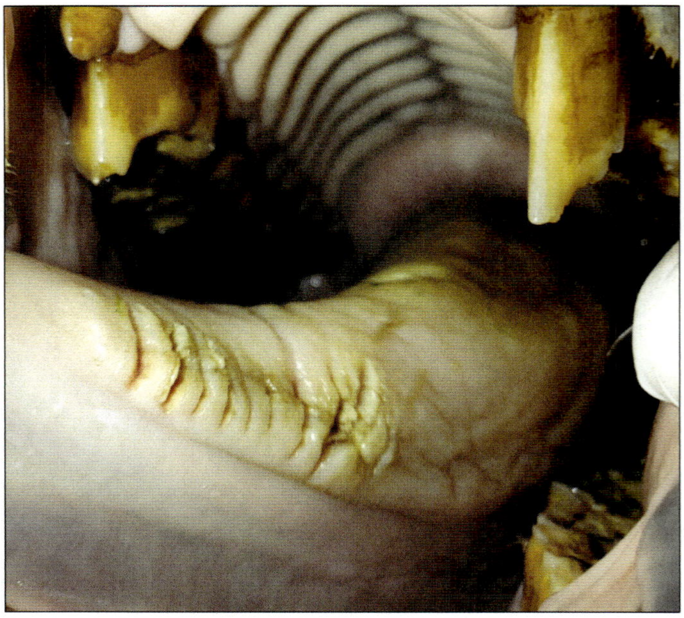

Severe tongue lacerations from sharp 206 hook and sharp enamel points. Image credit Dr Kirsten Jackson, Dental Vet.

The mucosa and musculature of the tongue can also be injured by a "tongue-tie", either placed too tightly, or left in place for too long. Horses have lost their tongues for this reason. One ***veterinarian*** recently reported to me that a horse had its tongue "amputated" when a trainer left the tongue tie in place and turned the horse out. The trainer's answer? He "must have forgot it was on". No photo was available. Even if a tongue laceration heals, the scarring can limit proper function.

Ulceration may also occur as a result of eating something caustic. Improvement of this condition will only occur following elimination of whatever caused the

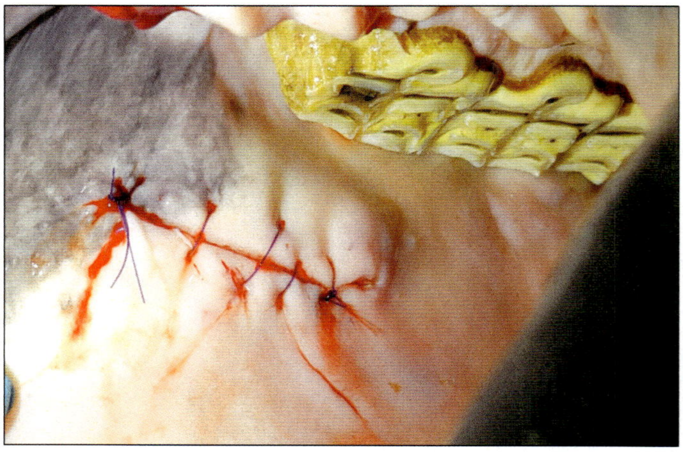

Buccal laceration requiring suturing. Image credit Cathie Heald Greenwell.

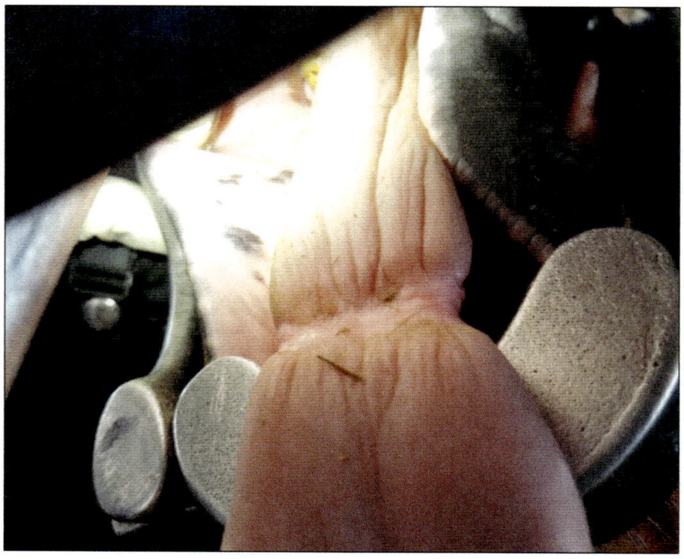

Long-term consequence of damage from a tongue-tie. Image credit Cathie Heald Greenwell.

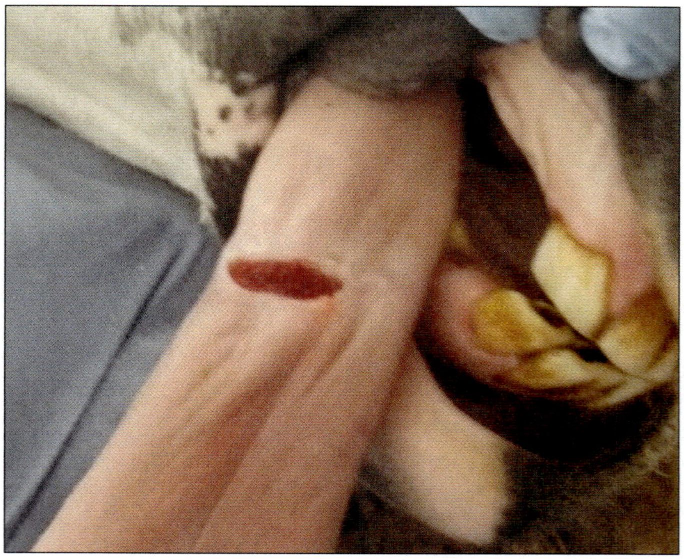

Tongue laceration. Image credit Cathie Heald Greenwell.

ulceration from the horse's environment and specific treatment for the caustic agent. See image to right:

Perhaps the most sinister and insidious (sneaks up on you) of mucosal ulcers are caused by crown elongations into the space where a missing tooth used to reside. These overgrowths, if not unchecked by regular odontoplasty, can erupt past the mucosa to protrude into the bone of the opposing mandible or maxilla, causing severe pain and reluctance to eat. Equids can starve from these elongations and the damage caused by them. The crown elongation to the right could not be reduced all at once without exposing pulps, but even the "safe" amount of reduction allowed this pony to eat again until enough time had passed for the pulp to retreat, after which we could reduce them more. See Chapter 9, Iatrogenic Disease, Iatrogenic Pulp Exposure or Near-Exposure.

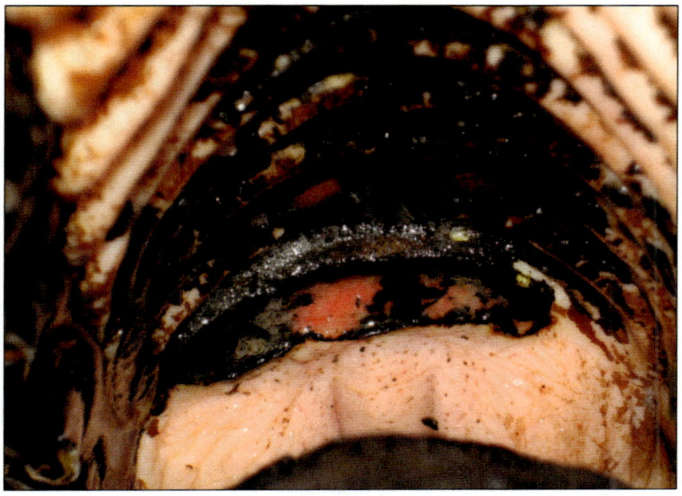

This horse sustained ulcers of the soft palate after grazing freshly "limed" paddocks. Type of lime unknown. Image credit Author.

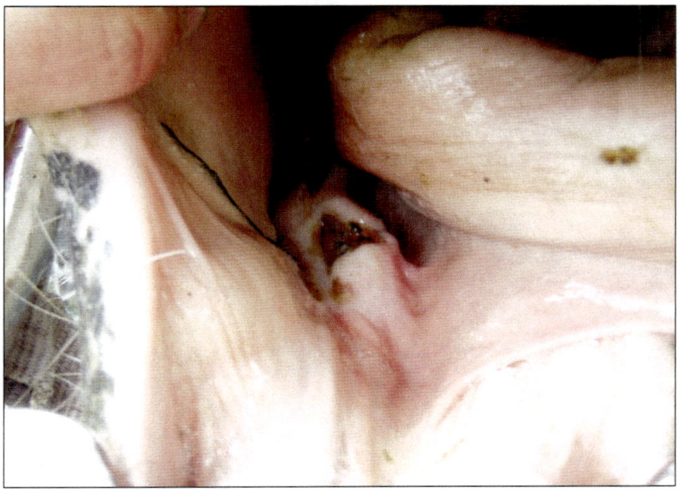

One of the two mandibular ulcers through the mucosa and into the mandibular bone due to impingement of the 106 shown above. Incredibly painful, the pathology in this mouth caused a starvation situation. Image credit Author.

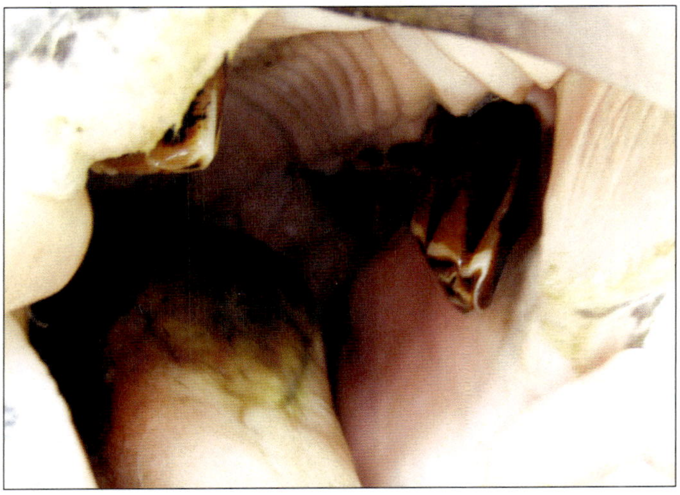

Severe crown elongations of maxillary '06s and mandibular '11s. Image credit Author.

How Do Horses Get Acquired Diastemata?

DIASTEMATA WERE COVERED in Chapter 6, Developmental and Acquired Conditions. Please go there.

Are Wolf Teeth Defined as Dental Disease?

WHILE ***WOLF TEETH*** are not a disease condition per se, their presence or partial extraction can cause problems for you and your horse. Wolf teeth are the small ***vestigial*** teeth usually found just ***mesial*** to the '06s (the first ***cheek tooth***), as described in Chapter 3, Anatomy of the Mouth. See Chapter 3.

What's the problem with wolf teeth?

First, because they are normally small and shallow-rooted, and second, due to their location mesial to the larger premolars and ***molars***, they tend to get hit by the bit with a heavy-handed rider or in an accident. A wolf tooth may fracture or loosen, causing pain to the horse. Have you even known anyone with a fractured (broken) tooth? It hurts all the time. Imagine having to go around an arena or over a cross country course, or even to eat, like that. Horses live with this constantly if they break a tooth, and usually no one knows until a good odontoplasty, which includes a thorough dental exam, is performed, perhaps years down the line.

Some lay dental operators file a wolf tooth to the gingiva. This creates ***pulp exposure***, and has the same painful effect. This tooth needs extraction. See Chapter 9, Iatrogenic Disease. Pulp exposure treatment pertains to wolf teeth as much as to ***incisors***, ***canines***, or cheek teeth. Just because it is smaller does not mean it doesn't cause pain.

For this reason, depending upon the bitting needs of the horse, the actual location, size, and structure of the wolf tooth or teeth, and the horse's intended use must be taken into consideration in deciding whether or not intact wolf teeth should be extracted. Discussions on the needs for extraction may be found in Chapter 15, Veterinary Specific Procedures.

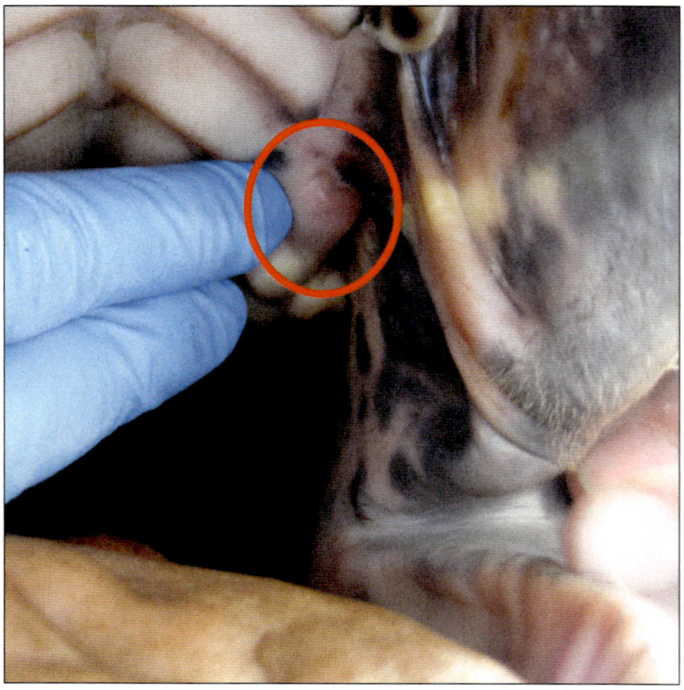

A "blind" or unerupted wolf tooth at the center of the circle. You could see how the mucosa over the tooth has been ulcerated, which must have hurt when was hit with a bit. These need extraction. Image credit Author.

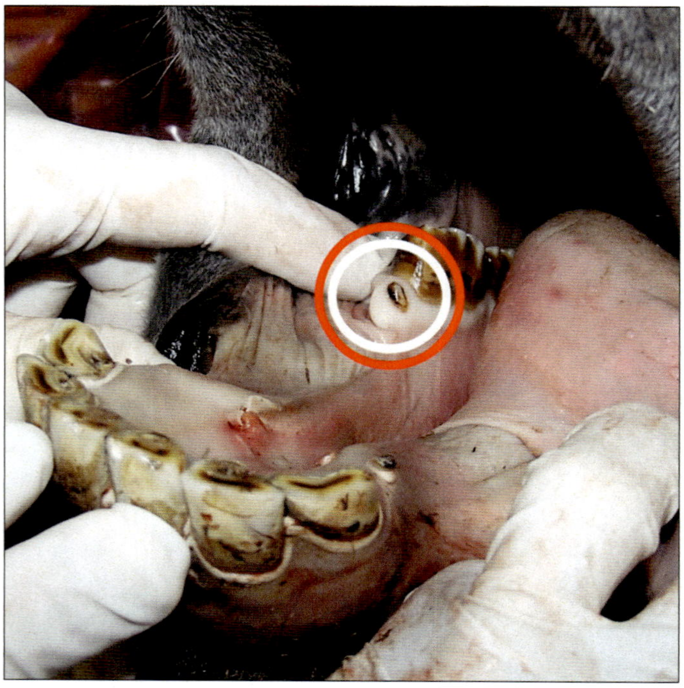

Mandibular (lower) wolf tooth adjacent to the 306 in a cadaver. This tooth may have been broken off or floated to the gumline in the past. Image credit Author.

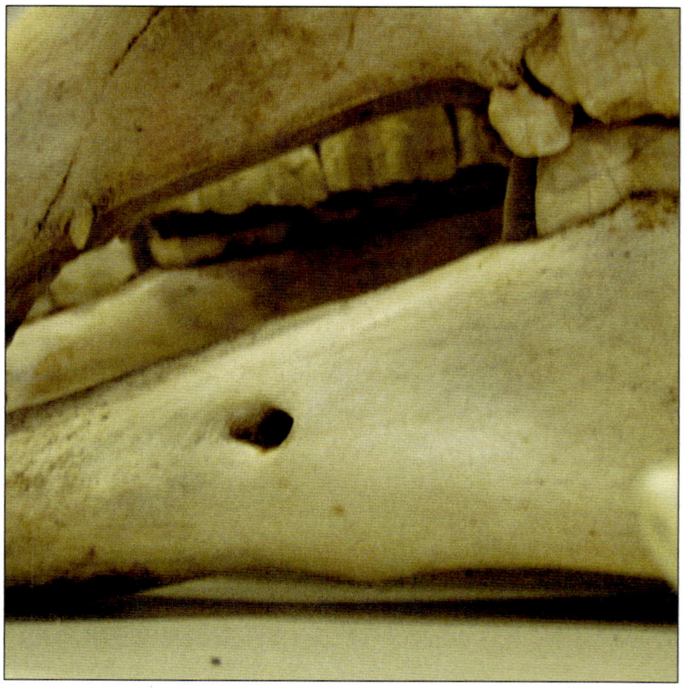

Molarized wolf tooth shown directly mesial to the 206 at the top right of the image. There is also a tiny canine to the top left of the image. Image credit Author.

If a wolf tooth is mesial to the first cheek tooth, but not directly in contact with it, that wolf teeth is at high risk of fracture, as it is not supported by the adjacent cheek tooth.

Unerupted, or "blind", wolf teeth have erupted from the alveolus but still lie under the gingiva. As you might expect, if a bit hits the gingiva over an unerupted wolf tooth, it can cause considerable pain and will likely result in ridden behavioral problems if it is allowed to persist.

Molarized wolf teeth are large, deeply rooted wolf teeth, often with more than one root. They may be quite stable, especially if they are directly apposed (snug against) to the first cheek tooth and may not require extraction.

Fractured wolf teeth may occur if they have been hit with a bit or from chewing an inappropriate object. While these teeth are small, they still have pulps, which contain nerves and are PAINFUL. These teeth need extraction.

The wolf teeth are usually found in the maxilla (105 or 205) but the rarely occurring mandibular wolf teeth (305 or 405) are almost always a problem if a horse will ever wear a bit inits lifetime. They must be removed in a horse which is meant to be bitted because they will cause a horse pain if it bitted... and one can never be too sure where one's horse might end up if the unthinkable happens.

Wolf teeth are often unerupted and these tend to lie flat along the bone, or may point buccally and mesially, amongst other presentations. Any of these can cause problems for bitted horses until they are extracted. Even if you never plan to ride with a bit, at some point your horse may pass on into another person's hands and they could well ride your horse with a bit. Because these unerupted teeth are relatively rare and often hidden from view, these mandibular wolf teeth may be missed by dental practitioners and can cause a horse misery in training issues before they are diagnosed and treated, if they *are* ever located.

Wolf tooth injuries may occur from jerking on the reins, a sign of poor horsemanship, and the wolf teeth may become fractured or loosened, both extremely painful conditions. This can occur even with large, molarized wolf teeth in the worst cases. Please call your vet as soon as anything like this is noted. Every horse presented for extraction deserves proper care with sedation, local ***anesthesia***, and post-operative ***analgesia*** (pain relief) for at least three days, or as advised by your veterinarian.

CHAPTER NINE

IATROGENIC DISEASE? NEVER HEARD OF IT!

IATROGENIC DENTAL DISEASES are those diseases caused by an operator, whether a ***veterinarian***, veterinary surgeon, EdT, or a lay dental operator, which is usually inadvertent (not on purpose), but may occur as a result of something they did while working on an equid.

What is Pulpar Exposure or Near Pulpar Exposure?

EXPOSURE OR NEAR exposure of the pulp may also be termed ***pulpar exposure***. This may occur due to iatrogenic (operator) causes, or accidental injuries. While accidental injuries such as tooth fracture or fractures of the skull involving fracture of a tooth can cause pulpar exposure, iatrogenic injuries are more common, unfortunately.

Iatrogenic injuries may result from:

- Excessive ***odontoplasty*** causing over- reduction of teeth, including overzealous profiling or "bit seating" of the '06s. Even the slightest pinkness over a pulp canal is ***pulp exposure***
- Overheating (hyperthermia) of teeth with insufficient water-cooling of teeth during power odontoplasty
- Cutting of teeth
- Damage from excessive pressure applied to teeth
- Damage from application of certain chemicals during restoration of teeth
- Injury to teeth or immature ***tooth buds*** during surgery to repair skull fractures

Pulp exposure and dentinal bridge formation

Any of the above injuries to the pulp may result in pulpitis, or ***inflammation*** of the pulp. Thankfully, not every pulp exposure or near-pulp exposure causes pulp death and resultant tooth death, because ***hypsodont*** teeth have

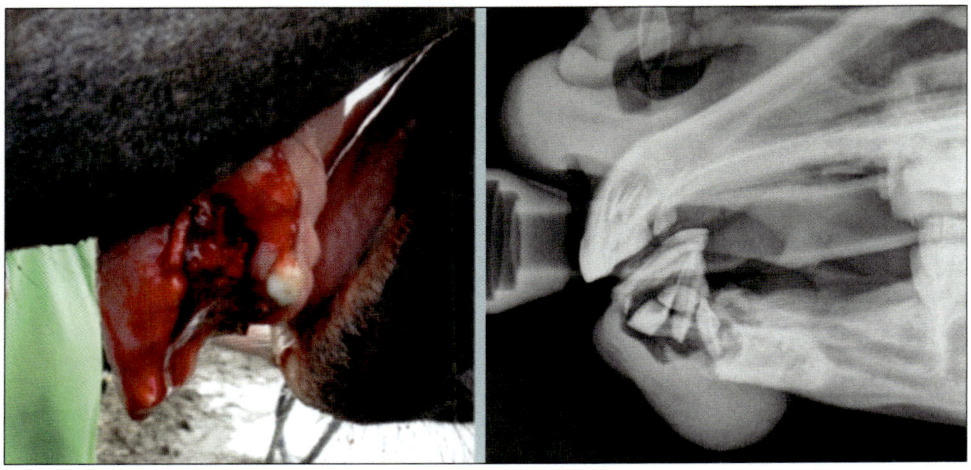

This horse's dental injuries were profound. Image credit Dr Maxwell Hall.

evolved a repair mechanism. This mechanism has evolved over many millions of years for gradual tooth ***erosion***—but unfortunately, not for rapid human-caused pulp exposure.

As horses evolved over the millennia, they became grazers. As grazers, they needed a system which would allow their teeth to repair while undergoing ***attrition***, being ground down against their opposing teeth in the while consuming hard and/or fibrous feeds contaminated by grit. At the same time, horses developed ***prolonged eruption*** of their teeth to balance this attrition.

Now the tricky bit. It's not enough to merely grind teeth against each those in the opposing ***arcade***, keeping a balance. To prevent exposure of the pulps as this attrition occurs, equids have also evolved pulps which can retreat away from the ***occlusal*** surface toward the pulp chamber, which is further into the tooth toward the ***apex***, or root tip, to get away from the insult and try to keep the tooth alive. If attrition of the occlusal (or other) surface of a tooth occurs slowly over time, the pulp is usually able to respond and keep the tooth alive. If attrition or exposure occurs too quickly, the pulp may not succeed in repairing it, and the tooth may die.

So how can a pulp save the day? The process is called ***dentinal*** bridging. Here's how it works: Cells inside a hypsodont tooth pulp possess fine extensions called odontoblast processes, which radiate away from the pulp proper toward the occlusal surface inside thousands of cylindrical ***dentinal tubules***. There are excellent images of these in the online link associated with the first item in the Bibliography, if you want to see them. Insults to the pulp listed above, e.g. sudden exposure to the environment, heat, pressure, vibration, drying, chemical exposure and bacterial infection, cause the odontoblast processes to retreat deeper into the dentinal tubules toward their pulp chamber and begin to form dentinal bridges, or bridges made of reparative dentin. These bridges serve as a blockade between the insulted portion of the tooth and the pulp in an attempt to keep the pulp, and thus tooth, alive. When these insults happen gradually, over months, the tooth can usually respond in time to repair the damage by creating a dentinal bridge.

However, when these insults occur in a shorter time, such as over minutes or seconds, rather than months, the pulp is in danger of becoming overwhelmed with inflammation or infection. It is up to the pulp's immune system to keep infection or inflammation from killing the pulp before a dentinal bridge can be formed. If the immune response is successful, the pulp inflammation may be temporary and the tooth might live. If, however, the pulp exposure is too

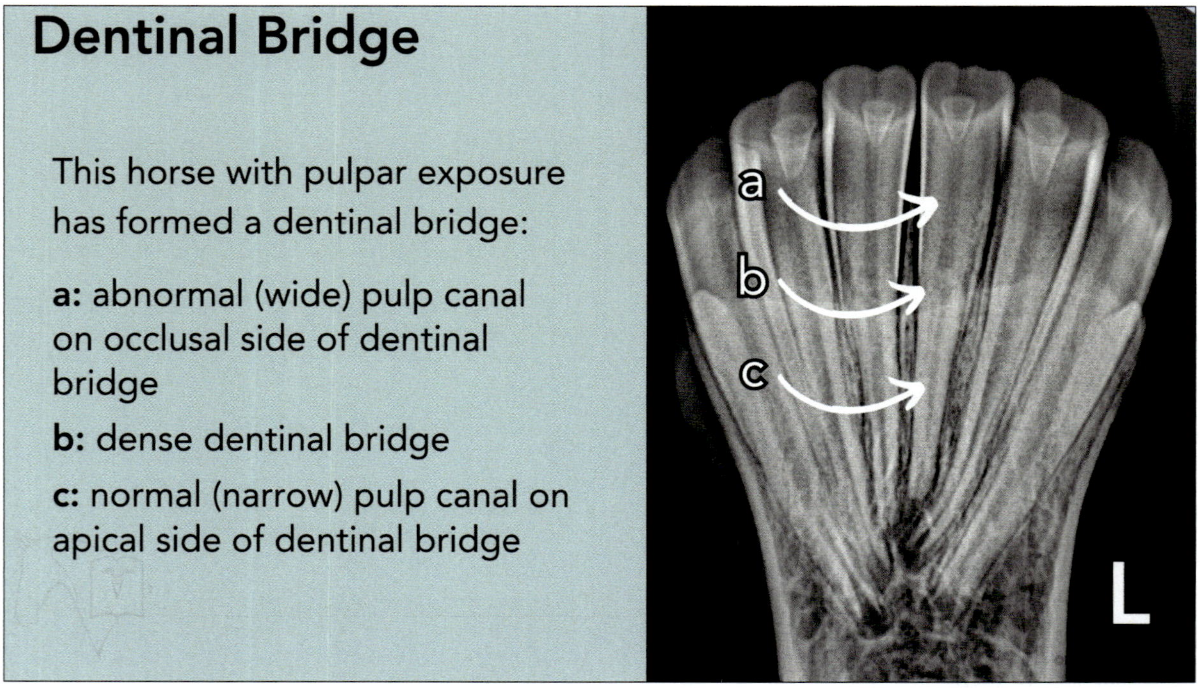

This horse had a pulpar exposure of his 301. Note the overly wide pulp at a) on the occlusal side of the radiodense dentinal bridge at b), which has formed to protect the normal pulp chamber at c), which is apical to the dentinal bridge. Image credit Dr Marieke van den Enden, graphic credit Author.

sudden or the insult too great for the pulp's ability to respond, the exposed pulps begin to bleed and become edematous and inflamed. Bacteria invade, if they did not before, and the resulting pulpitis may cause pulp, and thus tooth, death.

Non-vital pulp exposure

If the pulp is overwhelmed with pulpitis and the pulp dies, the secondary dentine (normally laid down both on the inside walls of the pulp) and the sub-occlusal secondary dentine (***SO2D***: the dentine overlying and protecting the pulp, which should fill in the pulp chamber with age as the pulp recedes), are no longer made. This leaves a wide pulp canal visible on radiographs. As the tooth undergoes attrition, the pulp is exposed. It starts as a pinpoint lesion, then enlarges as attrition progresses, to the width of the pulp canal when the pulp died. The defect now fills with feed material and becomes affected with secondary dentinal ***caries***. This is called a non-vital pulp exposure. This tooth should be treated with endodontic therapy or extraction, as it may be painful to the horse, depending upon when the insult occurred and when the pulp died.

What are Iatrogenic Odontoplasty or Occlusal Surface Injuries?

OVER-REDUCTION OF tooth from overzealous odontoplasty causes pulp insults to occur faster than the pulp can respond. This is where improved understanding of the thickness of the SO2D becomes important in prevention of iatrogenic pulp exposure.

How does pulp exposure relate to excessive odontoplasty?

If your operator is not carefully watching the teeth as odontoplasty is performed, nor frequently rinsing and cooling the teeth, he will not see the dentinal colors change, which could indicate to him how close to the pulp he is. If grinding or ***rasping*** continues, the cream-colored dentin will become pink, then red. Pink and red mean danger, that the odontoblast processes of the pulp have been directly exposed, or a pulp exposure has occurred. Without treatment, the tooth is at risk of pulpitis, pulp necrosis (pulp death), and tooth death. Many factors contribute to whether that tooth will die, but the best action at this time is for your veterinarian to perform a vital pulpotomy to try to keep the tooth alive.

Careful odontoplasty should not result in this situation. See Chapter 14, Odontoplasty... Occasionally, though, the pulps are extremely close to the occlusal surface, especially when the tooth is unopposed (doesn't have a tooth directly opposite in the opposing arcade).

How far can one reduce the tooth? Researchers have found the ***subocclusal secondary dentine (SO2D),*** the secondary dentin/dentine which is laid down by the retreating pulp and lies between the live pulp and the occlusal surface of a hypsodont tooth. The more occlusal portion of this SO2D stains brown in the presence of feed pigments and may be used as a "color coding" to help prevent pulp exposures during odontoplasty. SO2D has been found to be between 1.5 and 11.7 millimeters (mm) for the ***maxillary incisors*** and between 0.7 and 6.7 mm for the ***mandibular*** incisors. These are wide ranges, but look at the lower numbers: 0.7 and 1.5 mm are extremely short distances, requiring rasping of only a tiny amount of tooth before the risk of iatrogenic pulp exposure becomes real. Therefore, great care should be exercised by any practitioner during tooth reduction, and in particular, during reduction of incisors and any unopposed teeth.

How could one overheat teeth?

When power instruments are used by dental operators, they create heat when grinding the teeth. Pulpitis and tooth death may result from hyperthermia due to prolonged power grinding with inadequate water-cooling. I use a battery-powered dental odontoplasty unit with constant water irrigation of the burr and teeth to prevent hyperthermia. Preventing the grinding disc or burr from resting on the surface of a single tooth for more than a few seconds at a time and flushing with cool water frequently can help prevent hyperthermia as well, but I prefer constant water irrigation for my patients' tooth safety. Above is an example of a horse whose incisors were affected by direct pulp exposure from

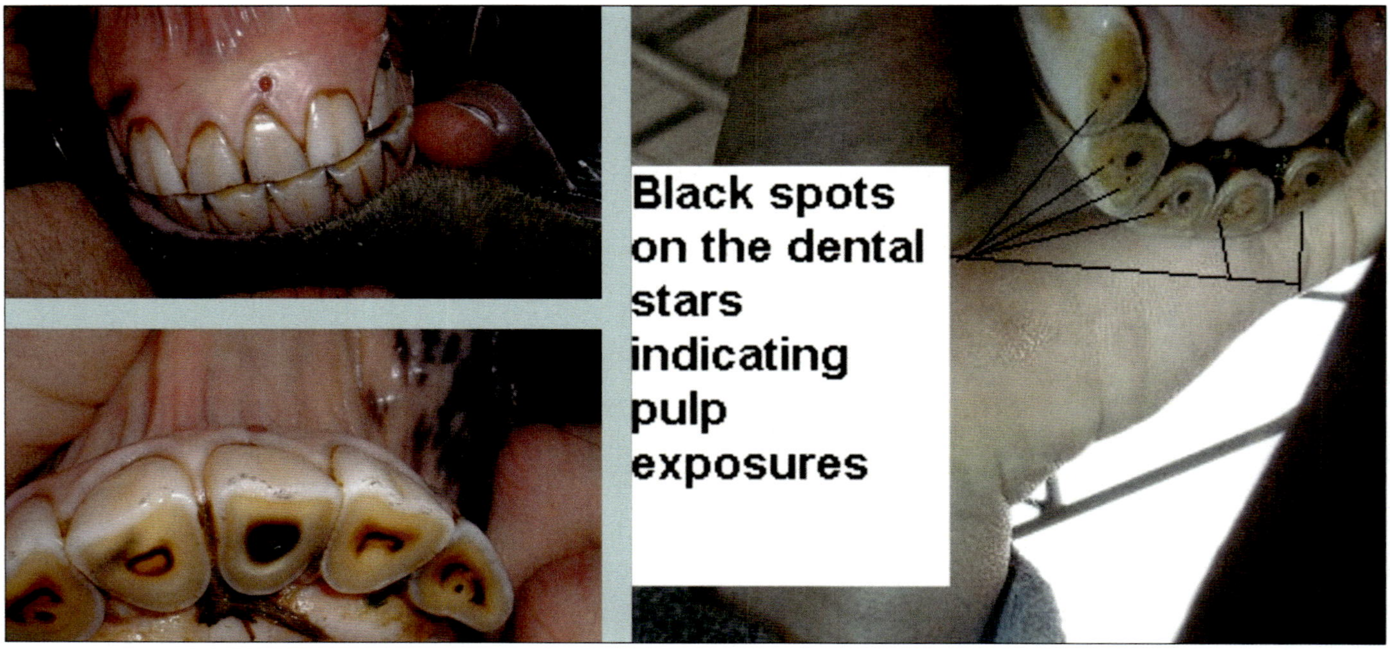

Exam findings which may indicate iatrogenic incisor disease. Original Images credit Dr Oliver Liyou, final graphic credit Author.

overzealous power floating. You may see this in horses which have had tooth length reduced too far, and/ or have not their teeth cooled in time to prevent pulpar injury.

What is indirect, or near-pulp exposure?

Even teeth that don't show the before-mentioned pinkness or redness may:

- be within three mm of the pulp, called an indirect- or near-pulp exposure, and be susceptible to pulp invasion by bacteria via the open dentinal tubules, or
- have had the smear layer removed (the protective layer of finely ground dentin present on the surface of each tooth), which may result in exposure of the sensitive odontoblast processes with subsequent infection of the pulp, or removal of the processes from their tubules. These may be extremely painful for the horse and initiate pulpitis, which can lead to pulp necrosis and tooth death. One of the biggest challenges with this form of tooth damage is that there may be no outward signs of injury until long after the operator is gone. A savvy owner or veterinarian may notice signs of pain, ranging from unwillingness to eat following dental treatment with power instruments (usually with

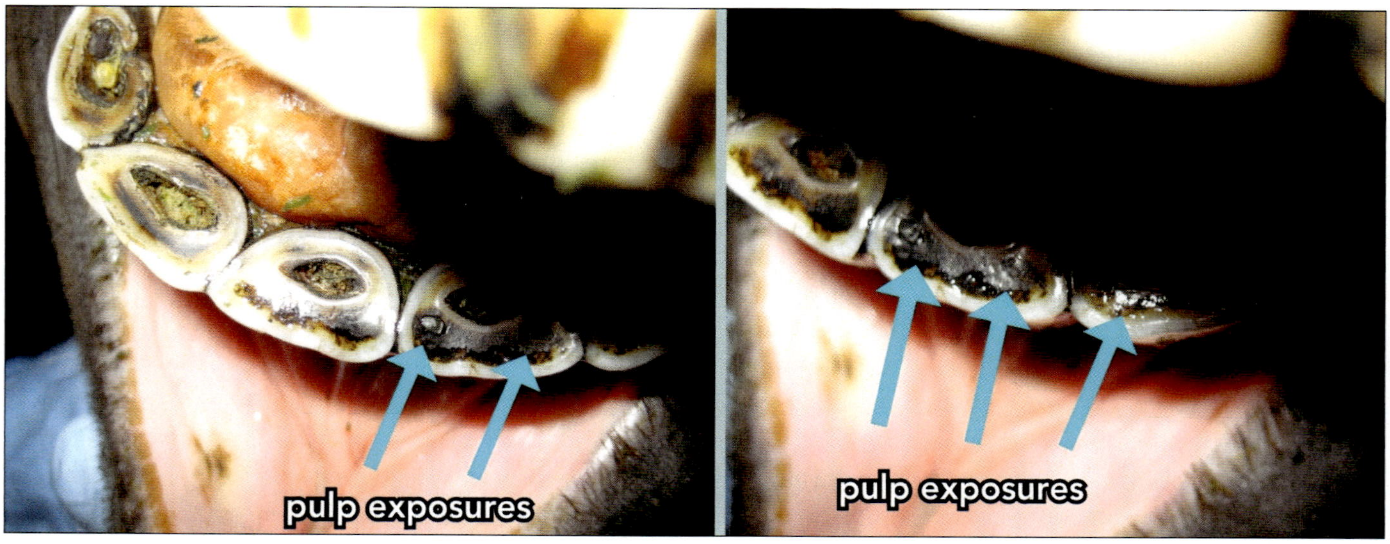

This young horse was examined after he was found to be obsessively chewing on his carpi, or knees, due to the pain from his incisors. He sustained near pulp exposure in multiple teeth from power dentistry without water cooling. The arrows point to the shiny, wet pulp exposures between the open infundibula (normal for his age) and the labial border of the mandibular incisors. Image credit Author.

insufficient or no cooling) to a horse obsessively sucking on her knees or other odd signs, which may be accompanied weeks to months down the line by evidence of the pulp exposure. On dental exam, your experienced dental vet may be able to place a probe into the ***dental stars***, or what have become exposed pulp chambers on the occlusal surface of the incisors or other teeth. It is tragic to see this in a young horse. These teeth may never recover, and if they die, they will be painful until they are extracted.

Why would you cut teeth? Really?

Direct pulp exposure easily results from the cutting of teeth, whether with molar shears (also called molar cutters) or by cutting incisors transversely (across the tooth) with a cut-off wheel. With these instruments, an operator isn't gradually and carefully grinding from the occlusal surface and cannot readily appreciate the dentinal color changes as the excessive length of a tooth is removed. Molar cutters tend to cause longitudinal (occlusal surface to root tip) and other fractures which split the tooth into multiple, difficult to extract, pieces. Pulps are readily exposed by these methods, and the operator risks pulpitis and tooth death in your horse. Some teeth cannot be saved after this kind of treatment, especially those with comminuted (multiple pieces) fractures, but some others may be saved by proper treatment from an experienced and well-trained equine dental veterinarian.

Damage from excessive pressure or application of chemicals

Excessive pressure applied to teeth, or the application of certain chemicals (such as during dental endodontic procedures) has been shown to cause damage to the odontoblast processes of the teeth and result in pulpitis, with possible subsequent tooth death.

Excessive profiling ("bit seats") of the '06s

Like ***wolf teeth***, "bit seats" aren't a disease condition, but they can become so if the operator removes too much tooth, exposing the dentinal tubules or the pulp itself. A bit seat is poorly named, as this name might suggest the bit is meant to sit upon it. Correctly used, the bit should not come into contact with the '06 (the first ***cheek tooth***) at all. Only when excessive force is applied to the reins does a bit actually touch them. When the reins are pulled back with great force, the cheeks or lips may be cut between the bit and the '06s if they are sharp on their ***mesial*** edges. Some operators mistakenly remove a large proportion of this mesial portion of the '06s, including cutting into or close to the pulp chambers. This is dangerous. See Chapter 6, Developmental and Acquired Conditions.

We properly "profile" the '06s, a better term than "creating a bit seat", by removing only enough of the sharp mesial edges of the '06s to prevent them from cutting the cheeks and tongue and always taking care to note the color changes of the SO2D as the '06s are rasped.

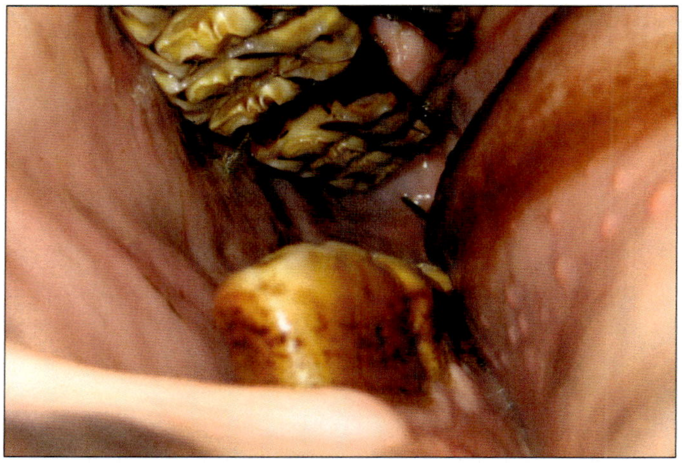

This 406 has been correctly profiled, not exposing pulp, but there is more pathology further back in the mouth. Image credit Author.

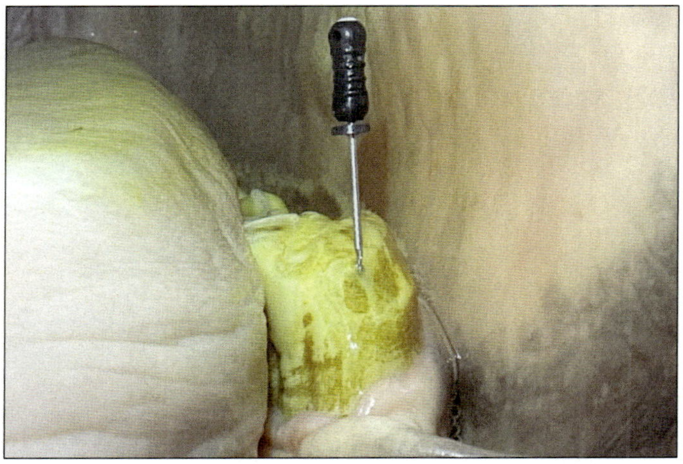

Excessive profiling or "bit seating" has been performed on this horse in the past and caused pulp exposure. The endodontic file penetrates into pulp horn 6 of the 306. There is no reason for such extensive profiling and it risks the life of the tooth, especially in an older horse. Image credit Dr Elke Pollaris.

If you notice that that '06 profiling appears to be is overdone on your horse, or is pink, red, or looks like dried blood, or if your horse seems uncomfortable, unhappy to eat, graze, or drink after dental care, call your dental veterinarian immediately because vital pulpotomy within about 48 hours will give teeth with pulpar exposure a better chance of survival. Remember, the teeth of older horses with their narrowed tooth apices are at greater risk.

What are Some Iatrogenic Wolf Teeth Considerations?

WOLF TEETH ARE discussed in detail in Chapter 8, Secondary forms of Dental Disease: Wolf Teeth and Chapter 15, Veterinary Specific Procedures: Extraction Considerations. Wolf teeth are the small ***vestigial*** teeth often found just mesial to the '06s. While wolf teeth are not a disease condition, partial or incomplete extraction can cause problems for both you and your horse!

Contrary to some people's understanding, these teeth often have long roots and should be completely extracted like other teeth, by careful elevation, rotation, and extraction. Many operators break them off and leave them, rather than extracting them properly. These teeth, although small, also have live pulps, complete with nerves, which equals pain. They should be completely extracted to prevent pain to the horse, if they are extracted at all.

Unerupted, or "blind", wolf teeth erupt from the ***alveolus*** but do not erupt through the ***gingiva***. It is painful for the horse when a bit hits the gingiva over the tooth. These must be surgically extracted with sedation and ***analgesia*** (pain relief) to avoid causing pain to the horse. Administration of sedation and analgesia are acts of veterinary medicine in most places and limited to veterinarians.

Molarized wolf teeth have large, deep roots, and often with more than one. They may be quite stable and difficult to extract, and many don't need extraction under normal circumstances. Roots have been known to be left in place.

Please call your dental vet if any of the above problems are noted. Every horse presented for extraction deserves proper care with sedation, local ***anesthesia***, and post-operative analgesia for at least three days.

My lay dental operator ("dentist") just files off wolf teeth

Rasping or filing any teeth down to the gumline, including wolf teeth, instead of extracting them is ***contraindicated*** and an iatrogenic disaster. All teeth, no matter how small, have live pulps. Filing them will cause pulp exposure. This will cause pain, likely pulpitis, and tooth death, coupled with ***periodontal*** disease and draining tracts from possible ***osteomyelitis***. This is a bad idea.

Can't you leave some wolf teeth in?

Sometimes they don't cause a problem and can remain in the mouth. If they reside against the first cheek tooth and are tucked toward the palate, they may never cause a problem to a bitted horse. If they are solid, molarized teeth against the first cheek tooth and you have good hands for riding, they also may not require removal. This is covered in the above-mentioned chapters.

How Do Iatrogenic Dental and Skull Fractures Happen?

IATROGENIC DENTAL AND skull fractures have various causes, such as during placement of a speculum on a horse with a previous issue, usage of a unilateral speculum, or during surgery.

During placement of a speculum: Equids with preexisting (unknown) pathology

As mentioned in Chapter 10, Head Trauma and Dental Pathology, it is vital to manipulate the ***mandible*** and ***palpate*** the ***temporomandibular joints*** (TMJ) for pain and mobility before placing a speculum. Placement of a speculum and opening it on a horse with a skull fracture can ***exacerbate*** an incomplete fracture or displace a previously non-displaced one.

Due to the use of a unilateral speculum...especially a "spool"...

These specula go by the name of Bayer, Schouppe, spool, coil, Landmeisser, wedge, and the like. They have a bite piece which fits between the ***cheek teeth*** made of either:

- cylindrical spring steel or a solid metal cylinder (the "spool" types), or

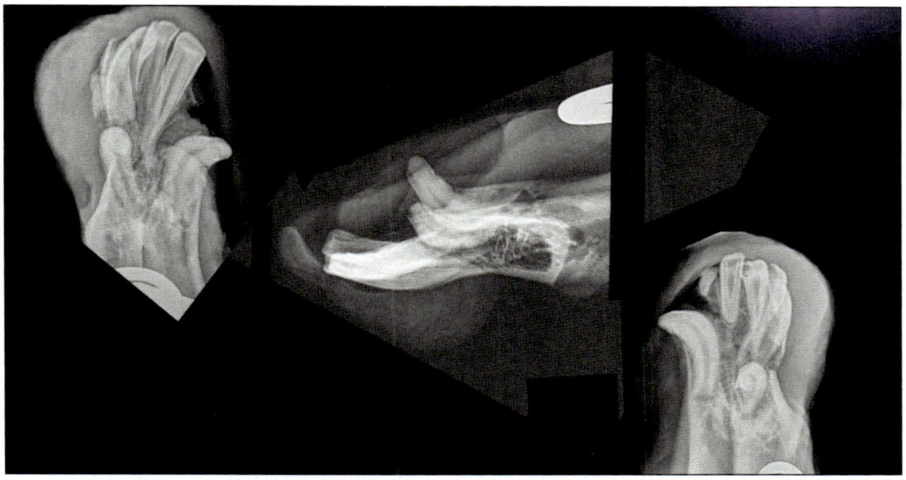

An accidental paddock injury caused this mandibular fracture of a previously-diseased mandible. This horse was presented because the owner thought he had broken his teeth. He did that, and more. Previous disease of the mandible had not been noticed until pulp exposures were noted by the emergency and referral veterinarians and post-fracture radiographs were taken. This case is presented as a caution: with a less obvious fracture, it may not be apparent that a fracture (displaced or non-displaced) is present, and disaster could result from opening a speculum when a horse has disease of the mandible. Original images credit Dr Barbara Hunter, graphic credit Author

- a wedge of metal, plastic, or rubber (the wedge types).

The only benefit from using either of these types of gag is slightly easier floating of the teeth because one side of the mouth held open to some degree. However, these gags are not recommended because at best, they do not significantly assist in examination or floating, and at worst, they frequently cause serious damage. The reasons for this are as follows:

- A horse ***masticates*** (chews) a lot with a unilateral (one-sided) gag in place. This makes it difficult to examine the teeth, which is the primary purpose of a dental examination, which should be performed before the teeth are filed.
- As the gag occupies mouth space on the side where it is placed, the tongue is pushed toward the other side where examination or floating is being attempted. This decreases visibility inside the mouth, already minimal at this level, and making floating more difficult.
- The ***temporomandibular*** or jaw joint, commonly known as the TMJ, may be damaged when a horse bites down hard on only one side at a time
- If the gag slips from *between* the teeth to *the inside* of the teeth, the palatine artery may be ruptured. It bleeds. A lot. For a *long* time.
- Most seriously, however, the danger of fracturing cheek teeth is very real. The cylindricalshape of the "spool" types causes the entire force of both sides of the strong masseter (chewing) muscles to be focused on a narrow line across two opposing teeth, which may lead to a fractured cheek tooth or teeth, with severe consequences. A fractured tooth needs to be extracted. A fractured tooth will cause your horse a lot of pain until the tooth is

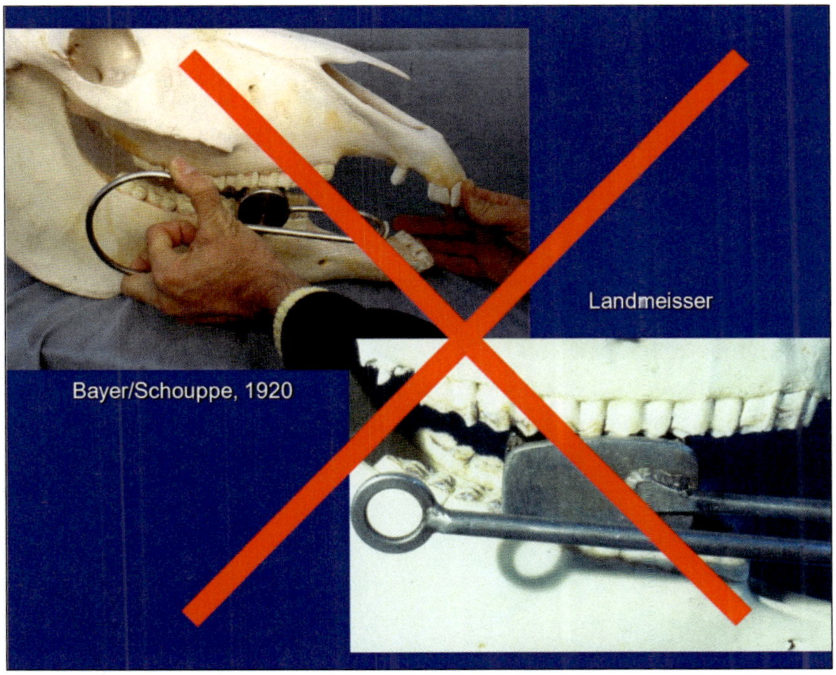

The image shows two of the many NON-recommended gags which are sometimes used at The Second Level: Shown are the Bayer/Schouppe (1920) and the Landmeisser. These can seriously damage teeth and other tissues, including the fracture of cheek teeth. Unmarked images credit Dr Jack Easley, graphic credit Author.

discovered and extracted. Make no mistake, this is a major surgery, especially because that recently-healthy tooth will be firmly stuck in place.

And the worst thing about a spool gag-created fracture? It never had to happen in the first place. Keep them far from your horse! The same goes for molar cutters and captive bolt percussion tools which fit over a tooth elongation and chop it off.

During surgery...

Dental and skull fractures may occur as accidental sequela to surgical treatment, especially when trauma has weakened areas of the skull. Skull and dental radiographs help identify weakened areas and assist in identification of all existing fractures and determining which structures are involved for treatment and prognostic purposes.

Avoidance of iatrogenic fractures is a significant reason why veterinarians now usually perform intraoral extraction instead of the older method of repulsion, or "trephination and repulsion". Intraoral extraction is extracting a tooth from within the mouth using long-handled instruments. As discussed in Chapter 10, Head Trauma and Dental Pathology: Evaluation for fractures of mandible, maxilla and teeth, trephination involves drilling a hole or holes in the skull into a sinus and then bashing the tooth out with a punch and mallet, usually under general anesthesia. Unfortunately, this can fracture and destroy the alveolus within which the tooth resided. Until only the past few decades, repulsion was the primary method used to extract equine ***cheek teeth***, but thanks to better understanding of the anatomy, the development of improved instrumentation, and advances in standing anesthesia, most teeth may be extracted by intraoral extraction. It is still possible to create fractures with intraoral extraction, especially as one is dealing with infected, weakened bone, but it is much less common than seen with repulsion.

Iatrogenic injuries which may occur during repulsion include fracture of the ***infraorbital canal***, damage to sinus structures, multiple fractures of the alveolar bone and surrounding skull, and creation of an extremely large oro-sinus (mouth to sinus) ***fistula***, which can be difficult to repair. What that means to you is a large, persistent (not going away) fistula between the mouth and the ***sinuses*** will cause a secondary sinusitis, and your horse will be draining extremely smelly pus from its nostril for a long, long time until it hopefully heals. Even with surgical intervention. Utilizing intraoral extraction techniques minimizes damage to other structures during extraction when compared with tooth repulsion. See Chapter 15 Veterinary Specific Procedures: Extraction Considerations.

Surgical repulsion should only be considered when intraoral extraction is impossible due to lack of access, a severely malformed tooth, or a horse with a temperament which would create a dangerous situation for the operators, horse, and handlers. In other words, repulsion should only be used as a last resort for extraction, after intraoral and minimally invasive extraction methods have failed.

Iatrogenic Trauma From Speculum Placement: Equids with EOTRH Have Painful Incisors!

IF A HORSE is found to resent the speculum, which may show by the horse waking up during sedation as soon as a speculum is placed or when the pain-relieving component of the sedation drug wears off, 5-7 minutes after injection, the horse's incisors should be checked for signs suggestive of Equine Odontoclastic Tooth Resorption and Hypercementosis (***EOTRH***). If the disease is suspected or horse is nearing fifteen years of age or more, it is wise to X-ray the horse to check for radiographic signs of the disease. See Chapter 7, EOTRH. EOTRH makes placement of a speculum extremely painful for an affected horse and their teeth may be fragile. Radiographs are required to definitively diagnose this disease. See images in Chapter 7, EOTRH.

CHAPTER TEN

HOW CAN HEAD TRAUMA CAUSE DENTAL PATHOLOGY?

TRAUMA TO THE head and teeth are common in horses, even if we don't always see it. In all the excitement of an emergency with bleeding wounds, upset horses, and stressed people, hidden damage to teeth or the bones supporting the teeth may go unnoticed unless your horse is carefully examined. Missing these hidden injuries can cause unnecessary pain, prolonged recovery, or permanent damage to your horse.

Examination of the Head Trauma Equid… or "Oh, There Were Teeth in There!"

External examination

Your ***vet*** will first observe from a distance to gain insights into the whole horse and not miss subtle problems, especially when confronted by excited onlookers. She will take a thorough history while making observations. Is the lower or upper lip drooping? Pulling in one particular direction? Tongue protruding from the mouth?

For your part, take even greater care around any horse which is obtunded ("out of it", seeming not to care or understand what's going on around them) or seizuring.

Your vet will likely perform a neurologic examination to assess injuries involving the brain or nerves, including checking for pupillary light reflexes, retinal detachment, and assessing zones of skin sensation to check for post-injury nerve function. The structures of the skull will be ***palpated*** while observing for symmetry and penetrating wounds. If the ***sinuses*** are penetrated, multiple ***fistulae*** may become established and become a problem for years to come. The vessels, nerves, and bones are under only a thin layer of skin, with the sinuses and teeth just under the thin layer of bone beneath *that*.

Get the idea? A hoof to the side of their face or smacking their head on a post can damage a lot of structures in a fraction of a second.

A penetrating wound to a sinus may require invasive investigation with a bone flap or drilling a hole in the skull to see inside the sinus with an endoscope. Your horse may have had an injury you didn't know about, so if you notice your horse suddenly has bad breath, difficulty or unwillingness to eat, drooling, or misalignment of its ***incisors***, there is sure to be pain involved, so let your vet know right away. It's vital.

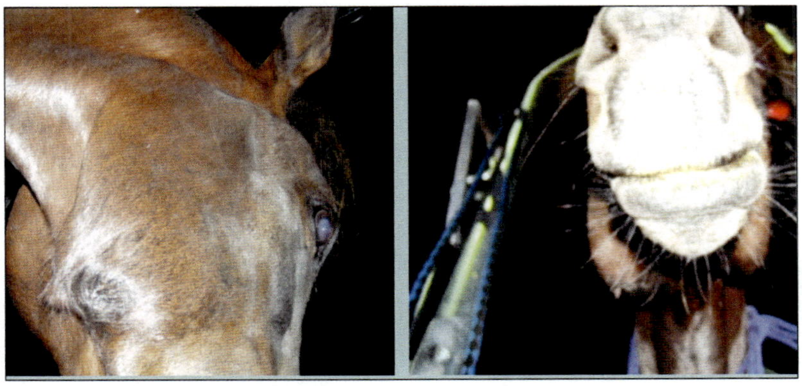

This stallion was kicked by a mare and sustained multiple fractured cheek teeth and subsequently, a mandibular draining tract, seen ventral to his 400 arcade. Image credit Author.

Examination inside the mouth

Before examining the ***oral*** cavity, your vet will fully palpate and gently manipulate the ***maxilla*** and the ***mandible*** to check for fractures before placing a speculum in the horse's mouth to thoroughly check the inside of the mouth. Even if no obvious maxillary or mandibular fractures are evident, they could still be present, and a fracture could be exacerbated by opening the speculum. Your vet will rinse the mouth so the feed material and clotted blood don't hide any injuries present.

If there *is* a fracture near the incisors at the front of the mouth, a speculum may still be used after your horse is sedated, but only if padded gum plates or a tube speculum can be placed ***distally*** to the fracture site on the ***bars of the mouth*** to evaluate the oral cavity.

Inside the mouth, your vet will look for any irregularities or asymmetry of the soft ***tissues***, including

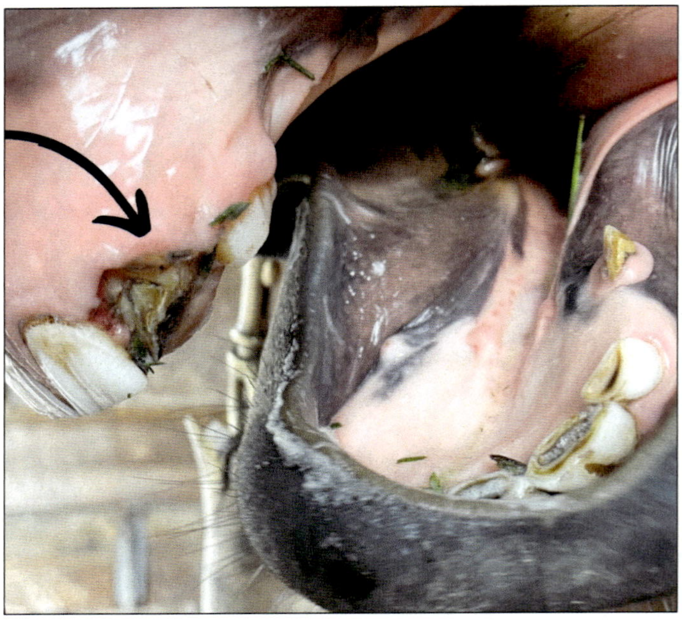

Fractured 202 in a young horse, presented for restoration of the tooth. Image credit Author.

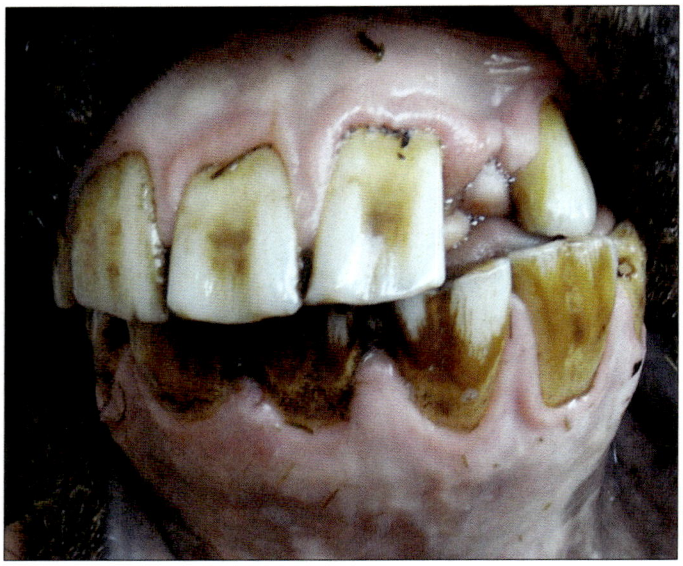

It is unknown what sort of trauma this horse encountered, but it caused major incisor and cheek tooth imbalance. Image credit Author.

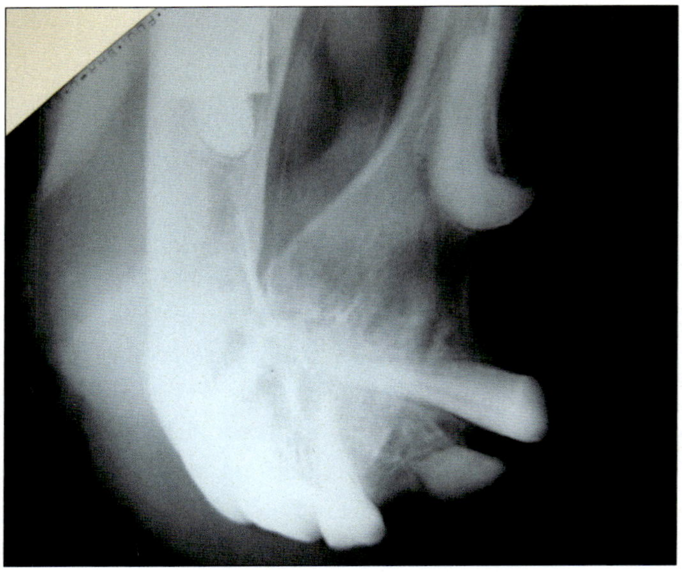

Another historical traumatic injury which left this horse with incisor damage. One partially resorbed piece of dead tooth is in evidence in this radiograph. Image credit Author.

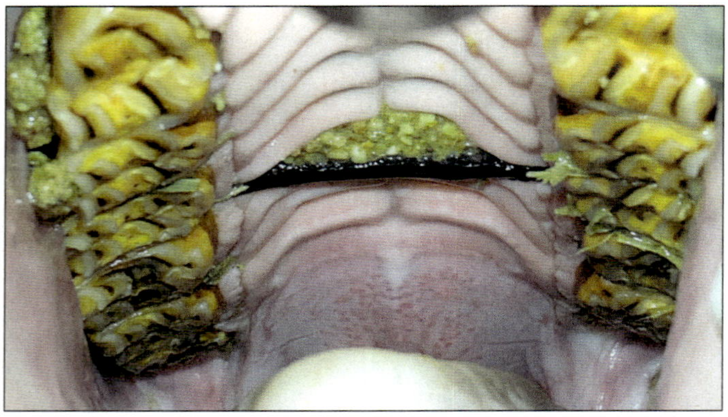

This horse had a stick jammed between two teeth of his maxillary arcades. Image credit Dr Kirsten Jackson, Dental Vet.

the palate, cheeks, tongue and frenulum for punctures or ***lacerations*** from objects gripped in the horse's teeth or from foreign bodies like sticks or pieces of plastic or wire, some of which may have lodged beneath the ***mucosa*** or within sinuses. See Chapter 3, Anatomy of the Mouth.

Full dental radiographs of a horse with a head injury can highlight problems which may not otherwise be found. CT may be an option if radiographs do not not help find the issue.

Evaluation for fractures of mandible, maxilla, and teeth

Your vet will carefully evaluate the supporting bones of the teeth for fractures and check for any loose or fractured teeth. He will note any dental fractures which have resulted in ***pulp exposure***. For the best chance of saving those teeth, these fractured teeth should be treated with vital pulpotomy as soon as possible after injury.

In the case sinus surgery or extraction is required, your dental vet or surgeon will take care to avoid destruction of the normal sinus anatomy, including using intraoral extraction techniques over repulsion if at all possible. If the mandible or maxilla is fractured, they may be able to be repaired with wires, which compared to plates and pins, which tends to conserve (save) the existing erupted teeth as well as the developing ***deciduous tooth buds*** still deep in the mandible and maxilla.

Sometimes no obvious mandibular or maxillary fractures are present, but the teeth have fractured. The images to the right are from a young horse who presented for a mandibular draining tract. He had long, well-fixed tooth roots which radiographs indicated had been fractured for quite some time before he was examined.

You know how some horses like to play with solid objects or ropes in their mouths? Well, sometimes that goes terribly wrong. You've seen them chew on something and then flick their heads up? Sometimes they forget to let go. Unfortunately, that can result in luxations (fractures) of the ***rostral*** mandible, maxilla, or bars of the mouth, especially when dental or bony ***pathology*** is already present.

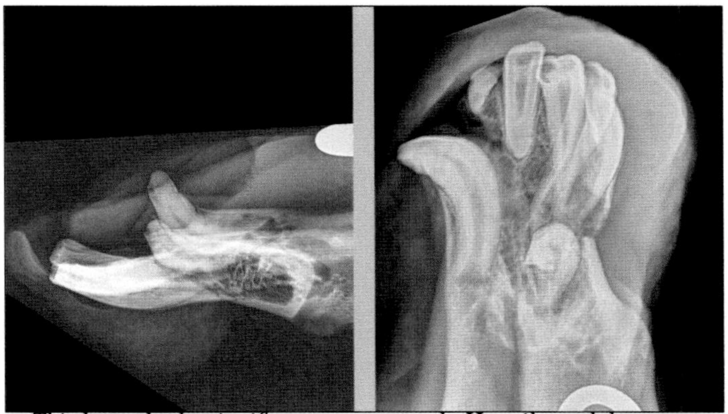

This horse had a significant parrot mouth. He cribs and the owner suspected he had caught his mandible on a gate. Post-injury radiographs revealed a complete transverse fracture of the mandibular incisor bone, along with significant older pathology of the incisors, including misshapen incisors, nonvital pulps, and abnormal infundibula. Due to the abnormal bone at the fracture site and the need to extract multiple teeth at a later date, the least painful course of treatment for the horse with the lowest likelihood of complications was removal of the mandibular incisors and fractured bone completely just rostral to the canines. The horse happily ate grass and whatever else he could find. Images credit Dr Barbara Hunter, graphic credit Author.

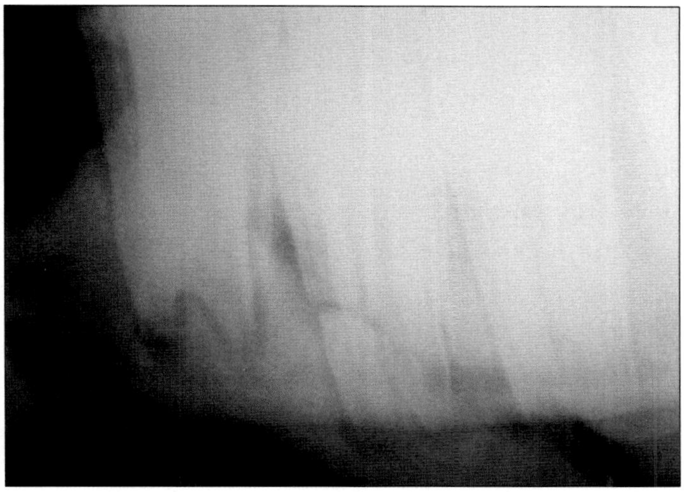

A young horse presenting for a draining tract at the bottom of the mandible. One tooth fracture is obvious, but the tooth distal to it is also in trouble. The mandible is likely fractured as well. Several problems are evident in this case. More radiographs are needed. Image credit Author.

The same horse, from a different view. Multiple views are needed to show detail. Notice how much displacement exists between the two parts of the fractured tooth. Image credit Author.

Those with appropriate training will understand that TEETH, potentially both ***permanent*** and deciduous, lie just beneath the surface of the skull. They will also know teeth are at risk when performing surgery in any areas which contain deciduous or ***permanent teeth***, or their precursors. Let me say that again in a slightly different way. When your vet is evaluating damage to the skull, surgically repairing fractures, or otherwise invading the skull, they will remember the ***tooth eruption*** sequences and times, as well as placement of all teeth and sinus locations, as they are so essential. See Chapter 3, Anatomy: Tooth Development and Placement.

The parotid duct runs just under the skin of the cheek before it dives deep and enters the mouth near the '08s. See Chapter 3, Anatomy of the Mouth. It is also susceptible to injury! From the same chapter, you might remember that the ***nasolacrimal duct*** runs from the eye to the inside of the nose. It is also just beneath the outer bones of the skull, running through the sinuses. It may also be in the path of damage in a concussive injury to the head.

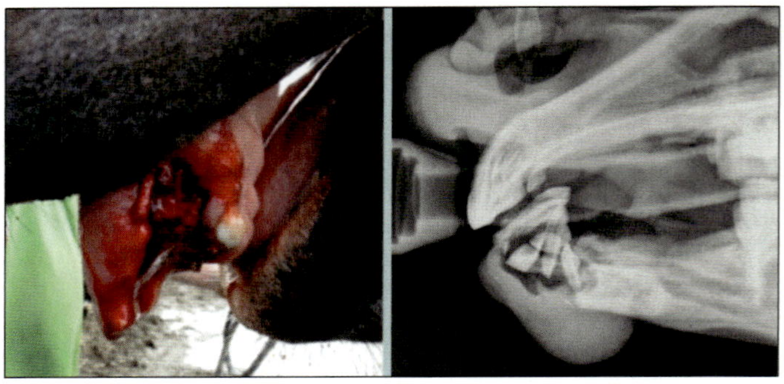

A maxillary and a mandibular fracture involving teeth. Note in the radiographs the deciduous teeth still present in the maxillary and mandibular bones. Image credit Dr Maxwell Hall.

Other diagnostic modalities

Endoscopy is useful to assess hard and soft palate injuries and identify foreign bodies in the pharynx. Their light and flush functions can be used to help clean the blood and debris from traumatized areas for better visualization. Ultrasound images help locate and determine the extent of soft tissue damage and helps identify foreign bodies in the tongue, cheek, or gums.

As shown above, radiography (X-ray) is essential to determine the extent of trauma to the teeth and supporting bones. It also helps identify foreign bodies (at least the radio-opaque ones like bone or metal) in the tongue, cheeks, or gums. Injecting a radio-opaque contrast dye into a draining tract can outline the tract on a radiograph, allowing the definition of the path taken by a foreign body or outlining an oro-nasal or oro-sinus fistula.

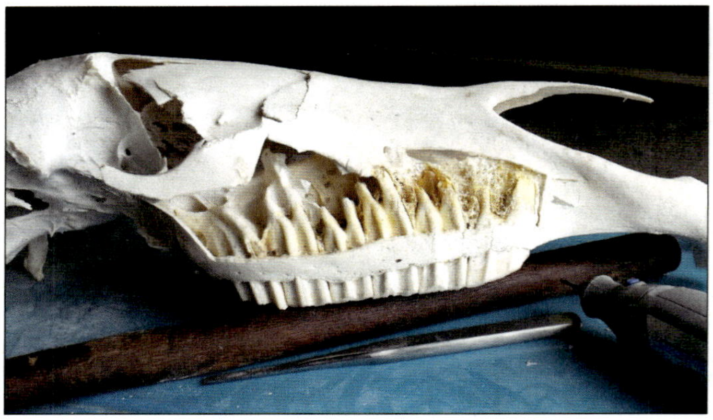

The openings in this skull show the apices of the cheek teeth and many other structures. Image credit Cathie Heald Greenwell.

General Oral Trauma Treatment and Repair

YOUR VET WILL treat the injuries they safely can, with respect to the mental and physical condition of your horse. This will generally involve antibiotic and anti-inflammatory drugs and tetanus prophylaxis, if not surgery as well. See Chapter 15, Extraction, Tetanus cover.

Taking teeth out of occlusion with a rotary, power float rather than via hand ***floats*** or reciprocating floats may help to prevent further destabilization of injury-caused tooth mobility, as the back-and-forth motion of hand floats or reciprocating floats may further loosen them.

Any exposed pulps require vital pulpotomy as soon as possible, ideally within 48 hours or so, to help prevent pulpitis, potential tooth death, and all its sequelae.

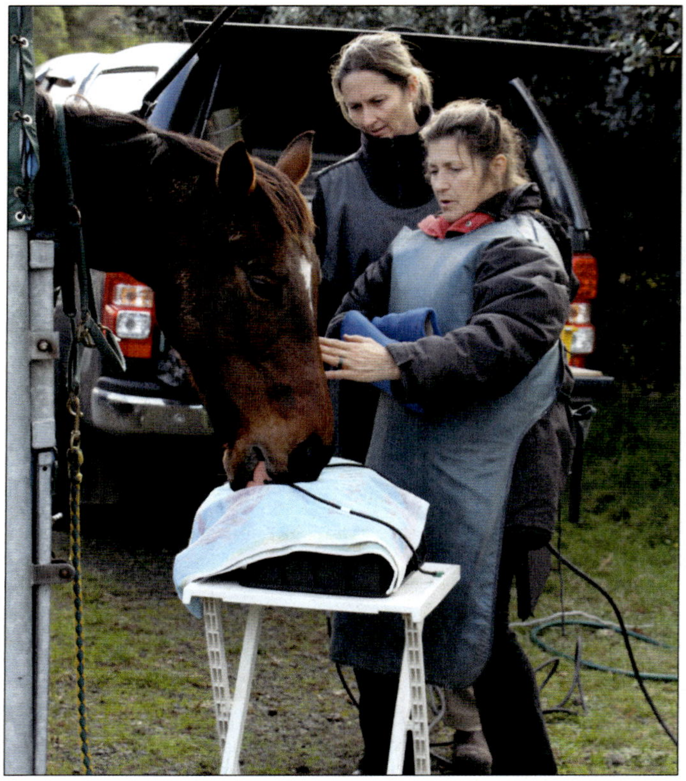

Radiographs are essential to discover the extent of bony trauma post-injury. Image credit Matthew Mole.

How Would a Horse Get Accidental Pulpar Exposure?

IT OFTEN SURPRISES people to see how close the tooth buds and apices lie to the bottom of the mandible in a young horse. I shudder to see young horses kicking out and catching each other beneath the jaws, because I know what's in there, only millimeters from the bottom of their jaw...

A kick to the bottom of the jaw can not only fracture the mandible in a young horse, but also can fracture deciduous teeth or injure the developing permanent ones. In an older horse, the permanents can be fractured or otherwise damaged. A kick to the incisors or onto the side of their face can easily fracture teeth and bone as well. These fractures may cause ***pulpar exposure***, with risk of pulpitis and possible pulp necrosis and tooth death. See Chapter 9, Iatrogenic Disease: What is Pulpar Exposure... or Chapter 6, Developmental and Acquired Conditions: Apical Infection...

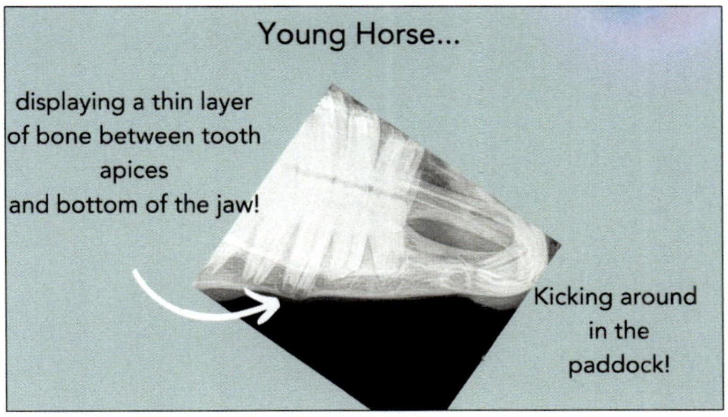

Don't you love the young horses kicking around in the paddock? You might not look at it the same way again! The tooth apices are a few mm from the bottom of the jaw! Image credit Author.

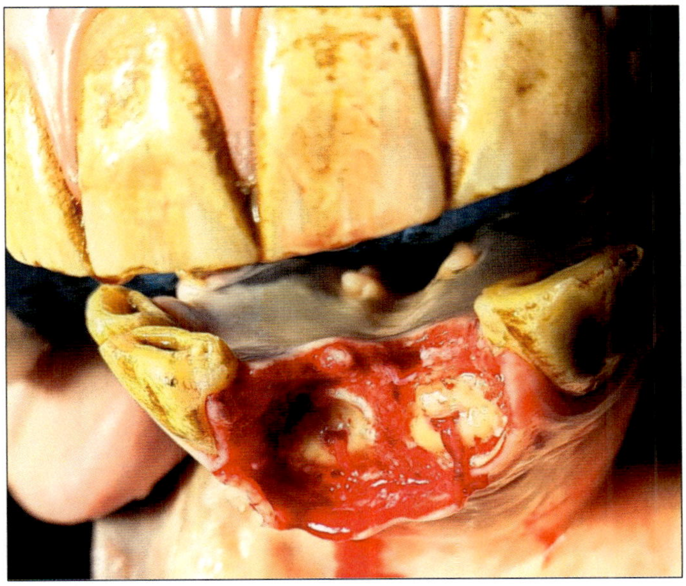

The 301 and 401 incisors have fractured near the gumline. Note the red pulps exiting the center of these two teeth. This horse will be in serious pain and is in need of vital pulpotomy as soon as possible. Image credit Dr Elke Pollaris.

What are Suture Periostitis and Exostosis?

THESE INFLAMMATORY CONDITIONS usually follow trauma. They have been covered in Chapter 6, Developmental and Acquired Conditions: Masses, Tumors, Lumps, and Bumps.

Suture periostitis

Suture periostitis is a thickened ridge along the suture joining two or more of the flat bones of the skull which may occur following a concussive injury to the head or muzzle, as when they trip or fall and hit nose-first. This most commonly involves the frontal and nasal bones.

Suture exostosis

A suture exostosis is a bony protrusion at any bony suture. May result in secondary problems if it causes blockages of ducts, etc.

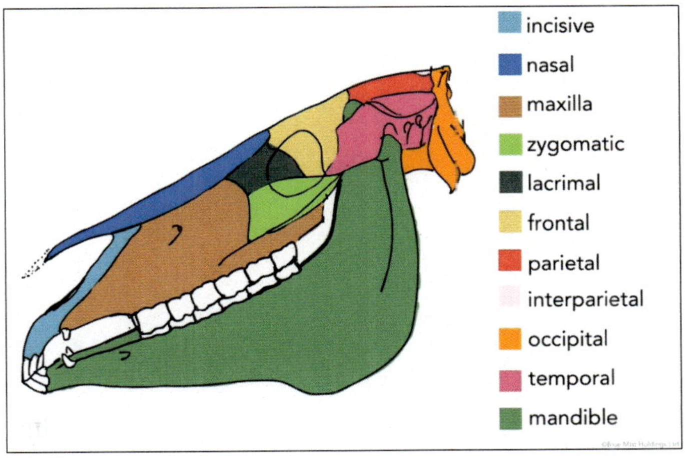

The lines where two bones join are called the "sutures". Note especially the suture between the nasal (dark blue) and frontal(gold) bones, a common site of suture periostitis and exostosis. Image credit Author.

CHAPTER ELEVEN

WHAT IS SINUS DISEASE?

DISEASES OF THE ***sinuses*** are simple to miss as they are even more hidden from view than are the teeth. Diagnosing them is important, as these conditions can cause untold suffering to equids before they are discovered and treated. If you have ever had a serious sinus infection, you may have experienced the pain from the increased pressure within your sinuses.

How Do Equids Get Sinusitis?

WHILE THERE ARE many causes of sinusitis in the horse, primary sinusitis, not an apical infection, is the most common.

Primary sinusitis

Primary sinusitis is a sinus infection which originates in the sinus ***tissue*** itself rather than as an extension of another infection (such as an infected tooth). Primary sinusitis is usually the result of a previous upper respiratory infection, caused by a bacterium such as *Streptococcus sp.*

Secondary sinusitis

The most common cause of secondary sinusitis is dental disease. It may also be caused by facial fractures, neoplasia, and granulomas. Secondary sinusitis tends to be more difficult to treat than primary sinusitis because it usually requires surgery to repair the initial cause.

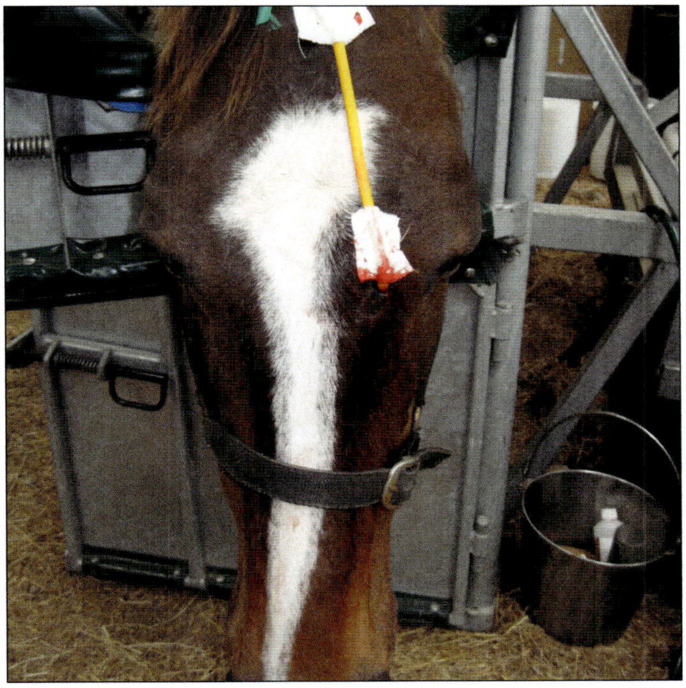

Following intraoral extraction of a maxillary tooth with large cementomas and an oro-sinus fistula, a flushing tube was sutured into place for repeat sinus flushing to treat this secondary sinusitis. The horse had displayed a chronic one-sided purulent nasal discharge before the surgery. Image credit Author.

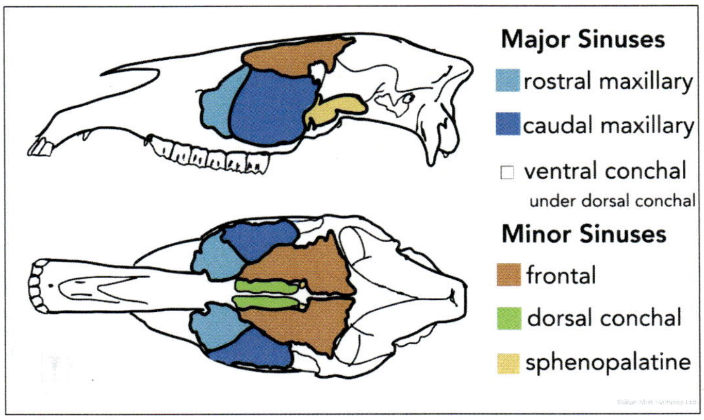

Here are the major and minor sinuses in the skull. The apices of the more caudal cheek teeth reside inside them, along with many other structures. Image credit Author.

The dental disease which causes this sinusitis is usually due to an ***apical abscess*** which has burst into the sinus in which it resides, creating an oro-sinus (mouth to sinus)

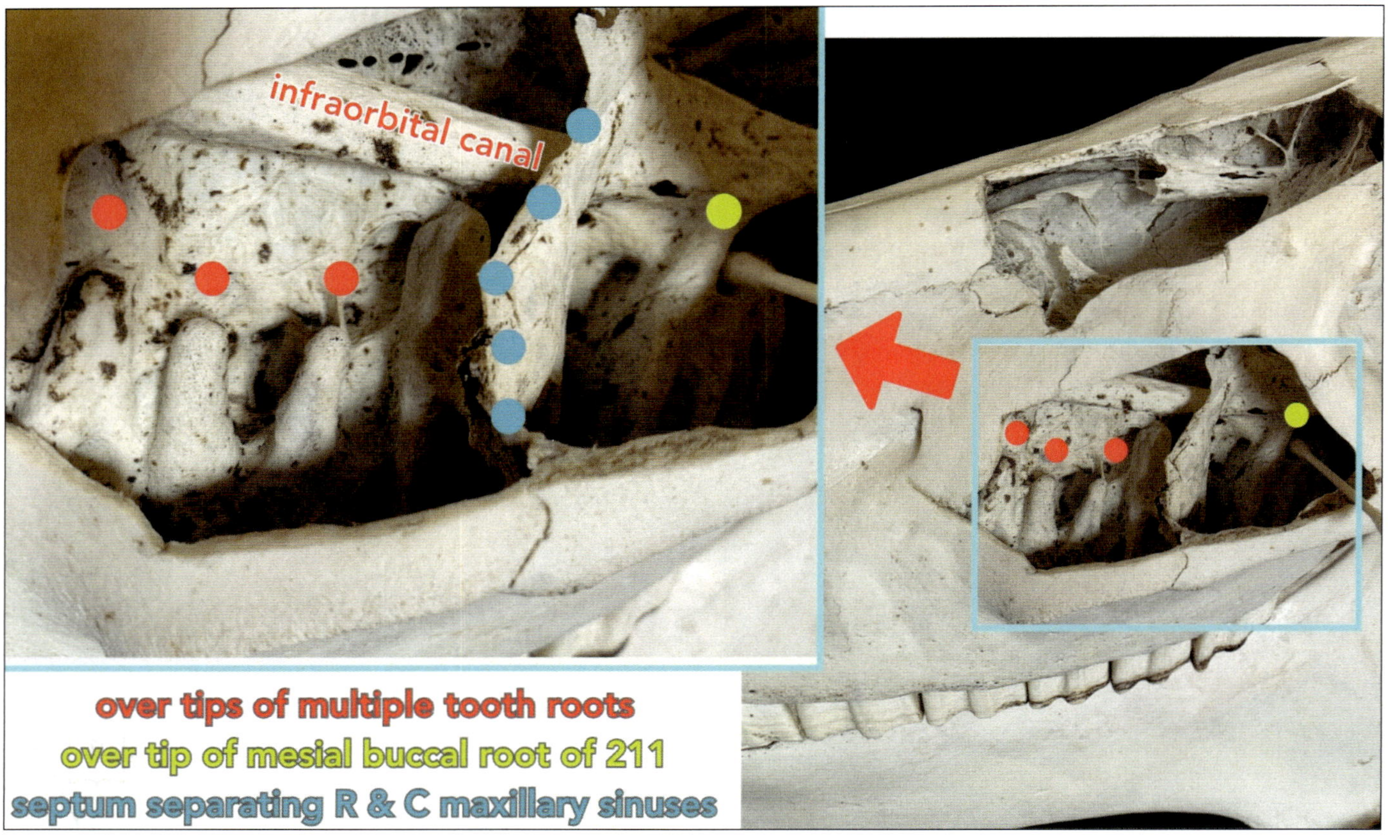

Distal maxillary cheek tooth apices reside in the maxillary sinuses for most of an equid's life. This graphic shows the opened rostral and caudal maxillary sinuses with the nasolacrimal duct and multiple tooth roots within these sinuses. This horse had only the 211 in the caudal maxillary sinus (the rostral buccal root of the 211 is marked with a yellow dot, just to the left of the cotton bud), while the 210, 209, and part of the 208 in the rostral maxillary sinus (red dots just over the root tips). These two sinuses are separated by the septum, marked with blue dots. Image credit Author.

fistula, and causing the infection of one or more sinuses. See Chapter 6, Developmental and Acquired Conditions: Apical Infection, Pulpitis,... When the affected tooth is extracted, there may be an even larger fistula. While your ***veterinarian*** will plug this or close it surgically, it can be extremely difficult to achieve proper healed closure in some cases. Clearing of the extremely nasty ***purulent*** material in the sinus will require repeated flushing and other pharmaceutical treatment. This is not pleasant for anyone involved, from the horse to the owner to the vet, but if your horse's sinus infection hurts anything like some I've personally had, the treatment sure beats your horse having its head pound with every heartbeat from the increased pressure within an infected sinus.

Secondary sinusitis is one of the most significant reasons veterinarians have moved over to intraoral extraction instead of the older method of trephination and repulsion. Trephination involves drilling a hole or holes in the skull, often into a sinus, then bashing the tooth out with a punch and mallet, usually under general ***anesthesia***. Unfortunately, this destroys the ***alveolus*** within which the tooth resided and results in multiple fractures of surrounding bone, leaving one or more large oro-sinus ***fistulae*** behind, which can be difficult to repair. Trephination and repulsion should only be used as a last resort after intraoral and minimally invasive extraction methods have failed.

What is an Ethmoid Hematoma?

ETHMOID HEMATOMAS ARE smoothly encapsulated masses which usually originates in the ethmoid turbinate labyrinth of one of the paranasal sinuses. See image on next page for its location. No one knows exactly what causes an ethmoid hematoma, but it seems to begin with bleeding under the mucosa of a sinus, which causes the mucosa to stretch and thicken, then continue to enlarge into other sinuses as it grows. It can even extend so far as the maxillary sinuses and nasal cavity.

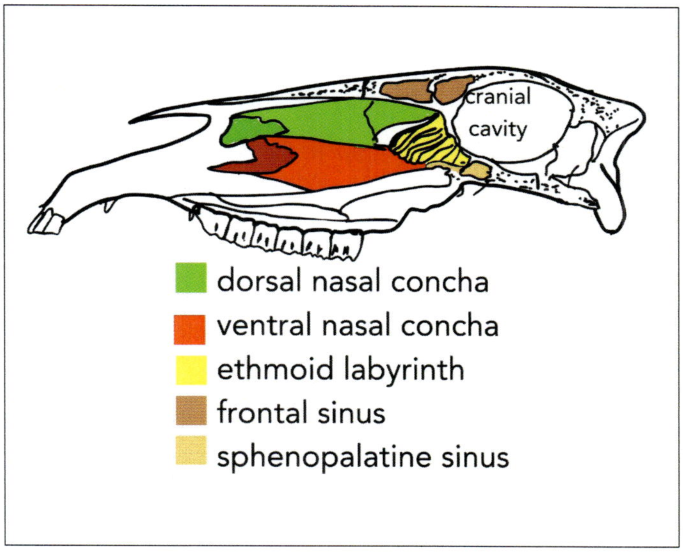

Interior view of the sinuses which may be significant in disease of the head, including the ethmoid labyrinth, or sinuses (yellow). Image credit Author.

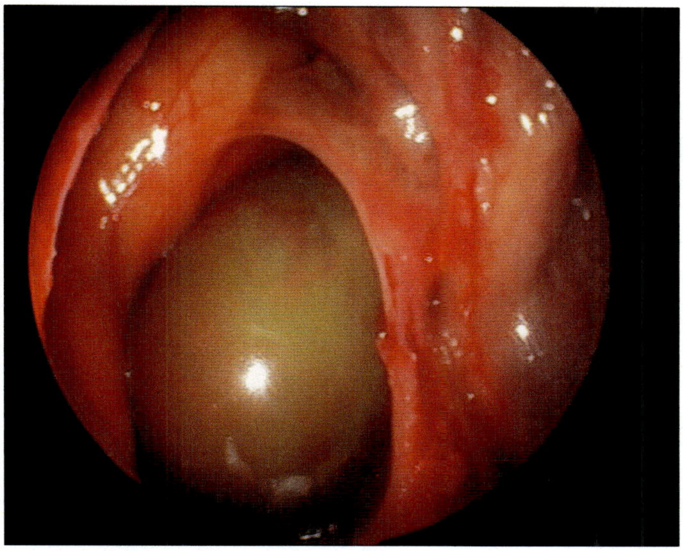

An ethmoid hematoma. This is a sinoscopic image (endoscopy in the sinus) taken following a trephination of the frontal sinus. The yellow circular mass is an ethmoidal hematoma that has expanded and protruded into the maxillary sinus. Image credit Dr Denis Verwilghen.

How do I know if my horse might have an ethmoid hematoma?

The most consistent sign is a unilateral (one-sided) bloody nose which occurs from time to time, sometimes after exercise. The horse's breathing may make excessive noise as the mass grows and partially fills the sinuses and nasal passages. You may notice foul-smelling breath, head shaking, facial swelling, and increasing head shyness.

Oro-Nasal or Oro-Sinus Fistulae

AS MENTIONED ABOVE, these fistulae may be extremely difficult to close, even after multiple surgeries. A new product has come available which gives new hope for some of these hard to heal fistulae, but it is still in the experimental stages. It is only for cases we cannot heal in a conservative way or surgically, with tissue grafts. It is not able to be used as a first-stage repair, and requires prior surgical attempts at closure of the fistula to achieve a solid granulation bed into which to fix the specially-made titanium or zirconium plugs, called Stoll Fistula Implants.

The procedure is only used by specialist dental veterinarians who perform minimally invasive transbuccal surgery. It is early days yet, but I wanted to mention it. Images below.

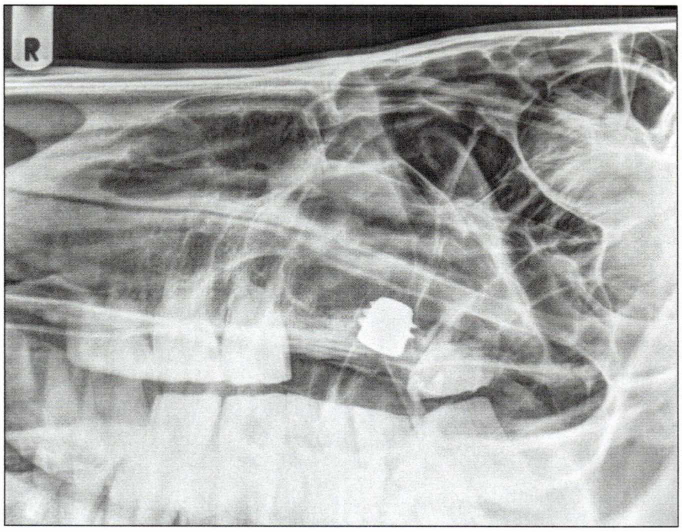

The Stoll Fistula Implant in place, visualized on radiograph. Image credit Dr Manfred Stoll.

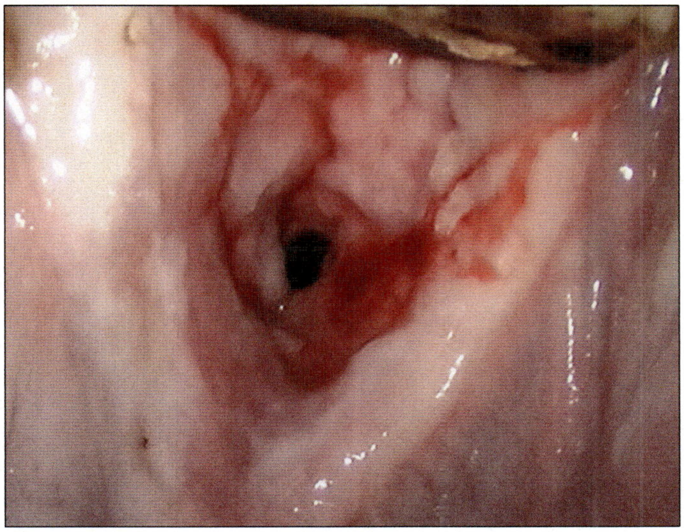

A problem fistula which hadn't closed after several surgical attempts. Image credit Dr Manfred Stoll.

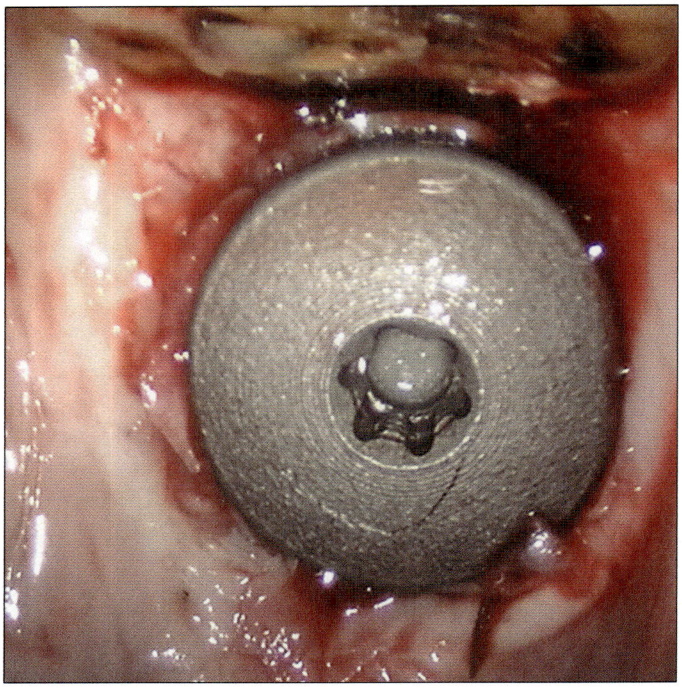

The Stoll Fistula Implant in place.
Image credit Dr Manfred Stoll.

CHAPTER TWELVE

HOW ARE GERIATRICS AND MINIATURES DENTALLY SPECIAL?

SOME HORSES ARE, if not more special than others, more of a worry than others. Come along and learn more about the special conditions and needs of geriatric and miniature equids.

Geriatrics, or the Oldies

OLDER EQUIDS NEED good dental care to live a comfortable life.

How do the oldies differ from younger animals?

As they age, they develop more irregular wear and ***calculus*** accumulation on ***incisors***, lower ***canines***, and the ***buccal*** side of the lower ***premolars***. Secondary to this calculus accumulation, they tend to suffer from ***gingivitis*** and ***periodontal disease***. Correction of the incisor and ***cheek tooth malocclusions*** can help prevent calculus accumulation.

Because horses are ***hypsodonts***, after ***eruption*** of a cheek tooth, it continues to grow in length until about two years after eruption, when its roots are fully developed and it stops growing. See Chapter 3, Anatomy of the Head. The tooth then moves toward the ***oral*** cavity (mouth) for a limited time until the tooth is worn out, or ***expired***, in a process called ***prolonged eruption***. Again, hypsodont teeth do not continue to *grow*, unlike rodents (e.g. rats) and lagomorphs (e.g. rabbits), whose teeth undergo ***continuous eruption*** and continue to grow throughout their lives. The equid incisors and canines are a little different in their development.

We see evidence of the aging process in the different stages of wear shown by teeth. The oldest ***cheek teeth*** in the mouth are the '09s, which show evidence of ***cupping*** when the horse is about 17 years old. Depending upon the feed the horse has eaten through its life, its dental care, and the environmental conditions under which the equid has lived (sandy, gritty desert or soft grassy ground), the wear levels of the teeth at different ages vary from horse to horse, but the sequence of wear in the teeth tend to be consistent. First, the teeth are abraded past the ***enamel***, and down to the softer dental ***tissues***, which quickly wear away, often breaking down and leaving tooth fragments and individual roots in the alveoli. Once the attachments are minimized, the teeth begin to loosen, and pain steps in. If the horse is lucky enough, he will gradually shed these loose teeth somewhere around 28-35 years of age. Unfortunately, any teeth still present in the opposing ***arcade*** may undergo ***crown elongation*** and cause soft tissue and bone trauma where the tooth has been lost, causing more pain and eating difficulty. Many horses are said to have "died of old age", when they probably starved due to neglected dentition. Horses can live well even if ***edentate***, or without teeth, if they are fed feeds appropriate to their condition. Generally, these include hay cubes, chaff (chopped hay), and complete feeds designed for geriatric horses. Your ***veterinarian*** can give you the best information regarding your horse's specific needs.

There are sedation protocols which assist in older horses to negate the need for heavy, more risky sedation using ***anxiolytic*** (anti-anxiety) drugs. See Chapter 23, How Can We Safely Sedate My Older Horse and Still Get the Job Done?.

Normal dental aging in the older horse

As normal ***attrition*** occurs, once the teeth have worn through the enamel, only the softer ***dentin*** is left. This dentin is yellow-tinted and feels smooth as glass when felt with the fingers, hence the association with the term "smooth-mouthed horse", which has historically been used for an older horse.

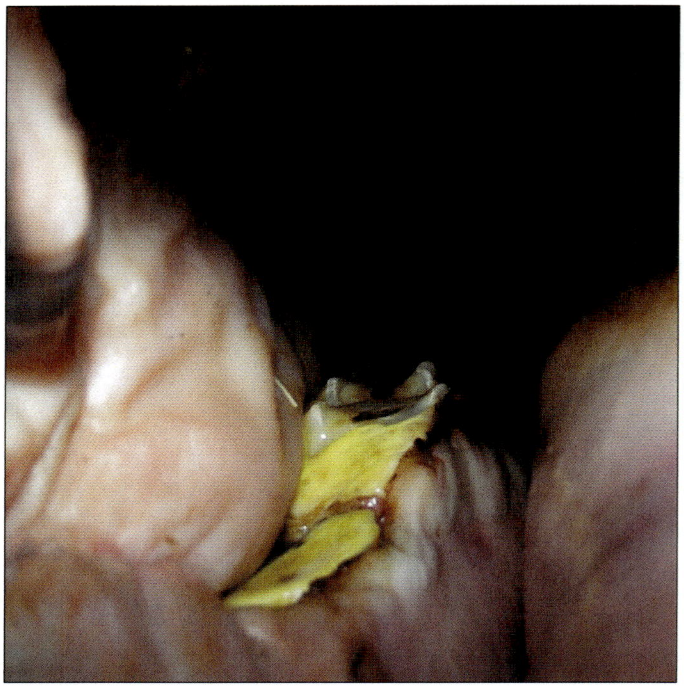

Good illustration of a "smooth-mouthed", or quite aged horse. The yellow portions shown feel smooth as glass, hence the name, because the tooth has been ground down past the sharper enamel. The most mesial tooth in the image and the mesial portion of the next tooth have undergone attrition past the enamel to the yellowed dentin. A little bit of white to ivory colored enamel is still visible on the tooth distal to this. Image credit Author.

Unfortunately, dentin is very soft and once the tooth wears down to the bifurcation of the root, the individual roots may be left behind as pictured in the X-ray above (right side). At some point they become mobile and painful.

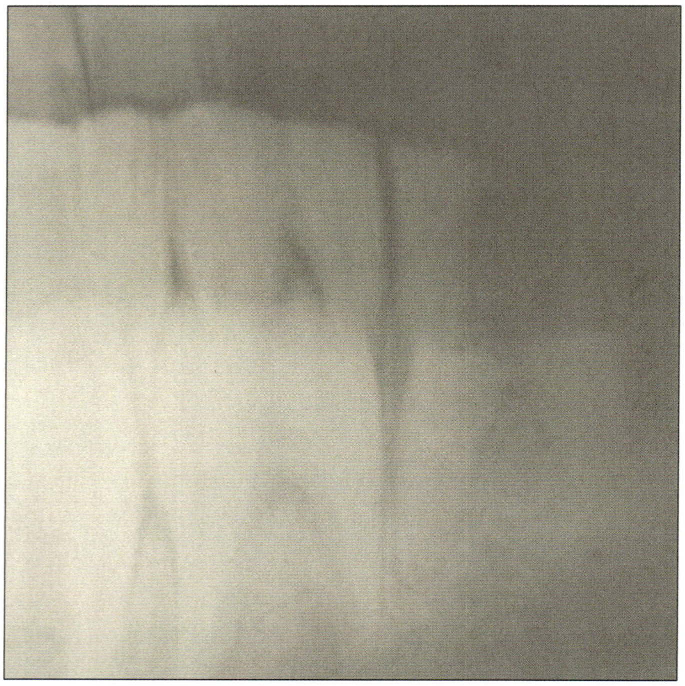

Retained dentinal roots (to the right) in an aged mare after rest of tooth has worn or fractured off. Image credit Author.

Malocclusions and mobile teeth

While attrition through the enamel to the dentin is normal as a horse ages, if malocclusions are permitted to exist, painful oral situations can arise quickly. If malocclusions such as crown elongations are allowed to remain when teeth are nearing the end of the life of their enamel, the elongated tooth will likely have more enamel, while the opposing tooth will likely have less and be worn

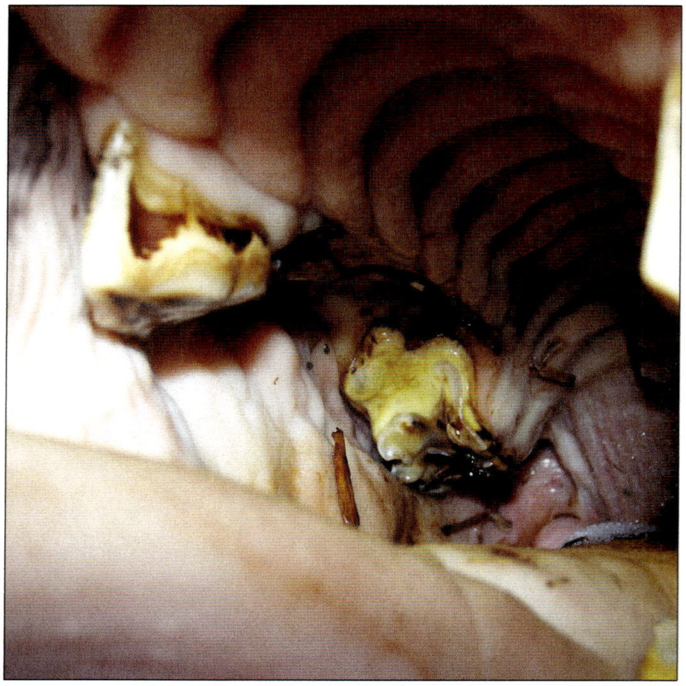

This is quite an aged horse with serious dental disease. 106 is present, but most of the 107 is now expiring. Malocclusion accompanied by attrition has eroded most of the enamel (the white part of the tooth) as well as much of the dentin (yellow) of the 108. Remaining teeth in this arcade are absent. Image credit Author.

away to dentin first. The enamel of the elongated tooth will quickly erode the dentin of the opposing tooth, and cause problems such as seen in the figures on this page. See also Chapter 14 for an excellent endoscopic view of another horse with neglected odontoplasty.

If your geriatric horses have been receiving thorough dental examinations on a yearly or six-monthly basis, they should not have significant crown elongations. They will have the best chance of keeping their teeth for longer, as ***sharp enamel points*** and malocclusions will probably have been eliminated long ago.

However, if this has been neglected, it's difficult to play catch-up once the horse has aged, but it is possible. In the older horse which hasn't been having effective dentistry, there may be many problems, such as large crown elongations, waves, ***diastemata***, mobile teeth, etc.

In this case, it may be a good idea to stage the treatment: I.e. to start by extracting the loose teeth and perform the ***odontoplasty*** on the first visit, and progressively treat the horse over several more visits. A major overhaul on an older horse all at once may cause so much damage there will be a high risk of post-treatment pain, which may be life-threatening. They may not be able to cope with irritation around teeth with short crowns and roots, ***inflammation*** of the ***temporomandibular joints***, possible dentinal exposure, and muscle inflammation.

Often an older horse's eating becomes slower or he stops wanting to eat certain feeds. If this occurs, a dental examination is indicated. There may be a malocclusion which was missed on a previous exam, a tooth which has become mobile and painful, or EOTRH may be present and becoming worse. Extracting these loose teeth or fragments, or removing the worst EOTRH-affectd teeth usually results in the horse bouncing back. Our horses need help from us to keep their teeth in a functional and pain-free state at any age, but for the elderly horse, it is even more important.

As mentioned before, I don't know of many horses who have died of what people term "old age". I have, however, seen plenty die when their dentition was so neglected they basically starved to death, likely because tooth elongations into opposing jaws caused so much pain, they couldn't eat enough feed to live. For more information, see Chapter 6, Developmental and Acquired Conditions: Malocclusions.

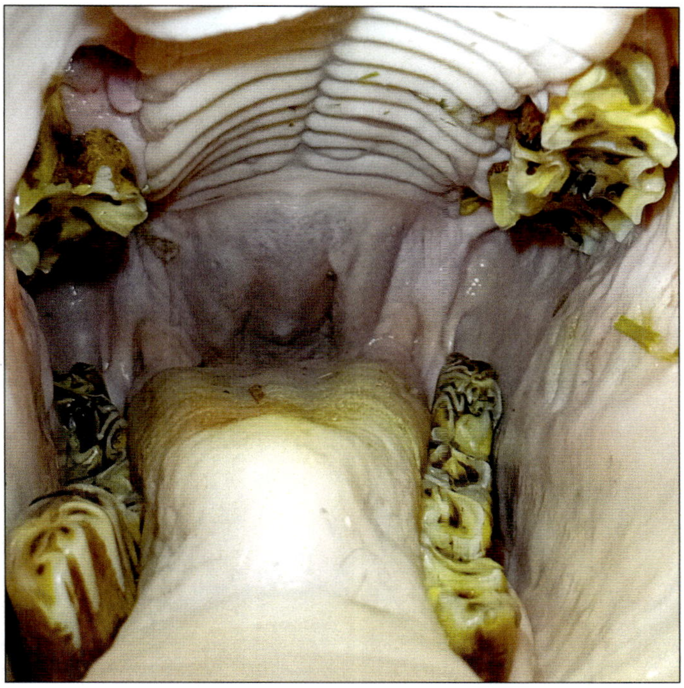

This geriatric horse's mouth has been unmonitored for years. Severe crown elongations of the 311, 406, and 411 are impinging upon soft tissue and likely bone in the absence of complete teeth in the opposing arcade, causing severe, painful injury in several locations. The "good" teeth and surrounding gingiva display a host of pathology: infundibular caries, periodontal disease, gingivitis, buccal ulceration from sharp enamel points due to the loss of cementum. These teeth are in varying stages of cupping and expiring. Image credit Dr Elke Pollaris.

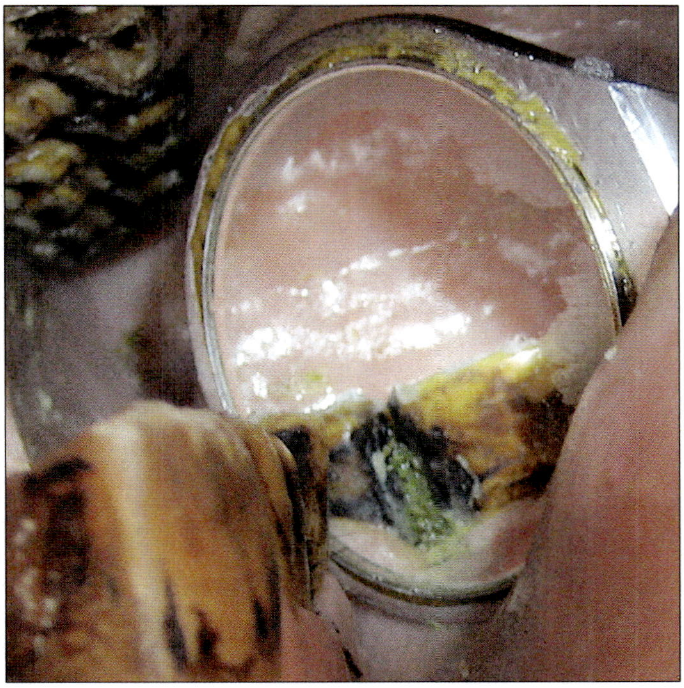

Diastemata may one of the most, if not the most, painful of all the dental pathologies. And they have to eat with those teeth sixteen hours per day. Here is a feed-filled diastema. The periodontal pocket was over 20 millimeters deep. Diastemata require pain relief (not just sedation) to treat effectively and painlessly. Image credit Author.

Equine Odontoclastic Tooth Resorption & Hypercementosis Syndrome (EOTRH)

Older horses are at risk of Equine Odontoclastic Tooth Resorption and Hypercementosis (***EOTRH***) as well. It is becoming more and more commonly diagnosed in horses 13-15+ years old as veterinarians become aware of this relatively recently described condition. The disease condition was in existence before it was described in the literature, but no one had named it before. A presumptive diagnosis may be made by clinical signs, but radiographic confirmation is needed for the diagnosis and staging. There are many ongoing studies examining this condition around the veterinary medical world. Veterinarians have been characterizing details of the disease and attempting to find a cure, but at this stage, the only definitive curative treatment is extraction of affected teeth. Luckily, horses do surprisingly well with no incisors. Certainly, better than they do with multiple painful incisors left in place.

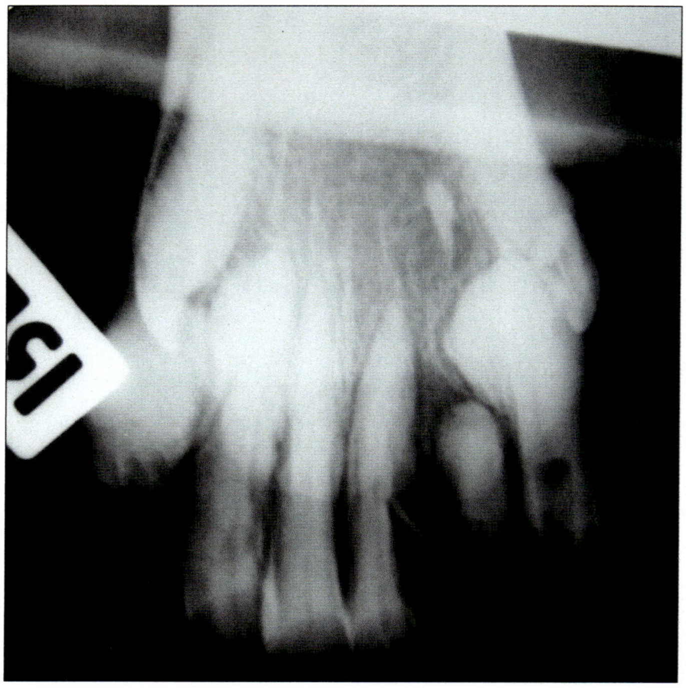

Radiograph of EOTRH patient incisors showing tooth resorption and hypercementosis. Different equids show these signs to varying degrees. Image credit Author.

To give you an idea of how painful EOTRH is, after the extraction surgery of one geriatric horse, I found him stripping the leaves from a stand of bamboo plants growing in his paddock the next day (thank you, Snow... glad you didn't take your sutures out...). He was eating his feed better than he had pre-extraction, despite having six incisors and seven mobile teeth extracted.

If you wish to learn more about this exceedingly painful condition, see Chapter 7, EOTRH, and learn about the "carrot test", which you can do with your own horses. For even more details, see the Bibliography and Further Reading for a survey article on EOTRH I published in a 2022 veterinary publication.

Diastemata and periodontal disease

While some diastemata occur due to anatomy, generally diastemata and periodontal disease can be kept in check and mostly prevented by consistent, regular, thorough examination and treatment. Correction of malocclusions, including sharp enamel points, help prevent these conditions from occurring or worsening. Because horses' teeth taper from ***occlusal*** surface to ***apex***, with increasing age and continued eruption and attrition, the diameter of their occlusal surface decreases, which results in the ***interproximal spaces*** becoming wider. This leaves wider gaps, or diastemata, where feed can accumulate and predispose to periodontal disease and tooth death.

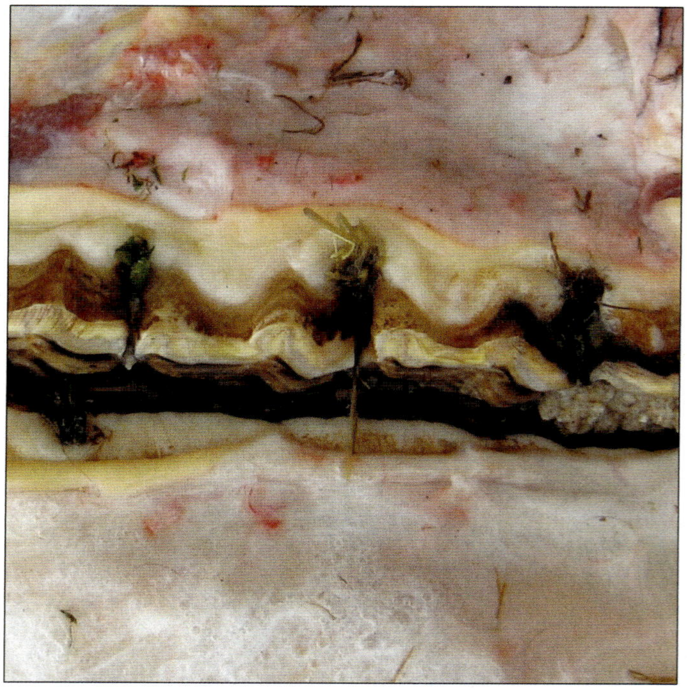

Widespread diastemata and likely PPID in this deceased aged horse cadaver. Image credit Author.

Feeding honey, sugar or molasses (this includes peppermints and other candies or lollies, as well as some commercial "horse treats" and horse feeds!) is detrimental to the health of your horse's teeth, no matter their age. In older horses with periodontal disease, feeding these sweet treats is especially ***contraindicated***, as metabolism of the sugar creates an acidic pH in the mouth which may contribute to periodontal disease. When periodontal disease is compounded with certain types of diastemata, such as valve diastemata, it becomes more difficult to treat. There are new ways of contouring the teeth adjacent to a diastema which are showing promise in diastema therapy. Frequent dental examination with judicious odontoplasty plus evacuation and flushing of the diastemata is essential to maintain your older horse's health if these problems are occurring. See more information about diastemata and periodontal disease in Chapter 6, Developmental and Acquired Conditions.

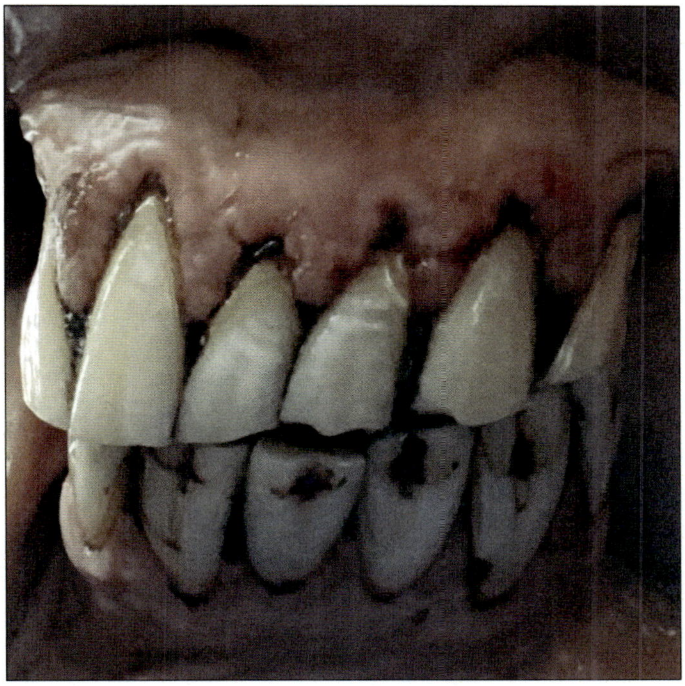

This mouth of this geriatric horse with PPID has some seriously painful periodontal disease and probably a lot more. EOTRH is a possibility, but radiographs are needed to confirm that diagnosis. Image credit Dr Elke Pollaris.

Pituitary Pars Intermedia Dysfunction (PPID)

The endocrine disease Pituitary Pars Intermedia Dysfunction (PPID), (also referred to as Cushing's Syndrome or Disease), causes high levels of the horse's own steroids to be released from the adrenal cortex into the bloodstream, causing immunosuppression, amongst other chemical changes from the disease. Some of the effects of the steroid release are inhibition of proper wound healing, impaired ability to fight infections, and initiation of other conditions such as laminitis. It is most common in older horses, and many of aged horses with widespread diastemata, non-healing wounds, or periodontal disease may be suffer from this condition, but not yet diagnosed. There are effective therapies for this condition now.

In an older patient it is wise to test for adrenal function before you get too far with extensive dental treatment. If the horse is positive for PPID, it may benefit by treatment first, then when immune function is restored, dental therapy is more likely to have a positive outcome. See more information about PPID in Chapter 6, Developmental and Acquired Conditions.

Preop and postop... Take special care of your oldies!

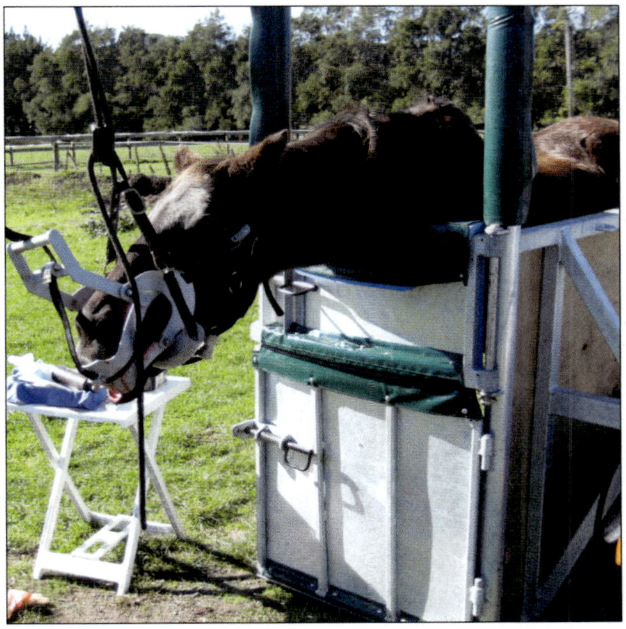

Take special pre-op and post-op care of your aged horses after surgery. While your veterinarian will take care as well with their sedation, likely including IV fluid support and stocks, your geriatric's organs are not what they used to be! Follow your veterinarian's feeding advice to get the best resolution of their condition. Image credit Author.

Miniature Horses... A Special Kind of Trouble?

MINIATURE HORSES (MINIATURES, or minis) and small ponies are special in many ways... and not always for the better. They might be cute and lovable, but they suffer if they don't get the dental care they may so badly need.

Their size makes them difficult to treat as well. Sheer logistics, including the proximity of their heads to the ground and the extremely small mouths make for challenging work. Before I had my portable ***stocks***, I used to do mini dentistry like this (below).

Luckily, the lowest door on the front of my Equi-Still Stocks is the perfect height for most minis to rest their chins upon.

When people breed for small ponies and miniature horses, the genetics which result in a smaller equid also result in a smaller mouth and jaw. Unfortunately, in this human-bred "evolution", the reduction of tooth size has been much delayed when compared to the decrease in size

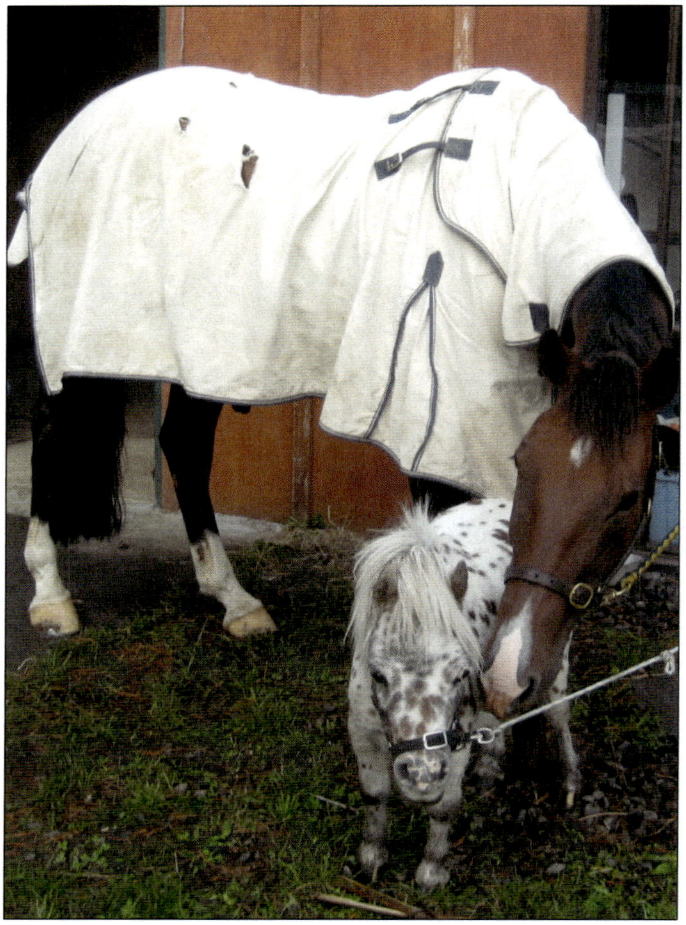

Adorable next to my big harness horse, but this little guy's mouth was... not. It was quite crowded, at best. Image credit Author.

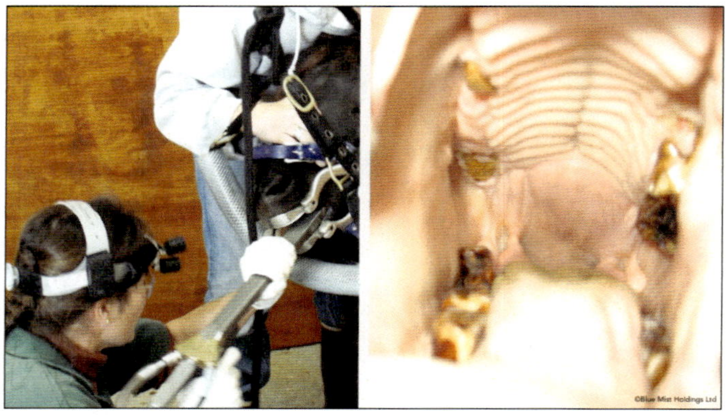

Mini dentistry on the floor, before the stocks! Image credit Author.

of the mouth. Hence, the bones of the jaw which support the teeth are very small, but the teeth are still overlarge... only marginally smaller than their larger horse counterparts. As you might imagine, this causes overcrowding of the teeth and resultant impactions and displacement. Think about this for a moment. See Chapters 3 and Chapter 6 for details about anatomy, eruption, impactions, and displacement of teeth.

This poor correspondence in size can create a lifetime of misery for miniatures if their teeth are not monitored from an early age and correctly and consistently cared for by an experienced practitioner. Even then, it's not all roses for them.

For these reasons, miniature horses and small ponies are at risk of delayed eruption, retained deciduous teeth, dental dysplasia (teeth improperly formed), oligodontia or hypodontia (developmentally missing teeth), dental

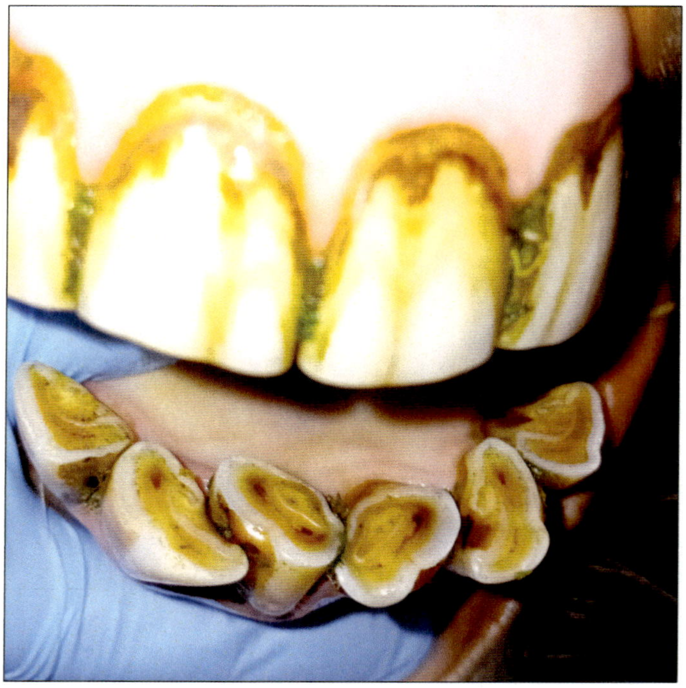

This miniature's incisors are crowded and misaligned. Since they are not correctly packed into a tight arcade, the diastemata between the teeth are packing feed and causing periodontal disease. Image credit Dr Elke Pollaris.

impactions (because of insufficient room for teeth to correctly erupt), maleruptions (teeth erupting where they should not), and the conditions which occur as a result of these, such as colic and choke.

Add in their extremely small size, which makes access to any of the teeth, much less the ***distal*** cheek teeth, difficult. Couple that with the requirement for miniature

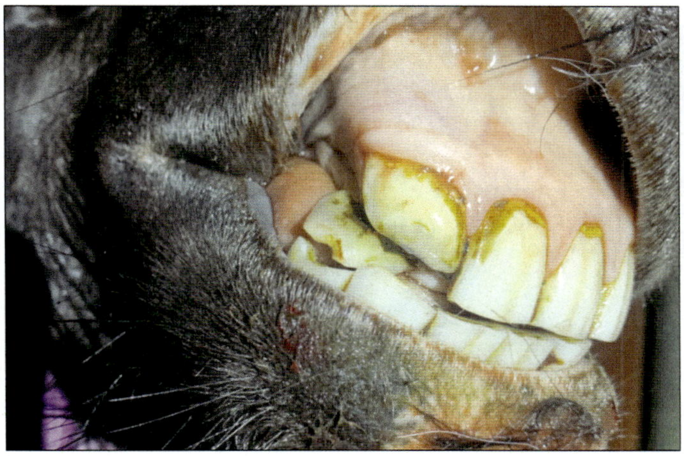

Retained deciduous incisor in a miniature. Image credit Author.

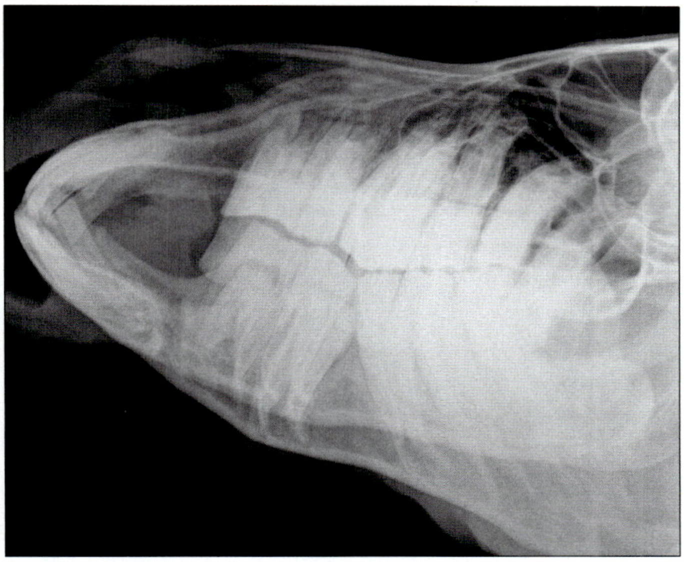

This mini has had some severe problems in its life so far, and without a lot of help, things will be getting worse. Several deciduous caps have been retained, there is oligodontia (developmentally missing teeth), crown elongations (overgrowths), and misalignments. Unfortunately, this is far from uncommon. Image credit Dr Amy Ardern

and strong equipment, and the challenges compound. In addition to these mini-prevalent challenges, miniatures have all the other malocclusions seen in full-sized horses as well.

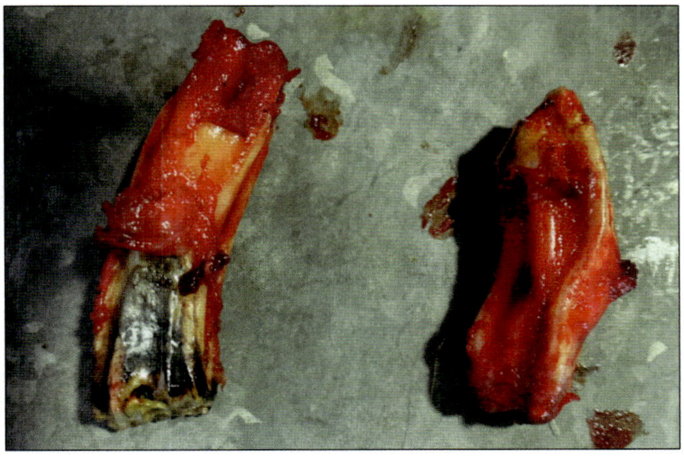

210 and 211 from a 6-year-old miniature horse. The 211 is dysplastic and was a challenge to extract, due to its shape as well as to the fact there was little room to work. They were both extracted intraorally. Image credit Author.

A recent study on 100 miniature horses has shed light on what were previously anecdotal reports in the literature, with no research to back them up. Full details are available from the paper cited in Bibliography and Further Reading. This study, recently published at the time this book is going to print, confirmed what so many of us already suspected from the examination and treatment of the miniature horses in our dental practices: namely, that as the breeders of these equids, we have created an extremely difficult situation for these small horses in our care. While this information might be new to some owners of miniature horses, most dental practitioners won't be surprised at the researcher's findings:

- Most common disease noted: crown elongation (74% of horses, mostly '06s and '11s) followed by oral mucosal ulceration (67% of horses), diastemata (34%), class 1 malocclusions (misalignments or displaced teeth) (34%), and hypodontia (12% with no history of tooth extraction had total of 19 missing teeth). (Note that while "sharp enamel points" were not regarded as a disease, the mucosal ulceration from them *was*.)
- 95% of the 100 miniatures had from one to five types of different dental diseases.
- Due to the high number of '06 and '11 crown elongations, the researchers suggested many miniatures in this population may have a mismatch in occlusion of the dental arcades despite matching mandibular and maxillary lengths.
- Of serious significance for miniature owners is the finding that body condition score (BCS) did not correlate with a decreased incidence of disease, on the contrary, the horses with a higher BCS had a higher prevalence of dental disease!
- 34% of miniatures in the study had one or more misaligned tooth. More than 50% of these are incisors. These misaligned teeth will predispose them to secondary periodontal disease, pain, and tooth loss.
- Prevalence of diastema and crown elongations increases with age of miniature horse.

- Hypodontia, especially of the '08s and the '11s, occurs frequently. 12% of these miniatures which have never had extractions (as far as the owners knew) had missing teeth— ten times the prevalence of that in non-miniature horses, which is 1%.
- The researchers hypothesized that the high frequency of hypodontia in the '08 positions and dysplasia of the '11s may be due to their proportionately large teeth and small skulls result in impingement, or overlap, of the denticles or tooth buds. As the '08s and '11s are the last teeth to develop, it makes sense these cannot properly develop because of sheer lack of space to grow.
- There was a significant correlation between increasing head width (not muzzle) and displaced teeth, primarily in the incisors.

And the conclusion? The researchers recommended early and frequent oral examinations as part of miniature horse preventative health programs to identify dental disease and effectively manage these potentially painful conditions. If dental disease is not identified, it cannot be treated. These wee creatures drew the short straw in life in terms of their teeth. Please look after them with regular six-monthly examinations and necessary treatment, just as you would after an extraction if any of the conditions we've just discussed exist and give them the best life possible.

Thank you for caring for them.

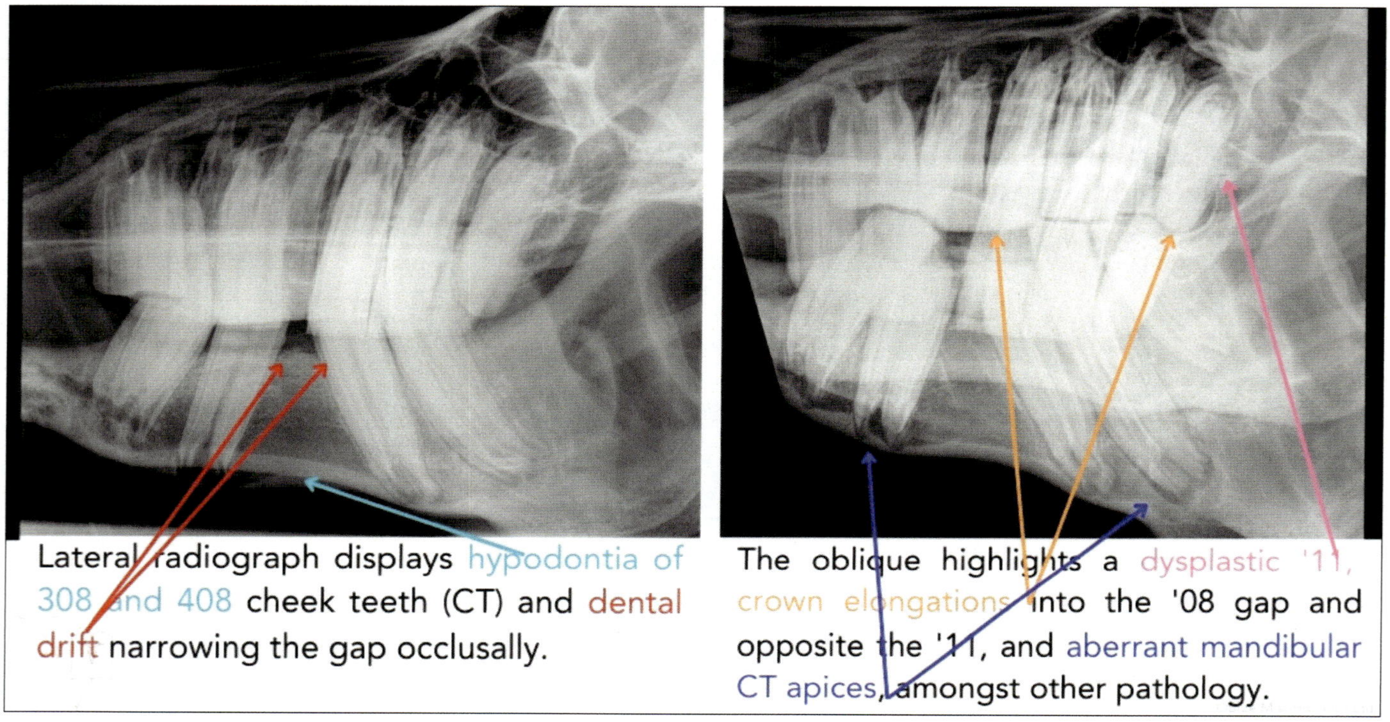

Quite a bit of the pathology we have just discussed appears in this image. Take a look! Image credit Author.

Cheek teeth

Have you ever noticed any of these small equids (miniatures or small ponies) with a very "boxy" head at around 3-6 years old, often with hard, bony bumps below and in front of their eyes, or under their ***mandibles***? These bumps are known as ***eruption cysts***, sometimes called "eruption bumps" or "tooth bumps".

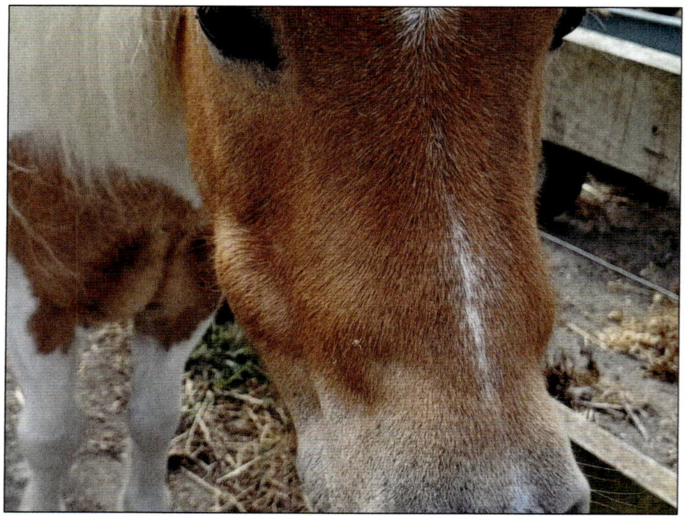

Mini's face bulging in so many directions... because the teeth are so large for their little heads...Image credit Dr Amy Ardern.

They form as a normal result of eruption, as long as they do not "persist", or continue to be present. Non-persistent eruption cysts are a normal part of eruption, as discussed in Chapter 6, Developmental and Acquired Conditions: Masses, Tumors... Normal eruption cysts are visible on radiographic exam and develop around the ***apices*** of the ***permanent teeth*** as they force the corresponding deciduous teeth out of the alveolus and into the mouth to enable the permanent teeth to erupt. However, as said before, eruption cysts are are "normal" until they are not... in some young horses, and in many miniatures and small ponies, delayed eruption and/or dental impactions make the eruption cysts persist long after they should. How does this happen? A "cap", or a remnant of the corresponding deciduous tooth, may be retained (stuck in place and not shed), or there may be an impaction due to a barrier to eruption, such as insufficient room between the '07 and '09 which won't allow the '08 to erupt into the mouth.

If an impaction occurs, a hard, bony swelling ***rostral*** to the eyes (for maxillary teeth) and/or on the ventral portion of the mandible (for mandibular teeth) may develop. This is due to the buildup of high hydrostatic pressure in the eruption cysts which isn't being relieved by eruption of the permanent tooth and possibly its unshed deciduous tooth.

If the impactions are not relieved and an anachoretic pulpitis occurs, extraction will be required to correct this painful and often messy condition. The miniature on the bottom right has just had his sinus flushed after extraction surgery involving the maxillary ***sinuses***.

So, in other words with many of these tiny equids, there simply isn't enough room in the mouth and thus the eruption pathway is blocked— not allowing the permanent teeth to erupt. This occurs in full-sized equids, but is found with much greater frequency in miniatures, resulting in several challenges. Because the eruption pathway is blocked, their unerupted permanent teeth may:

- enter the mouth but erupt rotated or displaced buccally (toward the cheek), palatally (toward the roof of mouth), or lingually (toward the tongue). This results in unopposed teeth (no tooth opposite to it to grind against), which causes crown elongations and trauma to nearby soft tissues in the horse's mouth. Incorrect tooth apposition also causes gaps between adjacent teeth, resulting in feed impaction and diastemata. If a conservative approach is selected, treatment may require frequent evacuation and flushing of these diastemata and six-monthly-for-life odontoplasty to keep overgrowths in check. If extraction of the affected tooth is chosen, six-monthly-odontoplasty-for-life will be required for same reason.
- not erupt into the mouth. As with other equids, normal eruption cysts develop around the apices of the permanent teeth as they try to force the corresponding deciduous teeth or any other barrier to eruption out of the way. In rare cases, periapical infections may occur at the site of these eruption cysts 6-12 months after eruption, even if the permanent tooth does erupt These usually result in infection and risk the life of the tooth. Discharging tracts out the side of the face or under the jaw are sometimes the first clue that there

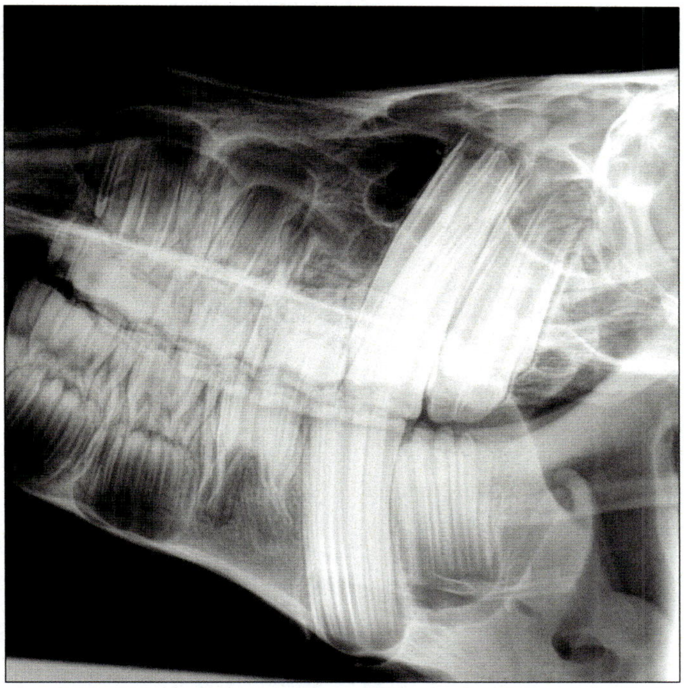

Those teeth on a mini fill up the whole head! Between the deciduous teeth stacked up with the permanents, the only place their skull over the teeth apices can go is outward, to create bulging little faces. Combine these overly large teeth and small jaws with the fact that the fourth premolar, the '08, erupts into the mouth last and must squeeze its way in-between the '07 and the '09, and it can be a recipe for apical infection and extraction. Image credit Dr Amy Ardern.

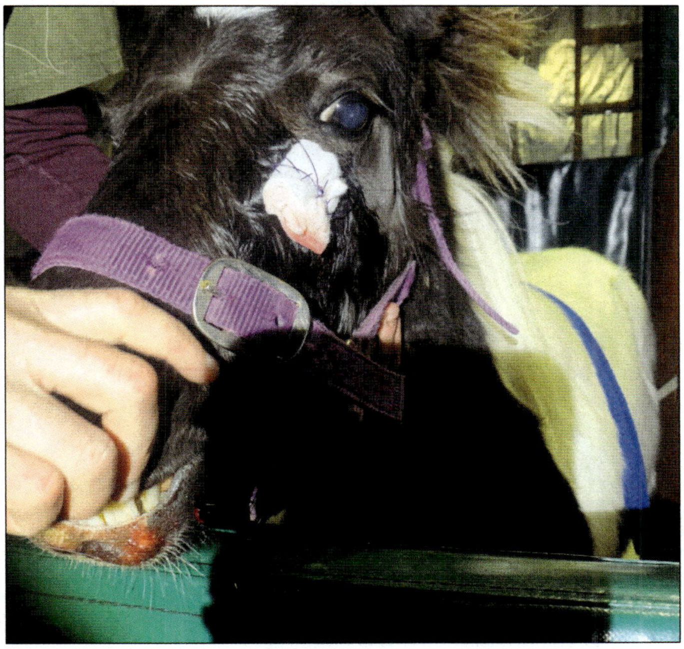

This miniature horse had a unilateral (one-sided) purulent nasal discharge, periapical infections, and an oro-maxillary fistula. He is shown in recovery with his chin on the padded bottom door of my stocks after his double extraction, including the dysplastic 211 shown above. A small tube has been inserted into his maxillary sinus (and a protective stent bandage stitched in place) for post-operative repeat flushing of the sinus. Their tiny mouths and massive teeth make extractions, even with specialized small equipment, challenging. I am grateful to have small hands on Mini-extraction days. Image credit Author.

is an infected, and probably dead, tooth requiring immediate treatment.

- erupt into a position which result in overly large interproximal spaces, which are "developmental diastemata" and trap feed to cause periodontal disease. Painful periodontal pockets form, and ascending infections work their way toward the apex, which if the causes are not addressed, can cause tooth death, and require extraction with its subsequent six-monthly-odontoplasty-for-life. See Chapter 6, Developmental and Acquired Conditions.

For more information about extractions, see Chapter 15, Veterinary Specific Techniques.

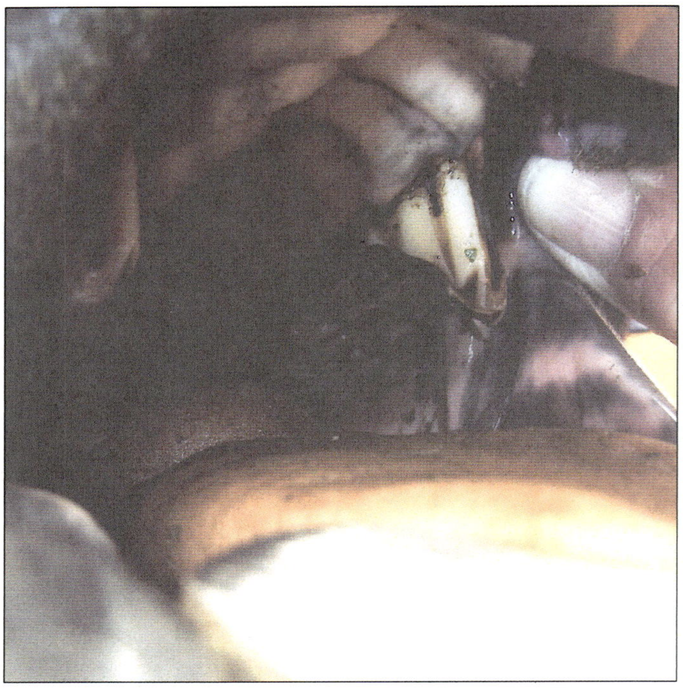

Severe 106 and 206 hooks in a mini. There were corresponding 311 and 411 hooks at the back of his mouth. Image credit Author.

Incisors

For many of the same reasons as in the Cheek Teeth section above, miniatures and small ponies have incisor difficulties as well.

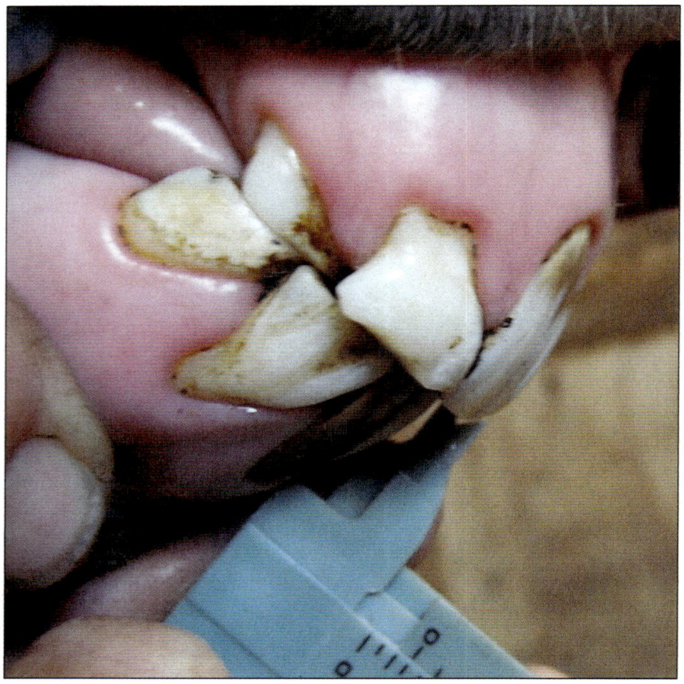

Brachygnathism in a young miniature horse. Image credit Author.

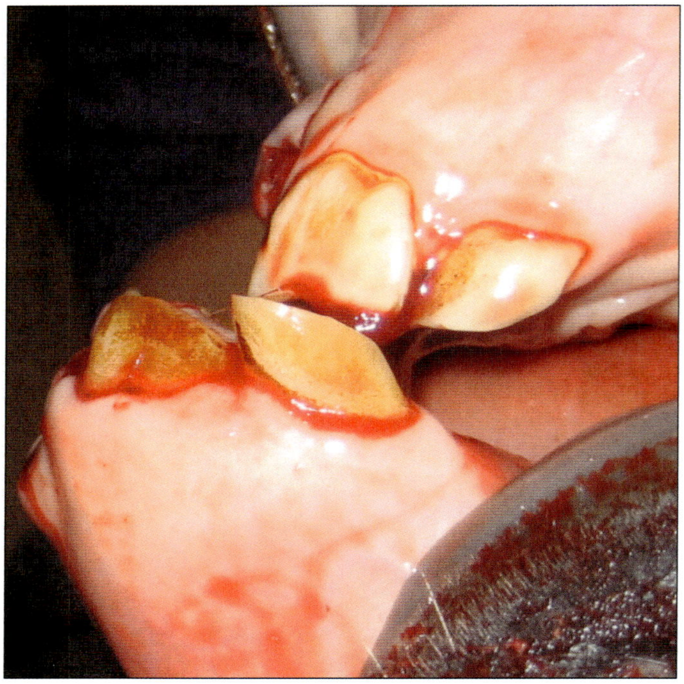

Prognathism, sow mouth, or monkey mouth with retained 101, 202, 301, and 401 in a young miniature horse. Image credit Author.

Their incisors often have malocclusions such as ***brachygnathism***, ***prognathism***, crown elongations, misaligned teeth, retained or impacted deciduous teeth, diastemata with feed impaction and periodontal disease. Many of these cause pain and lead to tooth death. See Chapter 3 and Chapter 6.

In miniatures and small ponies, certain incisors (often the '03s) may erupt in a reverse or otherwise abnormal direction (malpositioned), which causes not only tooth impaction, but also diastemata accompanied by feed impaction with subsequent periodontal disease. These cause constant pain and if these malpositioned teeth are not extracted, may result in pain, tooth death and the need for subsequent extraction.

An incisor diastema is a gap between incisors, often packed tightly with feed. Portions of opposing teeth may erupt unchecked into the diastema and further widen it.

Those individuals who breed horses, especially miniatures, can benefit the horses of the future if they begin to take oral conformation and prevalence of disease linked to this conformation into consideration when making decisions regarding which horses they select to breed or not to breed. This would prevent unnecessary pain and suffering.

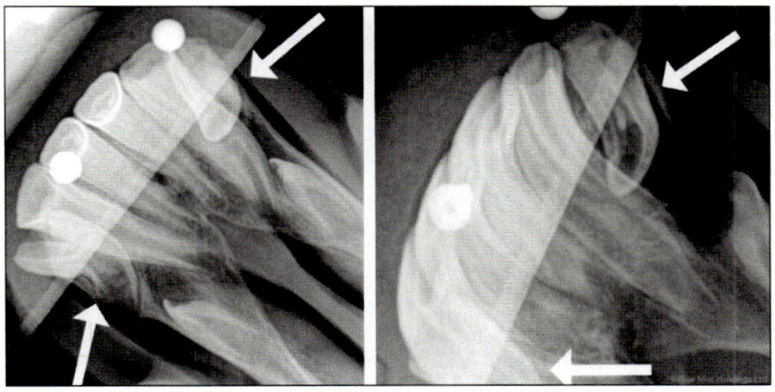

Malpositioned 303 and 403 (corner incisors) in this miniature horse with a Class 1 MAL (malocclusion). Image credit Author.

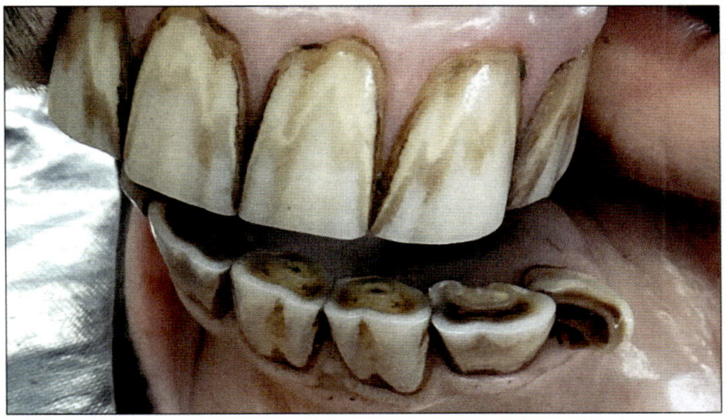

Malpositioned 303 in this miniature. Image credit Dr Elke Pollaris.

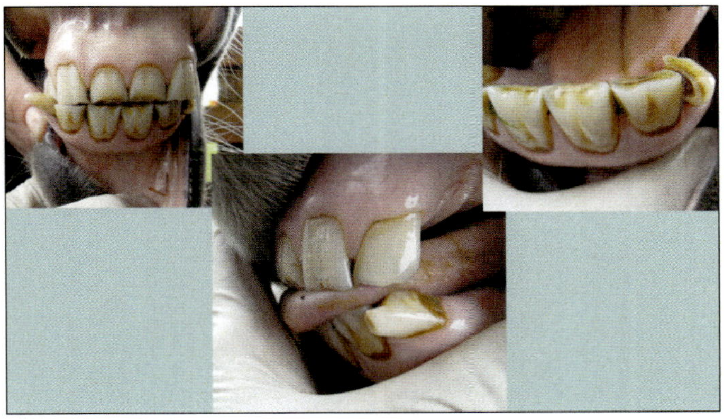

The same miniature horse in radiographs above. Maleruptions can lead to painful lives. Image credit Author.

In conclusion, there *are* ways to make mini dentistry more fun! Even tiny miniatures can be treated in stocks, for their comfort and safety!

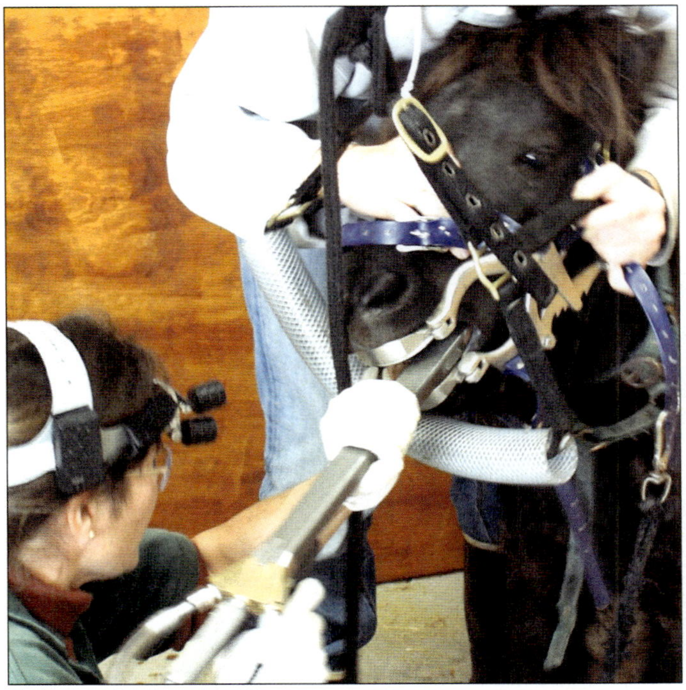

Yes, it can be tricky, but you can do it! Image credit Author.

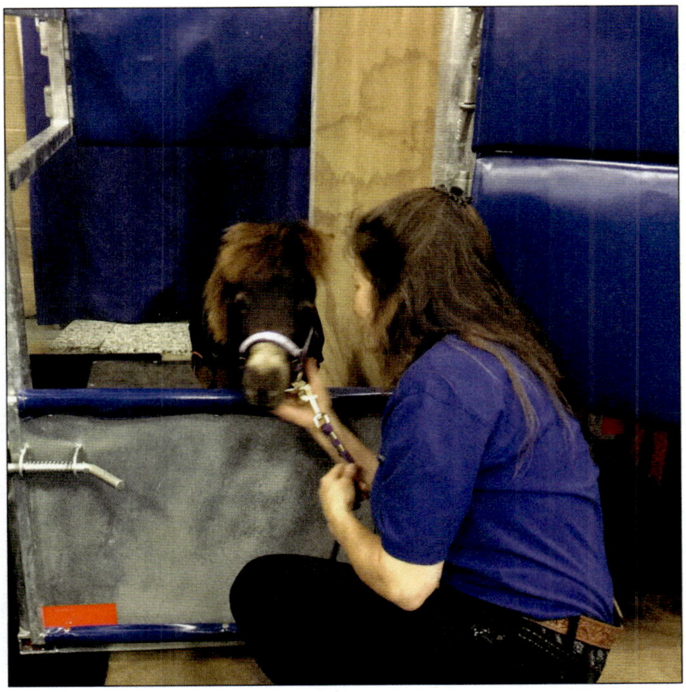

This tiny mini at AAEP veterinary meeting wanted to check out the stocks! He fit perfectly on the first door. Image credit Matthew Mole.

CHAPTER THIRTEEN

SUMMING UP PATHOLOGY… IT'S YOUR TURN

NOW THAT YOU'VE been through the ***pathology*** which may occur in horses' mouths, please go back to the Chapter 2, Eight Levels of Dentistry. Look at the images and descriptions of the eight levels and think about the pathological conditions you've seen in the past chapters. At which levels can you see this pathology, and at which levels will the pathology will be missed during an examination?

Now You Can Ask YOURSELF the Big Questions From Chapter 2 and Most Likely Come Up With Some More Informed Answers:

(and maybe write them down!)

1 – ***What are some types of pathology which may be missed at each of the Eight Levels of Dentistry?***

2 – Which level of examination do I desire for my own horse, and why?

____

____

____

____

____

____

____

____

3 -- Which level of examination should my horse have before I decide that his behavioral problem isn't due to oral or dental pain?

____

____

____

I'm not trying to tell you which level of dentistry you must choose. My purpose in writing this book is to offer you the opportunity to make an informed choice. I know which I would choose, but as I've always done in my equine veterinary practice, I offer people enough information to make informed choices, then find out which way they want to go. It's up to them. They must live with their decisions, as I must live with mine.

Now it's your turn to decide.

CHAPTER FOURTEEN

ODONTOPLASTY vs. "FLOATING? WHAT'S THE DIFFERENCE?

NOW WE'RE DOWN to the ***odontoplasty*** itself. It's important to know what odontoplasty really is, what should happen when odontoplasty is about to begin, and what should (and should not) happen afterwards!

What ... and is not... Odontoplasty?

WHILE SOME DEFINE "odontoplasty" as identical to "***floating*** ", I prefer to define odontoplasty as the *informed* redefining, contouring, or ***rasping*** of the teeth. To achieve the "informed" portion of this definition requires a thorough ***oral*** examination to be performed prior to rasping or filing, otherwise it is simply waving a rasp around in the darkness. "Floating", or smoothing down the sharp ***buccal*** or ***lingual enamel*** points (generally these locations, but may be needed in other areas) of the ***cheek teeth*** or ***incisors*** of horses with a rasp (either hand floating or power floating), can be done in the absence of an examination, but as you may have gathered throughout this book, ***pathology*** will be missed. Further, unnecessary reduction of teeth can shorten a horse's life. While floating has been performed for over hundreds of years, there is little to no scientific-based evidence to support general floating. The enamel ridges, ***sharp enamel points***, and transverse ridges may likely improve your horse's ability to chew forage, but sometimes as they become more pronounced, they can become "malocclusions" and cause problems such as interference with other teeth or injury to soft ***tissue***. This, then, helps further define "odontoplasty" as specific ***crown*** reduction dictated by a thorough examination which tells the operator which teeth should have their crowns shaped and reduced, and exactly how this should be done. See Chapter 2, Eight Levels of Dentistry, and Chapter 4, Examination of the Mouth for more details on thorough examinations.

Informed Consent in the Equine Dental World? How Do I Get That?

READERS MUST GAIN enough clear, understandable information from their registered and licensed ***veterinarian*** or lay dental operator/EDT to give their informed consent before attending at any dental procedures or allowing any dental procedures to be performed on their horses. Other medical professionals must gain informed consent from their patients or their patient's guardians as well. What is informed consent? In a nutshell, informed consent is that consent given after the reader has been given specific details on sedation, the dental examination, and treatment in a clear and understandable manner. The reader must have the opportunity to have their questions answered and have any aspects of the upcoming procedure clarified if they wish. The transparency and choice provided by all of the above empower the reader to make informed choices regarding their equids' care. It is essential to understand the potential risks and benefits associated with such procedures and to be able to make informed decisions based on professional advice. See the DISCLAIMER section for a more detailed discussion of requirements for informed consent.

What is a Pre-Odontoplasty Check?

AS MENTIONED IN Chapter 10, Head Trauma and Dental Pathology, it is vital that your veterinarian performs an examination of the head, heart, lungs, etc., as discussed in Chapter 4, Examination of the Mouth. Before placing a speculum into the mouth and opening it to perform an oral examination, it is especially important to manually examine the head for any pain and mobility, including manipulation of the ***mandible*** and evaluation of the ***temporomandibular joints***. This is especially important after a fall while jumping or after other trauma. Opening a speculum on a horse with a fractured skull can ***exacerbate*** a fracture. If the fracture was an incomplete one, opening a speculum may make it complete, or it may displace a not-previously-displaced one. If a fracture is suspected, radiographs are essential before progressing. The ***incisors*** should be examined for signs of ***EOTRH*** before placing a speculum, as any pressure on those teeth can cause severe pain to the horse.

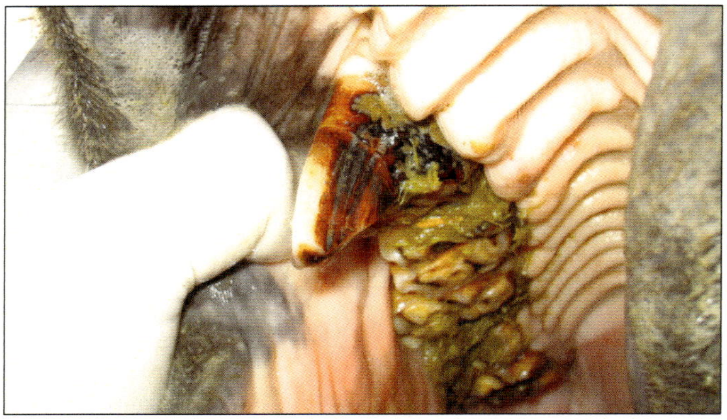

Severe crown elongation of the 106 into the opposing mandible itself. This horse must have severe osteomyelitis and incredible pain. Image credit Prof. Padraic Dixon.

Below three images: severe maxillary cheek teeth crown elongations into the space of the opposing mandibular arcade and mandible itself and periodontal disease. Images credit Dr Manfred Stoll.

What is Odontoplasty?

ODONTOPLASTY IS THE informed filing of teeth (meaning a thorough exam has been performed, problems diagnosed and noted BEFORE any rasping begins) to create a mouth that is comfortable and anatomically correct for the specific horse by removing only the pain-causing sharp enamel points and correcting malocclusions so as to eliminate interference with other teeth. Odontoplasty is not the wholesale destruction of occlusal angles nor over-reduction of incisors or cheek teeth. It is not overheating the teeth with a power instrument and not cooling teeth appropriately. Only excessive tooth which is creating problems for a horse should be reduced. The images on this spread show horses displaying the results of neglected odontoplasty.

In the Chapter 6, Developmental and Acquired Conditions, we discussed the damage some ***sharp enamel points*** (SEPs) can cause when a horse opens its mouth or moves its mandible sideways to chew. The ***maxillary*** cheek teeth come into increasing contact with the buccal ***gingival mucosa*** as the mouth is opened further or the jaw is moved sideways. SEPs on these teeth

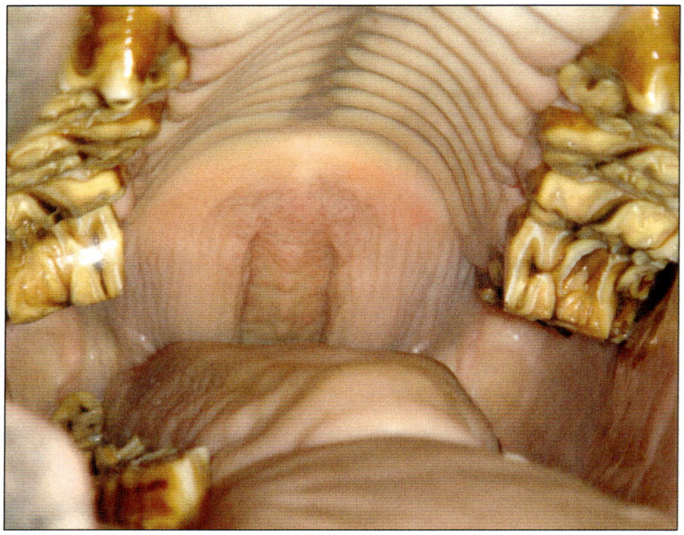

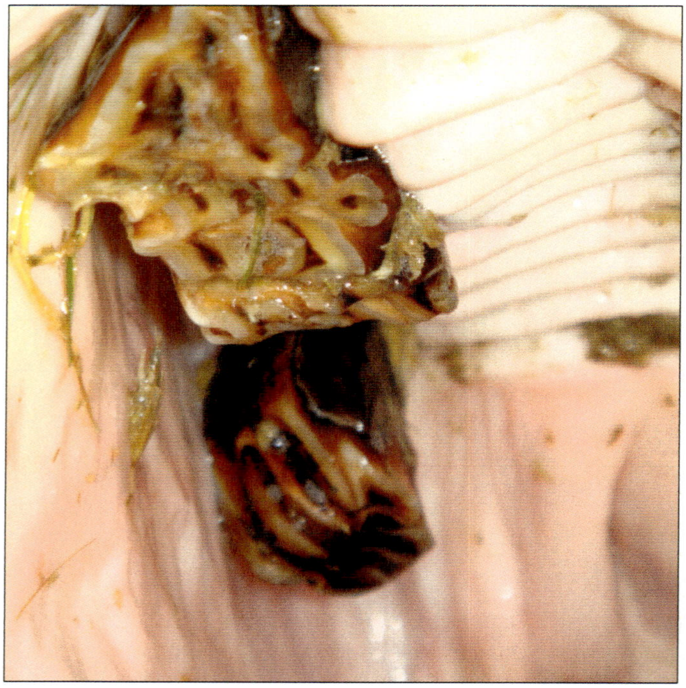

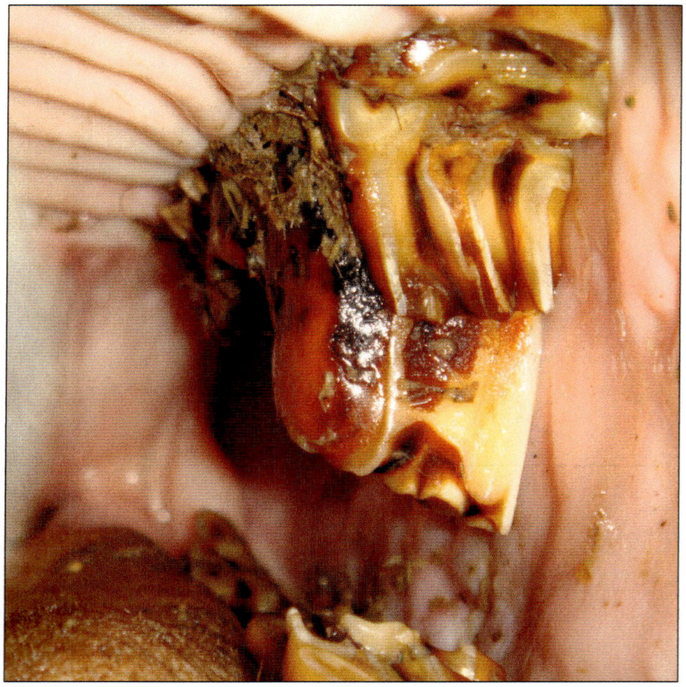

can ***lacerate*** the gingival mucosa lining the cheeks as they are pulled tightly over these projections, causing oral ulcers. Any of you who have experienced an oral ulcer know how painful it is, and that's without your tooth edges cutting into it every time you open your mouth or chew!

Because of the oral ulcer pain as they draw their mandible sideways, a horse may begin to keep their mandible from traveling the full excursion from side to side. As this occurs, the SEPs buccal to the maxillary cheek teeth and lingual to the mandibular ones begin to undergo ***crown elongation*** because there is no opposing tooth material to grinding it away on those furthest buccal and lingual edges, or said another way, little to no ***attrition*** occurs on the buccal maxillary and lingual mandibular edges. The result? The horse must chew abnormally, which can be uncomfortable for them, and is increasingly more painful as the imbalances increase and the SEPs become even longer.

When a horse's horizontal mandibular excursion decreases, it also leads to food packing. Food may not be flushed out by the abnormally short sideways movement and may pack into the narrow buccal cavity between the sharp points of the cheek teeth and the cheeks. As the crown elongations lengthen, the horizontal excursion decreases even further, and gradually affected horses begin to chomp up and down, rather than chewing sideways, which is not as effective in chewing grasses, hay, and grains, either. The food stasis (food remaining in one place beside the gingiva) leads to development of ***periodontal*** disease and worse, if the horse is not treated, and so, odontoplasty is indicated. There may be crown elongations, but can it all be corrected in one go? See the next section.

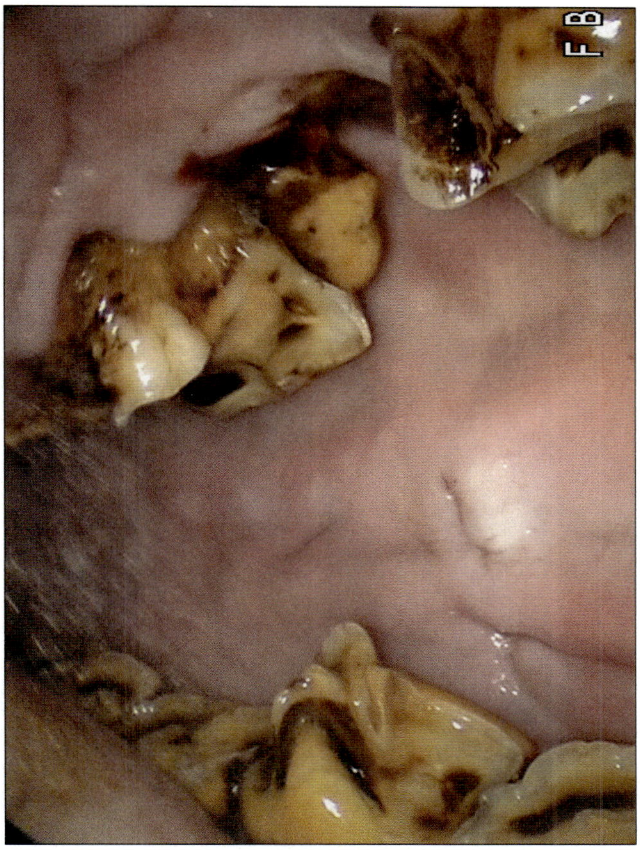

Endoscopic view of an older horse with neglected odontoplasty. Note crown elongations of the few teeth still containing enamel which have elongated into the opposing cupped teeth. Opposing the elongated mandibular tooth (centre of lower arcade shown, adjacent to the buccal ulcers), the the maxillary tooth above it exhibits gingival recession and has either fractured or the mesial root/s have undergone attrition past the gumline. Radiographs indicated to view status of the tooth, looking for fractures and/or osteomyelitis.Image credit Dr Manfred Stoll.

How much tooth is it safe to remove from the occlusal surface?

So, how far can one reduce a tooth with a ***crown elongation***? Researchers have found the thickness of the ***subocclusal secondary dentine (SO2D)*** to be between 1.5 and 11.7 millimeters (mm) for the maxillary (upper) incisors and between 0.7 and 6.7 mm for the mandibular (lower) incisors. A wide range for both but look at the lower numbers: 0.7 mm and 1.5 mm are extremely short distances, an extremely tiny amount of tooth to file off before the potential for ***iatrogenic pulp exposure*** starts. Great care should be exercised by any practitioner during reduction of any tooth. This is where over-reduction of teeth, over-zealous odontoplasty, or overheating rear their ugly heads. These insults to the pulp which occur during excessive odontoplasty happen too fast for the pulp to respond appropriately. This is where increased understanding of the thickness, or rather

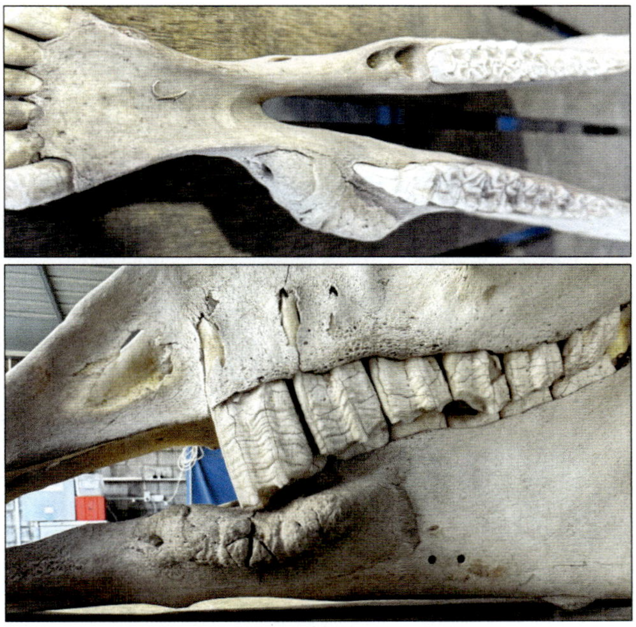

Severe crown elongations have driven into the bone and caused mandibular osteomyelitis. The horse must have had severe, incredibly painful osteomyelitis. Images credit Dr Oliver Liyou.

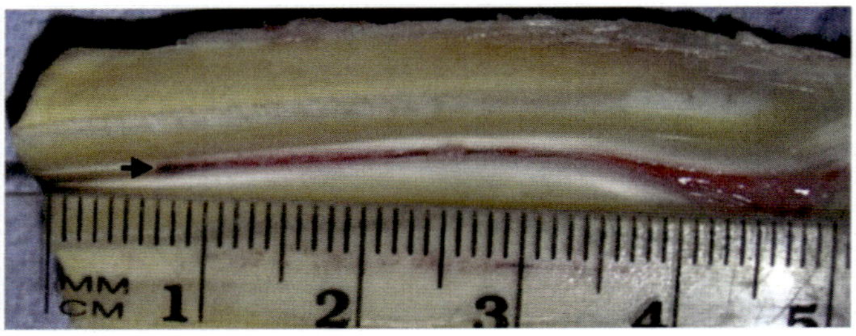

This cheek tooth has been longitudinally sectioned and shows the extent of the pulp (red) from the apex (to the right) toward the occlusal surface (to the left). To the left of the black arrow is 7 mm of subocclusal secondary dentine extending from the occlusal surface on left to the pulp. Image credit Dr Pearce C. (2020). Image originally published in Pearce C. Recent developments in equine dentistry. New Zealand Veterinary Journal 68, 178-86, 2020. ©NZVA

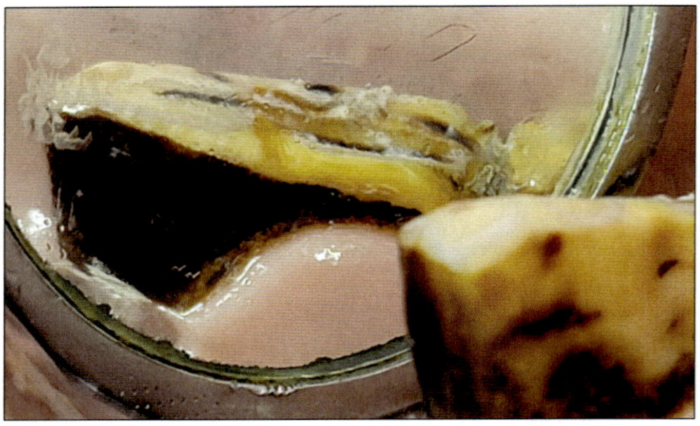

Here is a lower ramp and diastema. The ramp on the '06 has been reduced and profiled to a safe degree, where the SO2D covering the pulp horn #6 on the mesial end of the tooth is still light brown to tan. Image credit Cathie Heald Greenwell.

thinness, of the SO2D becomes vital to the prevention of iatrogenic ***pulp exposure***. See Chapter 9, Iatrogenic Disease. The ***cheek tooth*** below has been cut longitudinally to display the extent of the pulp, as well as its proximity to the occlusal surface on the left of the image. There is less than 7 mm of SO2D before the pulp officially begins. See Chapter 3, Anatomy of the Mouth.

The amount of occlusal surface your operator can safely remove when at one time is limited. As we have just learned, the pulps may reside only less than one mm to over six mm from the occlusal surface, and therefore only a small amount can be removed at once. Thankfully, the staining of the sub-occlusal secondary dentine (SO2D, the dentine overlying and protecting the pulp) serves as a form of color coding for careful operators as they perform odontoplasty. To understand this, consider the structure of the tooth as described in Chapter 3, Anatomy of the Mouth.

The hard enamel is resistant to staining by feed pigments and remains white. The softer ***cementum*** and dentin are more porous and pick up the brownish pigment from feed materials, which stains these softer calcified ***tissues*** brown on their exposed surfaces. That staining is darkest on the occlusal surface and grows paler as it leaches into the deeper structures. For your dental operator, it is significant that as dentin is removed along with the other components of the tooth during odontoplasty, the wide strips of dark brown dentin (overlying the pulp horns) on a cheek tooth fade to a lighter brown and become smaller and more circular. As one progresses, the dentin loses more of its staining to become cream-colored. This color change indicates the rasp is getting closer to the live portion of the tooth. If your operator is not rinsing and checking the teeth as

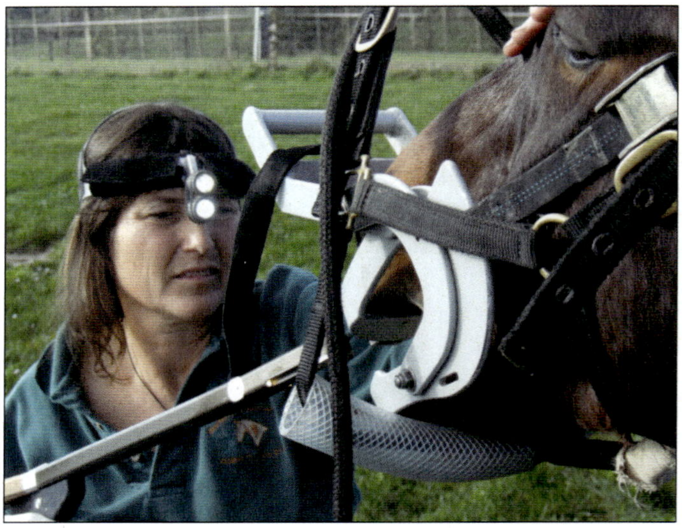

Odontoplasty in stocks with a dental halter helps horses maintain stability and comfort. It's a dental chair for horses. Image credit James Hewitt.

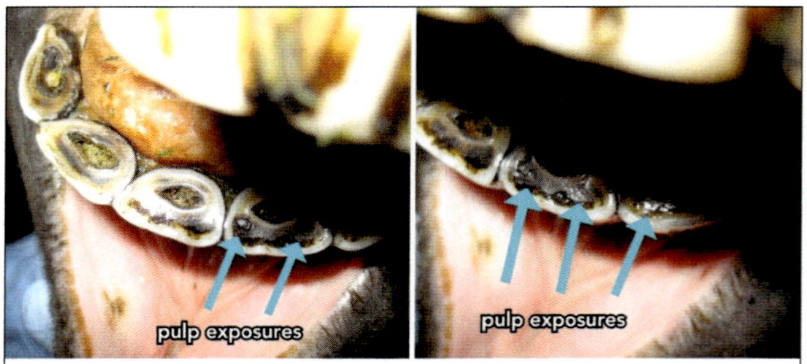

The incisors on this young horse were severely overheated and not cooled with water, causing pulpitis and severe pain. This horse was obsessively sucking on his knees (carpi).

This young horse was examined by Dr Elizabeth Thompson after he was found to be obsessively chewing on his carpi, or knees, due to the pain in his incisors. He sustained near pulp exposure in multiple teeth from power dentistry without water cooling. The arrows point to the shiny, wet pulp exposures between the open infundibula (normal for his age) and the labial border of the mandibular incisors. Image credit Author.

odontoplasty is performed, he will not see these color changes. If rasping continues, the cream-colored dentin will become pink, then red. Pink and red mean danger. Even the cream color is getting into the danger zone for ***pulpar exposure***. See Chapter 3, Anatomy of the Mouth and Chapter 10, Head Trauma and Dental Pathology.

Unfortunately, the pulp horns in unopposed teeth (those not in occlusal contact with another tooth) or teeth with unopposed portions, possess pulps which are very close to the occlusal surface, probably because they are not subjected to the trauma of ***mastication*** (chewing) and therefore have not pulled back their odontoblast processes toward the apex and laid down SO2D in their place.

Understanding this and knowing that SO2D may be only two to three millimeters thick (which means the extensions of the live pulp may be only one to three millimeters from the occlusal surface) these indicators are extremely significant. In incisors, the live pulp may be as little as less than ONE mm from the occlusal surface and therefore liable to be at risk of pulp exposure with only minimal rasping. If an unopposed tooth is overgrown, the horse can be made more comfortable with odontoplasty by reducing the long tooth incrementally, carefully monitoring the staining of the occlusal dentine. As the pulps retreats in response to the normal occlusal forces of chewing feed, SO2D fills the pulp chamber occlusally to the pulp, preventing pulp exposure. Clearly, the teeth in the image to the right would not have been able to be reduced all at once without exposing pulp!

Only after this SO2D is laid down to protect the pulp may more tooth be floated from the occlusal surface. This SO2D then stains with feed pigments and can be used as an aid during the next odontoplasty, but it can take two to three months to gain enough "safe" tooth to reduce crown elongations further.

The long-term goal is to have the previously elongated crown and the previously over*ground* tooth in apposition, and level with the rest of the teeth around it, to prevent further malocclusion.

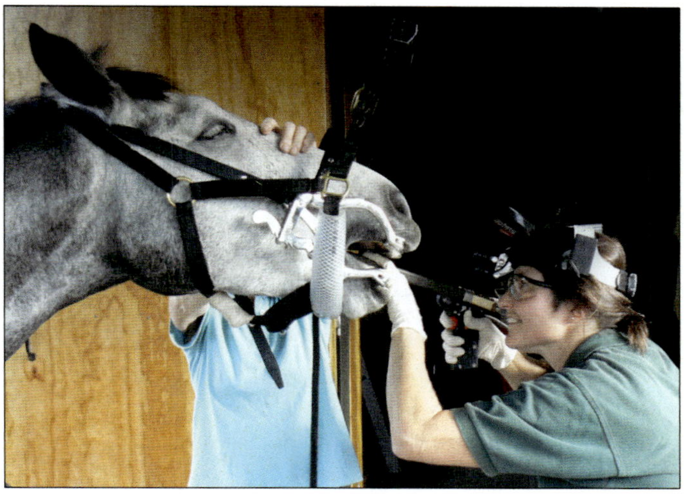

Using a floating system with a constant water irrigation cooling system to prevent thermal damage to teeth. Image credit Joan Gilchrist.

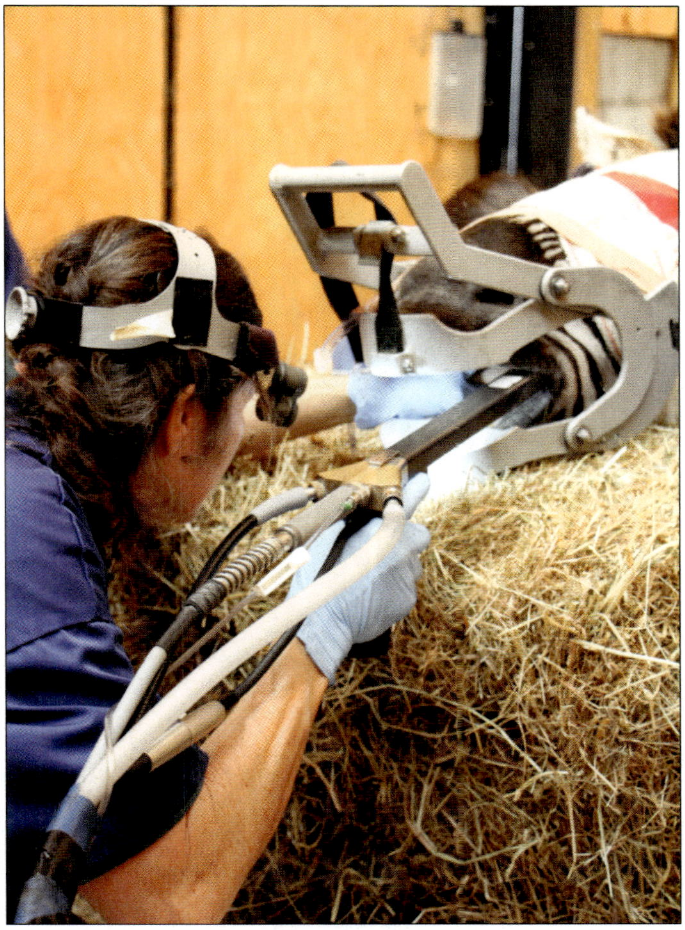

Sometimes you don't need to hold their heads up, but you need to get down to their level. Here is Itika from Auckland Zoo under general anesthesia for her planned dental examination and odontoplasty. The zoo goes to great lengths to ensure the comfort and safety of the animals under their care. When working with animals of infinite value such as these, it is vital to give them the best and safest instruments the world has to offer, like this water cooled floating instrument. Image credit Vanessa Marsh, used with permission of Auckland Zoo.

So why are we so concerned with over-reduction of teeth?

When excessive ***occlusal dentine*** is filed off or teeth sustain thermal or heat injury, see Chapter 9, Iatrogenic Disease: What are Iatrogenic Odontoplasty or Occlusal

Surface Injuries), and a pulp exposure or near-pulp exposure occurs, pulpitis can result.

Pulpitis is infection and/or ***inflammation*** of the pulp, which can kill a tooth if the pulp is unable to effectively fight off the infection and inflammation. If the pulp is able to survive, dentine may form a protective wall between the live pulp and the pulp exposure site. This is termed a ***dentinal bridge***.

Your vet may float incisor malocclusions, but the goal is to never create a situation where the cheek teeth and the incisors are ***in occlusion*** at the same time (Remember the lateral excursion test? It is used to test for this.).

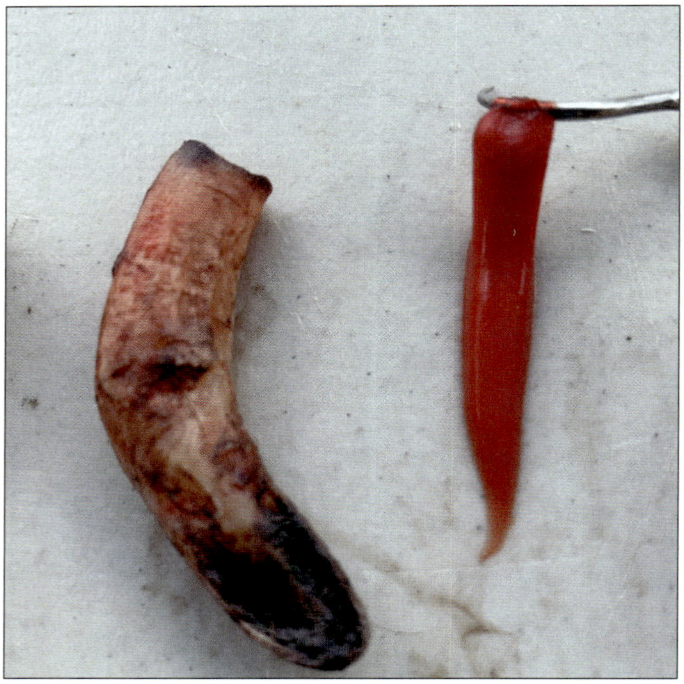

This is an equine canine tooth extracted from a cadaver. Notice the length of the pulp, nearly as long a the tooth. This is why we do not cut teeth, whether they are canines, cheek teeth, incisors, or wolf teeth. Teeth can have live pulp tissue from 1-3 mm beneath the occlusal surface, and in unopposed teeth, such as crown elongations, they may be even closer. Image credit Author.

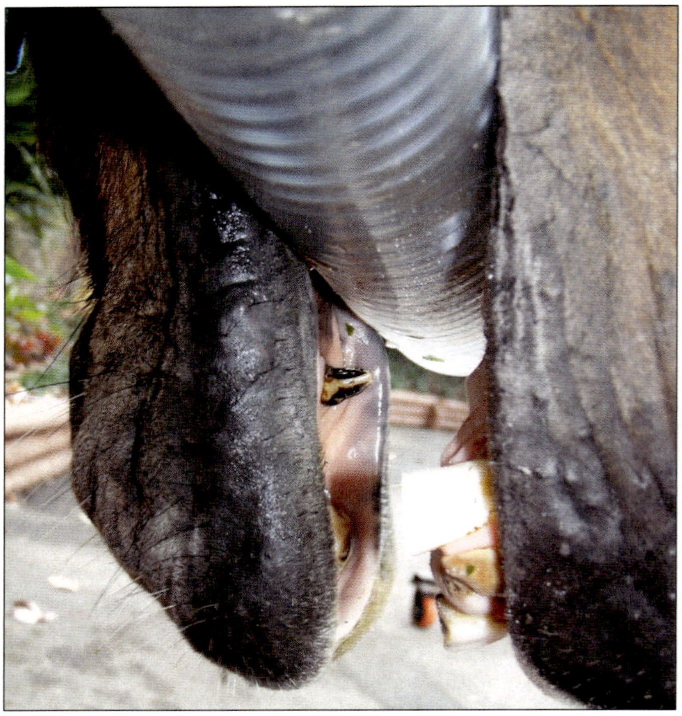

Tube speculum in place for incisor work. Image credit Greg Miller-Hard.

Odontoplasty or floating which results in cheek teeth and incisors being in contact at the same time is ***contraindicated***. Some non-veterinary schools of dentistry originated in places where horses are stabled and not on full-time grass, and thus perhaps grow excessive incisor length, but this is not common. What these programs term "rebalancing" can be severely detrimental due to excessive reduction of the incisors. Removing too much incisor length can cause the cheek teeth to be in occlusion at the same time as the incisors. At best, this causes pain and reluctance to eat, and at worst, severe, debilitating pain, pulp death, and requirement for extraction of affected teeth. See Chapter 9, Iatrogenic Disease.

But how will we ever fix anything if we can't take much tooth at once?

Your veterinarian can return in two to three months, by which time the pulp's reparative function will have usually caused the pulp to retreat toward the apex. SO2D will form in its wake, filling the gaps left by the pulp's retreat. This new dentin will stain with feed pigments, leaving its own color coding again, which your operator may use to deduce how far from the occlusal surface the pulp is, by incremental careful rasping, rinsing, LOOKING, then deciding if they can proceed. Dark brown to light brown to neutral to pink to RED. It's wise to stop at the light brown.

Why use water-cooling for power instruments?

Cooling the teeth with water during power odontoplasty is essential to prevent thermal (heat) damage to the live portions of the tooth, the pulp and its odontoblast processes near the occlusal and other surfaces. Your dentist would never drill into your teeth without water cooling. I prefer odontoplasty equipment with constant water irrigation, which sprays a constant flow of water onto the teeth being filed.

Constant water cooling ensures I don't overheat the teeth and cause a thermal-induced pulpitis. If non-water-cooled instruments are used, the teeth should be cooled with a jet of water as soon as possible, ideally as much as twice per minute of grinding. Rather than grinding on one tooth for prolonged periods, constantly moving the float over the teeth can help reduce the risk of thermal damage, but water cooling is non-negotiable if you want the teeth to remain alive in the long term.

Incisor reduction

Most incisor malocclusions are not primary, that it, they are secondary to malocclusion or pathology of the cheek teeth. The cheek teeth malocclusions should be addressed first, then your vet may lightly even out incisor malocclusions, but the goal is never to create a situation where the cheek teeth and the incisors are in occlusion at the same time. This is definitely contraindicated. Some schools of lay dental operators unfortunately promote incisor reduction to this extreme level. Remember we have discussed that the incisors and cheek teeth are not meant to be in occlusion at the same time? If a lateral excursion test reveals that the incisors do not separate as the mandible is slid sideways, a huge problem has likely been created for your horse.

Cutting of teeth

Cutting of incisors and other teeth is specifically contraindicated (i.e. should never be done) because of the danger of pulp exposure. Instruments such as cut-off wheels (the sharp edge, not the flat surface) and molar cutters risk the life of every tooth upon which they are used. It is impossible to cut the occlusal surface of any tooth without a significant risk of pulpar exposure. Even a near-pulp exposure is at risk of infection from bacteria accessing the live pulp tissue and heat from the cutting instrument. Case reports show painful periapical abscesses and death of incisors and canines result from reductions with motorized cut-off wheels. The only reason a tooth should ever be cut is during its own extraction, by your veterinarian, and then only because it is too long to extract with the extra length in place. This is especially significant in young horses with extremely long reserve crowns.

LIVE PULPS are why we cannot remove too much tooth at once during odontoplasty.

How Should My Horse Act After Odontoplasty or Floating?

AFTER ODONTOPLASTY, IT is ***not*** normal for your horse to suddenly begin to:

- Show signs of pain
- Refuse to eat for a day, much less a few weeks
- Shake and sweat
- Rub their face
- Chew or suck on their knees
- Drool
- Look miserable

After odontoplasty, horses should:

Enthusiastically rip into their feed or grass (usually better than pre-dentistry)

Look happy and relaxed

If they have had an extraction, they may be uncomfortable, but even post extraction it would be rare indeed for a horse to not be keen to eat after an odontoplasty, unless they have had excessive odontoplasty.

Anything else is extremely abnormal.

If your horse has recently undergone odontoplasty and you notice discomfort, drooling, or unwillingness to eat, check her teeth carefully. Pinkness or bleeding of an occlusal surface or pulp tissue coming out of a tooth indicates obvious pulpar exposure and constitutes an emergency, requiring timely treatment by a dental veterinarian. If you know power dentistry was done without frequent or constant water-cooling, pulpar compromise leading to tooth death may occur without displaying any visible signs, unfortunately. Even post-odontoplasty teeth which don't show this pinkness or redness may have had the smear layer, or the protective layer of dentin, removed, which has exposed the sensitive odontoblast processes of the pulp, or removed them from their tubules. This is painful for the horse and initiate pulpitis, or inflammation of the pulp. See Chapter 9, Iatrogenic Disease: Iatrogenic Pulpar Exposure... for more details. This is a serious situation and your dental vet should be contacted as soon as possible.

CHAPTER FIFTEEN

WHAT ARE VETERINARY SPECIFIC PROCEDURES, AND WHY?

WHILE PEOPLE MAY or may not agree about whether equid dentistry should be vet-only or not vet-only, (and your state, province, or country might have something to say about it, too), there are procedures which lie fully in the realm of veterinary medicine.

Why is Sedation Limited to Vets?

SEDATION IS NOT something to be taken lightly. Administration of sedation and ***analgesia*** are acts of veterinary medicine in most places, and limited to veterinarians for many reasons:

- In untrained hands, sedation drugs and the potential results of sedation in an animal that outweighs us by ten times can be lethal—not only for your horse, but for those around him, including you and yours.
- Sedation is not the same as pain relief. Your vet knows the difference.
- Particular equids have a compromised ability to metabolize and eliminate sedation drugs. Your vet knows how to compensate for this.
- Anxious horses can overpower the effects of drugs, then when the fear stops, they can "crash" and collapse, because the drugs are still in the horse's body. Your vet knows how to deal with the situation and can hopefully prevent it.

Can We Effectively and More Safely Sedate Older, Anxious, or Painful Horses?

EFFECTIVELY AND SAFELY sedating anxious, extremely painful, and/or older horses can be tricky.

I used to struggle with this, but a board-certified veterinary anesthesiologist helped me out and those disastrous old-horse and anxious-horse sedations rarely occur now for me.

Anxiety in these horses, usually due to a combination of moderate to severe long-term ***oral*** pain plus the smarts which old horses usually acquire, causes the release of chemicals in their bloodstream which help them override standard sedation drugs. You may have seen these sedated horses seem alert, while they're ataxic (wobbly). There are several problems here:

- Geriatrics may have compromised (poor) ability to metabolize and eliminate (clear out) sedation drugs
- Anxious horses' sympathetic (fight or flight fear) response may let them overpower the drugs
- Combined, the drugs are still there... and when the fear goes, the horse may crash. Not ideal in a geriatric.

These horses may become very sleepy and probably more ***ataxic*** (wobbly) when the vet stops working in their mouth. I use this technique with most of the anxious or elderly horses in my practice.

Twenty minutes before your vet expects to begin work, your horse may be injected intramuscularly in their own paddock near where the dentistry will be performed (but be sure other horses cannot push it around) with an ***anxiolytic*** (anti-anxiety) drug and a small dose of the standard sedation and pain relief drugs. I leave it alone without stressing it for the next 20 minutes. The anti-anxiety drug keeps the horse from working itself up and overriding the other drugs.

After this time, the horse can be quietly led to the ***stocks*** or working place and standard sedation drugs at a low dose administered. Giving the anxiolytic after they have become wound-up hasn't been effective in my hands.

Horses sedated with this regimen appear quite awake, but they don't seem to care what you're doing, which differs vastly from sedation without the anxiolytic. It's important that everyone takes their time and does not stress the horse at any time to achieve the longest-lasting sedation time with less anxiety and ***ataxia***.

How Do We Treat Periodontal Disease and Diastemata?

PERIODONTAL DISEASE WITH ***diastemata***, or gaps between teeth which should fit together like bricks in a wall but have widened and become impacted with rotting feed material, are extremely painful to treat. For effective treatment, they must be thoroughly evacuated (cleaned out) to the very bottom of the sulcus, or pocket, which may go a considerable way down the tooth, well flushed, and measured to monitor response to therapy. This is a painful procedure and is working below the gumline, therefore in most places it is regarded as the practice of veterinary medicine. Effective therapy of this disease requires sedation and usually, ***perineural anesthesia*** (nerve blocks). The evacuated sulcus may be packed with an appropriate material and allowed to settle for a short period of time or the diastema widened, according to your veterinarian's preference. There is a promising new technique where the diastema is widened, but only for the first 3 mm of particular edges of the ***occlusal*** surfaces.

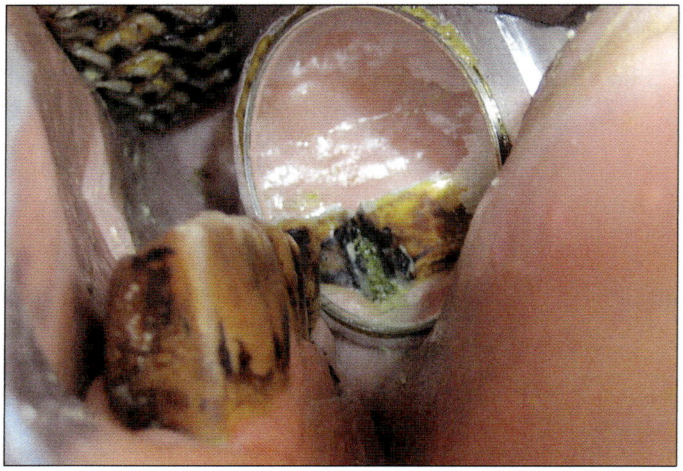

Feed-filled diastema in the 400 arcade. These are extremely painful and require sedation and perineural anesthesia (nerve blocks) to treat effectively. They should be treated as soon as possible. Image credit Author.

Ask your dental veterinarians how long they wish to wait to recheck. Diastema therapy will usually require more than one treatment to attempt resolution. They won't always resolve, but with dedication on your part, it improves the likelihood of a full recovery. Closed diastemata can be difficult to fully resolve due to their ability to hold feed, but discuss this with your veterinarian.

What Must We Consider Before Deciding to Extract Teeth?

CHEEK TOOTH EXTRACTION is most commonly indicated in the horse to treat conditions such as severe injury or disease of the dental ***crown*** or ***apices***, severe periodontal disease, tooth death, supernumerary teeth, neoplasia, endodontic disease with secondary ***osteomyelitis***, sinus disease secondary to dental disease, or as a surgical consideration in the management of oral fractures.

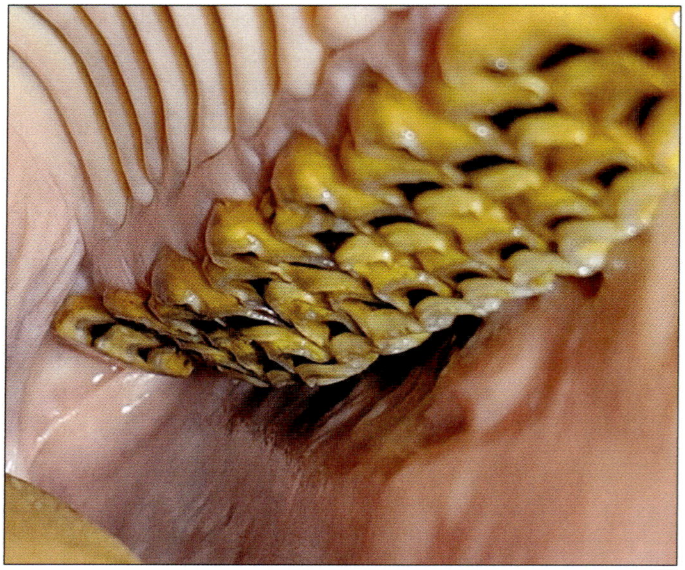

Count the teeth! There is a supernumerary tooth in the 200 arcade. If this tooth is unopposed, it may cause this horse grief if examination and treatment are neglected. Image credit Dr Tracy Tinsley.

Due to the serious long-term consequences of tooth removal in the horse, the decision to extract ***incisors*** or ***cheek teeth*** should be made only after an accurate diagnosis is obtained by physical and radiographic examination and only when there is no other reasonable alternative Some negative consequences of extraction include:

- wear abnormalities from continued ***eruption*** of the now-unopposed tooth
- disruption of the dental arcade
- ***dental drift***
- ***diastema*** formation with periodontal feed pocketing
- periodontal disease

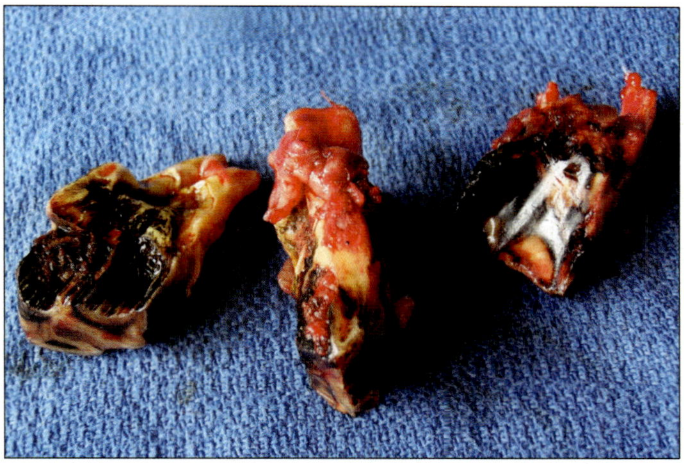

Extraction of two teeth, one with a sagittal fracture in a tooth with Grade 4 infundibular caries. This was a longstanding condition in a horse in full work, noted on a routine dental exam. Image credit Author.

The extraction

Ideally, your vet will perform these extractions intraorally, (only with instruments inside the mouth), rather than by repulsion (hammering them out with a mallet and punch through the sinus or side of the maxilla or bottom of the mandible), which should be reserved for teeth which cannot be extracted by intraoral extraction. Extraction is best performed in stocks, using sedation and pain relief in the form of local and regional anesthetics and pre-operative anti-inflammatories. Extraction of any tooth, no matter how small, is surgery, whether it's a wolf tooth, an incisor, canine, or a cheek tooth. It is an extremely painful procedure and when your practitioner is working below the gumline, it is surgery. Surgery is in the realm of veterinary medicine, and for your horse's health and safety, is best left to a veterinarian. Sedation is not the same as pain relief. Your vet knows the difference.

But wolf teeth can just be broken off, right? No.

Some people believe it is all right to file a wolf tooth to the gingiva or just break off the clinical crown. While this was done in the past, it is no longer acceptable today. ***Pulp exposure*** will most likely result. A wolf tooth which has been filed down may need extraction if a pulp exposure has occurred, which you may not know for many months if it is not bleeding at the time. See Chapter 9, Iatrogenic Pulp Exposure.

This discussion pertains to ***wolf teeth*** as much as it does to incisors, ***canines***, or cheek teeth. Just because a wolf tooth is smaller does not mean it does not cause pain to the horse! Have you ever had a fractured or broken tooth? It hurts all the time. Imagine having to go around an arena or over a cross country course, or even to eat with that pain.

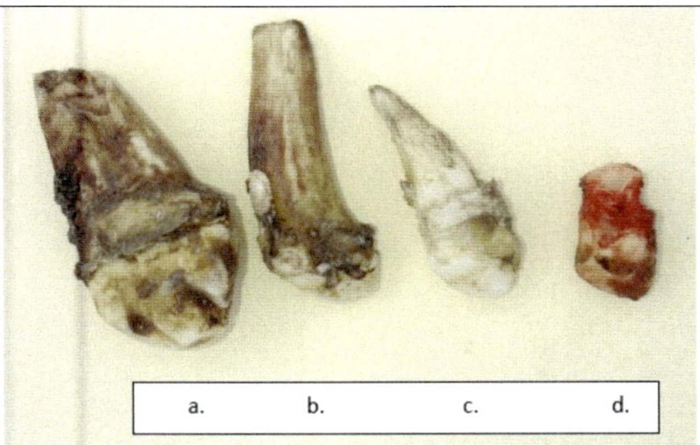

Figure 1. various morphology of wolf teeth. a. Wolf tooth with a flat root, showing a root tip fracture without pulp exposure. b. flat root, blunt apex. c. curved root d. showing a small simple crown and short fractured root, suggesting that the majority of this root is still in situ. Notice that the appearance of the crown does not predict the size or appearance of the root.

Various morphology of Wolf teeth ('05s). a. Wolf tooth with a flat root, showing a root tip fracture wit pulp exposure, b. flat root, blunt apes, c. curved root, d. showing small simple crown and short fractured root, suggesting that the majority of this root is still in situ (in place). Notice that the appearance of the crown does not predict the size or appearance of the root. Wolf teeth need complete extraction. Image credit Dr Marieke van den Enden.

If your horse is subjected to this, they live with this pain constantly. While we might moan and grip our cheek, an equid just won't do that, because first, a horse is a prey species, and second, if they figuratively do that, we likely won't understand, but it hurts them all the same. See Chapter 1, How do I Know My Horse has Dental Disease? After your horse is sedated, its mouth will be rinsed and flushed with an appropriate disinfectant before beginning. The wolf tooth will be carefully elevated from the ***gingiva*** with sharp, clean elevators, taking care to avoid the palatine artery. The ***periodontal ligament*** will be stretched with elevators until the tooth is visibly loose, then the entire tooth with its long root should slip from the ***alveolus*** with only the pressure of the vet's fingertips. Wolf teeth sometimes have curved roots which are extremely tricky to remove in their entirety.

As with all extractions, patience and time are essential. Tooth roots can be extremely long compared to the tiny portion of exposed crown we see in the mouth, so be patient with your operator— rushing breaks roots, which takes even more time.

The alveolus will be flushed with a disinfectant solution and possibly packed to prevent a painful "dry socket", and the horse's tetanus status assessed and remedied if needed. Do all wolf teeth need extraction? See Chapter 15, Veterinary Specific Procedures: Don't All Wolf Teeth Need Extraction?. Your vet will advise of anything else they wish you to do post-operatively.

Are canine teeth easy to extract? They're so little.

The canine teeth are actually extremely long and the vast majority of their length is well-buried in the bone of the mandible. See the image below. A is the clinical, or exposed, crown. All of B up to the black line of A is hidden from our regular view. This, plus their curvature, makes them challenging to extract. A flap of the gingiva must be surgically "raised" over the ***reserve crown*** of the tooth to be extracted, after sedation and anesthesia are in place. The bone overlying the canine must usually be removed before the canine tooth can be elevated and mobilized. The gingival flap will usually be sutured closed after the extraction is complete. General extraction procedures as discussed for incisors and cheek teeth apply.

What is cheek tooth intraoral extraction? (vs. trephination and repulsion)

Trephination and repulsion should only be used for extraction as a last resort after attempts at intraoral extraction, minimally invasive extraction, and even buccotomy have failed. Trephination and repulsion were once the preferred method of cheek tooth extraction. This involved drilling a hole or holes into the bones of the skull, often through the skull into a sinus, then bashing the tooth out with a punch and mallet, usually under general anesthesia. This technique

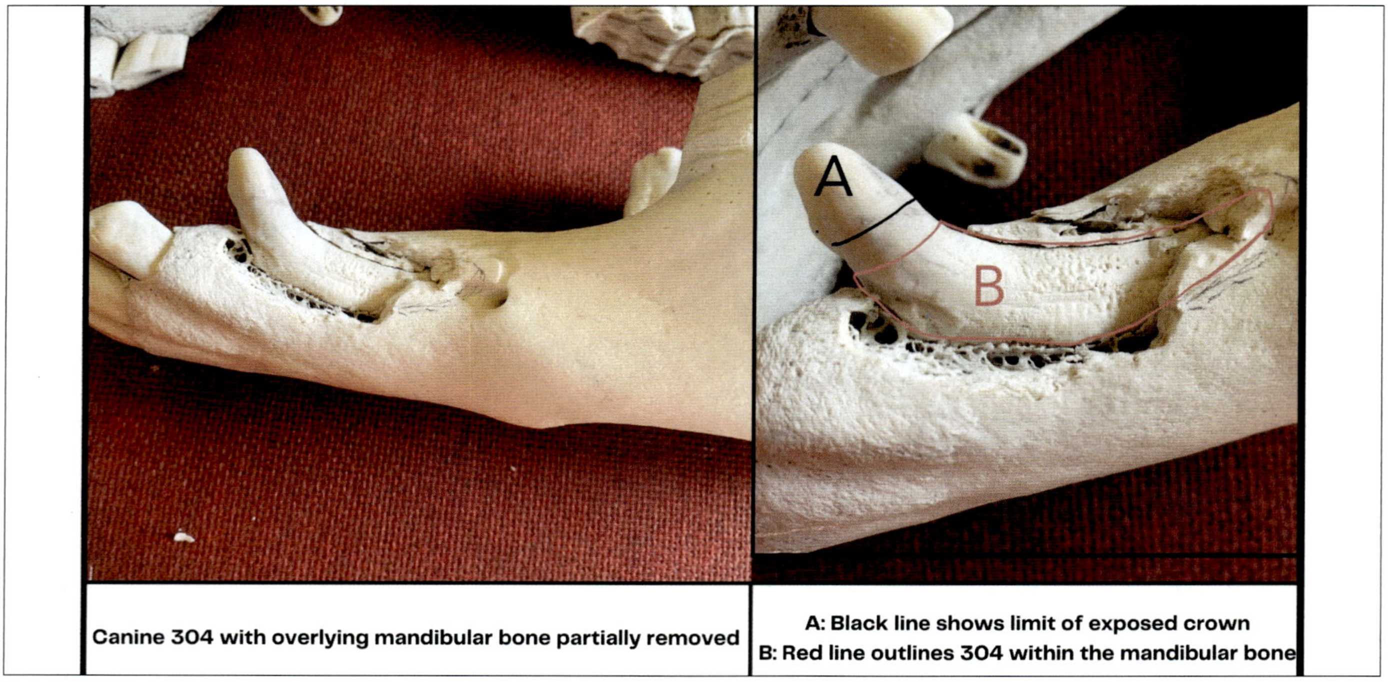

Equine canine tooth 304 with overlying mandibular bone partially removed, showing the extent of reserve crown (B) vs. the small clinical crown visible above the gingiva (A). Image credit Author.

has a few challenges. First, it can be difficult to be sure one was bashing out the correct tooth, especially before the advent of vets carrying X-ray machines in their vehicle. Second, unfortunately, this technique tends to destroy the bone of the alveolus within which the tooth resided, as well as causing multiple fractures and fragments of the surrounding bone, plus leaving behind an extremely large oro-sinus ***fistula*** (a hole between the sinus and the mouth), which can be difficult for even a board-certified surgeon to successfully repair. Research has consistently shown that intraoral extractions have lower complication rates than trephination and repulsion. Minimally invasive Steinmann pin repulsion, while still a form of repulsion, requires only a tiny opening, and has low complication rates. It may be used by your veterinarian when it is indicated.

Again, to emphasize, trephination and repulsion should only be used as a last resort for extraction, after intraoral, minimally invasive and buccotomy methods have failed.

Prior to extraction, your vet will have radiographed your horse's teeth, and evaluated all views for any disease or potential challenges with the upcoming extraction.

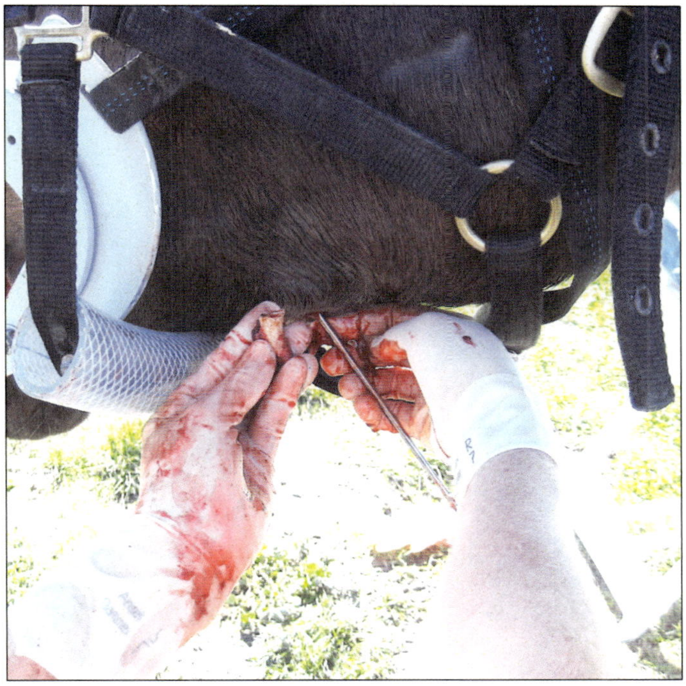

Steinmann pin repulsion was used to extract this root tip in an older mare who already had a draining tract to the tooth. Image credit Author.

Plan on this procedure taking considerable time. Depending upon the ***pathology*** of the tooth and the alveolar bone around it, extraction can take from one to eight hours or more to remove a cheek tooth, and some extractions may require a second visit for complete extraction, or even referral to a surgical facility. The bone of the alveolus must deform enough to allow extraction to proceed, and that can take time. Getting forceful can fracture not only the ***clinical crown*** of the tooth (which you need to grip to extract the tooth), but also the ***mandible*** or ***maxilla***.

Sometimes a vet may work faster and with more force, but I've been taught that with patience and controlled force, the tooth will eventually come out. If one loses patience and forces the tooth excessively, roots break off or the clinical crown will break apart, especially in a diseased tooth. This makes everything take even longer. Not ideal.

As extraction usually requires a long, standing sedation with repeated doses of drugs, or a continuous rate infusion of drugs, I support my patients with pre-operative analgesia which will last for the whole surgery as well as administering intravenous fluids. IV fluid therapy is especially important for older horses or those with compromised health, but all my patients receive it.

As with wolf tooth extraction, the mouth will be flushed as above. The cheek tooth to be extracted will be elevated with sharp, clean elevators. Even this takes time. Various instruments will be used around the tooth to stretch the periodontal ligament in all directions and then slow sustained rocking of the tooth begins. And goes on for quite some time.

There is new instrumentation available which allows minimally invasive extraction in the case that the tooth is broken off at the gumline. See Chapter 16, Advanced Techniques...: Minimally Invasive Extraction....

At some point, the tooth will loosen and can be taken from the mouth. Once the tooth is out, your veterinarian will take post-operative radiographs to ensure every bit of tooth has been removed, then the alveolus will be curetted and cleaned, and depending upon your veterinarian's choice, packed, or not packed, with a plug.

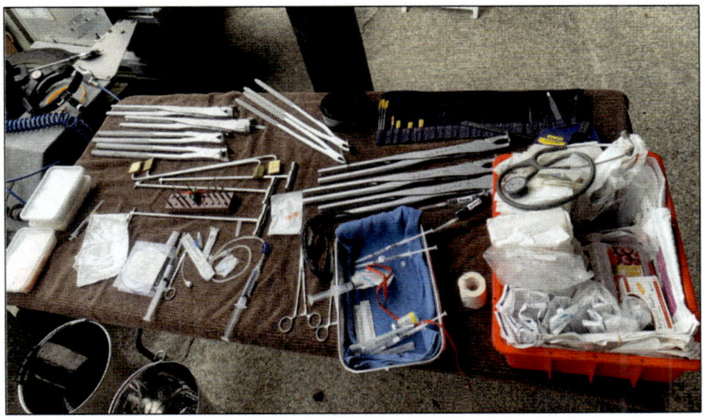

It is necessary to have significant instrumentation before proceeding with a cheek tooth extraction, as there is always a degree of uncertainty about exactly what one will find, even after preoperative radiographs. This is only part of the equipment I set out during extractions. Image credit Author.

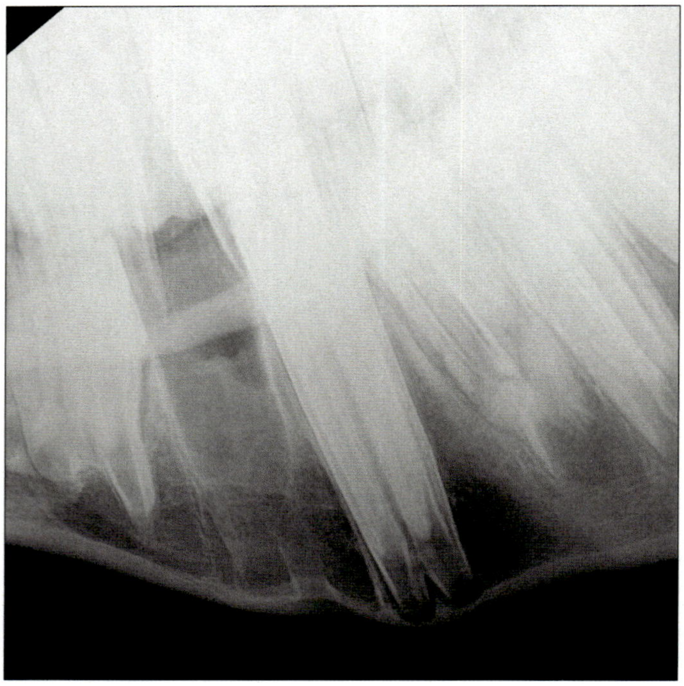

Post-op radiographs will be taken to ensure all parts of the extracted tooth have been removed from the alveolus. The 407 has been completely extracted. Image credit Author.

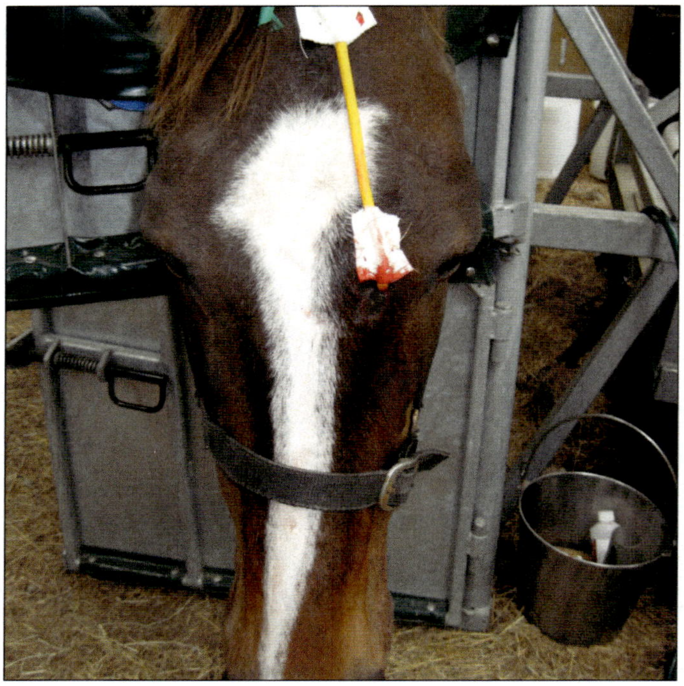

Drain tube sutured in place for sinus flushing therapy following intraoral extraction of a tooth with a severe apical infection with large cementomas and an oro-sinus fistula. The horse had displayed a chronic one-sided purulent nasal discharge before the surgery. Image credit Author.

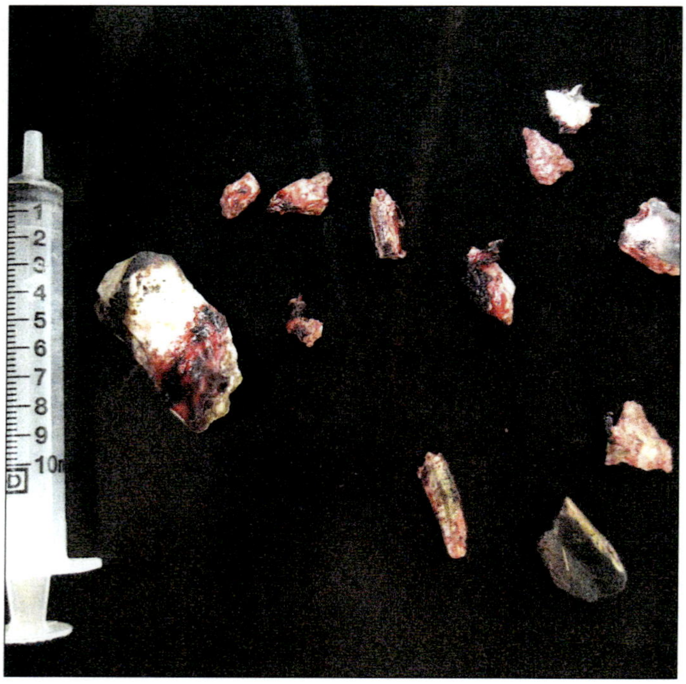

These are the tooth fragments extracted from the horse with radiographs on the left. No post-op radiographs had been taken at the time of extraction. They were definitely taken after extraction of these fragments! Image credit Author.

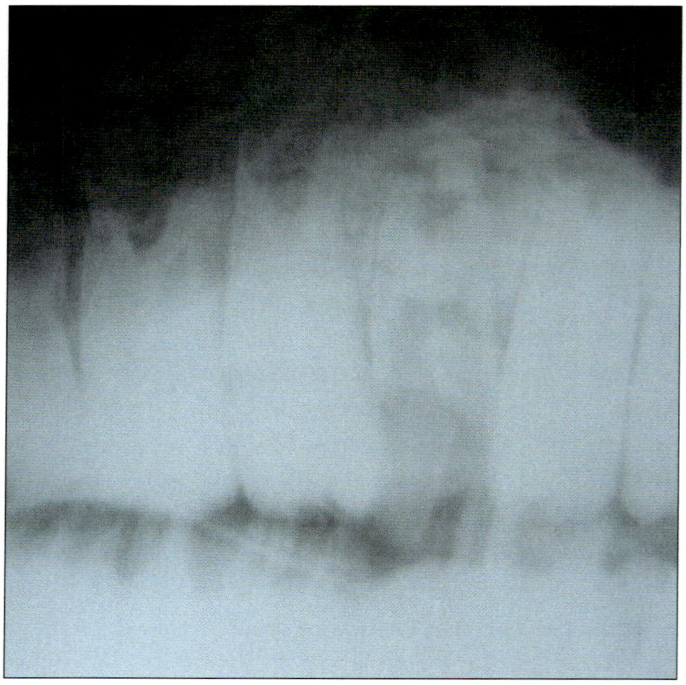

Illustrating the importance of post-op radiographs, this horse had an extraction overseas several years prior to my first examination. No post-op radiographs had been taken, or shown to the owner, anyway. The owner had no idea any tooth material had been left in the alveolus. Note the dental drift of the '08 and '10 into the space left by the extraction of the occlusal portion of the '09. Apologies for the quality of the radiographs on this page, they were taken in the old days when one had to take the cassettes into town for developing, so quality wasn't always what we have grown to expect with digital radiography. Image credit Author.

If the tooth to be extracted has an oro-sinus (mouth to sinus) fistula and an accompanying sinus infection, the sinus will need to also be treated by evacuation (cleaning out) and flushing to clear the sinus of ***purulent*** material (pus), which ranges from very liquid to solid, or a combination of both. This may require surgically opening the sinus to properly evacuate all that material. ***Sinuses*** containing ***apical abscessation*** are usually infected with anaerobic bacteria, which give off a very foul odor. Even after the extraction, the sinus will require flushing over at least the next several weeks to clear the infection.

Your vets may or may not place your horse on antibiotics, but will likely provide pain relief for several days post-op and will advise you of post-operative care. Grass is usually the preferred post-operative feed to avoid impaction of small bits of feed into the alveolus or around the plug if one is in place. A revisit may be planned in one to three weeks to check the alveolus for healing and to remove or replace the plug, if one was used, and to check for any sequestra, or pieces of dead bone which sometimes form post-operatively within the alveolus. If sequestra are present at that time, your vet can treat those areas.

Successful healing of an oro-nasal or oro-sinus (oro-maxillary) fistula can be extremely tricky. You will have to work closely with your veterinarian to get this pathology satisfactorily concluded and it may take many treatments to get it healed. A word about nomenclature of these fistulae: the term "oro-antral" was previously used, but as "antrum" is already a term for the maxillary sinus... you would be repeating yourself. Use oro-sinus. Thank you for that, Dr Padraic Dixon!

Occasionally a tooth is unable to be extracted intraorally or via minimally invasive means and must be referred to a surgical facility for general anesthesia and buccotomy or trephination and repulsion. In a buccotomy surgery, the tooth is extracted surgically through the cheek. Trephination and repulsion, as mentioned before, involves drilling a hole or holes through the bones of the skull into the bone or sinus directly over the path of the tooth roots, and then bashing the tooth out with a punch and mallet, usually under general anesthesia. Unfortunately, this can fracture and destroy the alveolus within which the tooth resided, as well as parts of the maxilla or mandible.

Here are a few case studies:

Case Study #1

THE NEW OWNER of this horse were concerned about this swelling on the side of this horse's face. The sellers told them it had been present for several years and that their previous dental operators had told them they needn't worry, as there wasn't a problem with it.

A thorough examination revealed feed impaction and a fractured 207, which was in numerous pieces. One large fragment was ticking straight buccally (into her cheek), causing a large, deep ulcer.

X-rays showed that the tooth had likely been dead for many years. Severe infection at the tooth roots had caused them to significantly remodel and become blunted (red arrow in radiograph on the next page).

Due to the length of time this fracture and its associated disease processes had been present, the teeth ***mesial*** and ***distal*** to 207 had begun to migrate together via dental drift, making the opening at the mouth (orange line) narrower than the remaining tooth, which added to the difficulty of the extraction. The tooth had to be extracted in pieces but was removed in its entirety, and was checked via post operative x-rays. This horse would have been in excruciating pain for years and this all could have been prevented by a thorough oral examination and appropriate treatment.

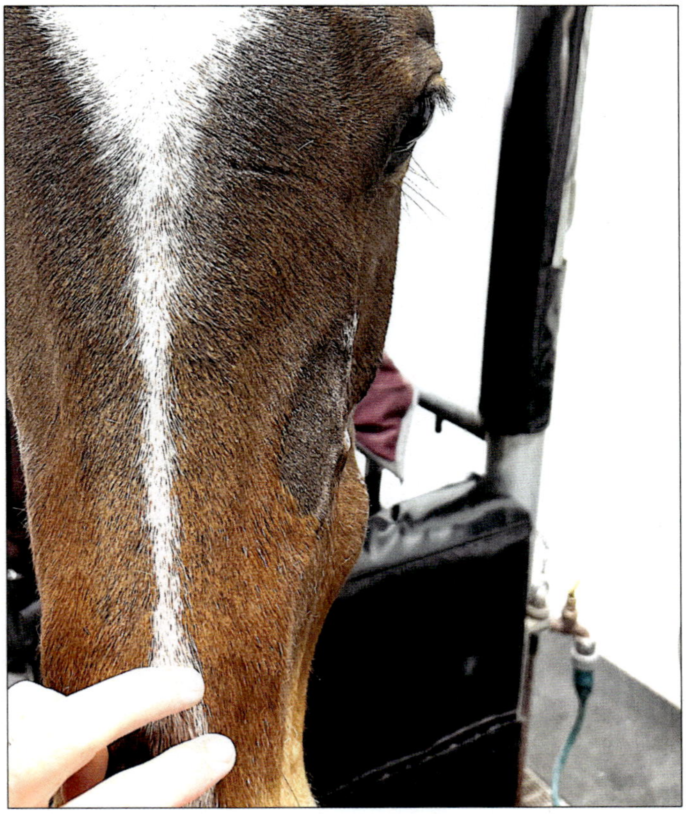

Image of the swelling on the side of this horse's face. Image credit Dr Kirsten Jackson, Dental Vet.

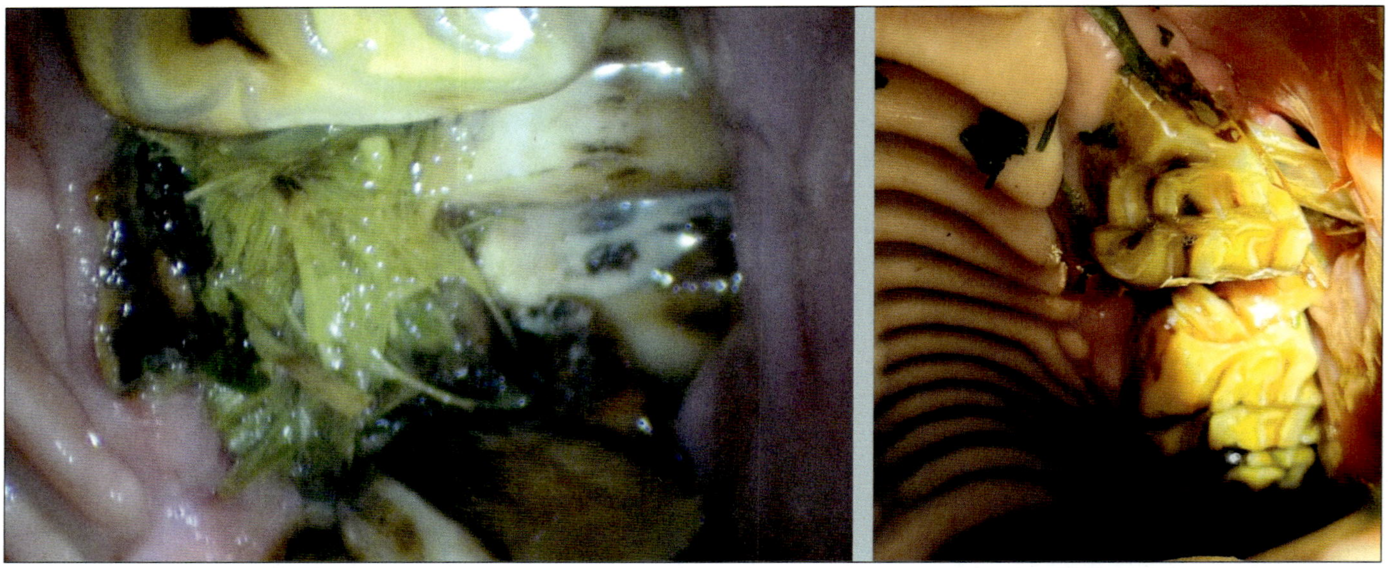

Appearance of the 207 before and after evacuating feed from around the tooth. Note the long tooth fragment protruding into the cheek in the image on the right. Image credit Dr Kirsten Jackson, Dental Vet, graphic credit Author.

Here are images from the oral examination, with preoperative, as well as postoperative, radiographs.

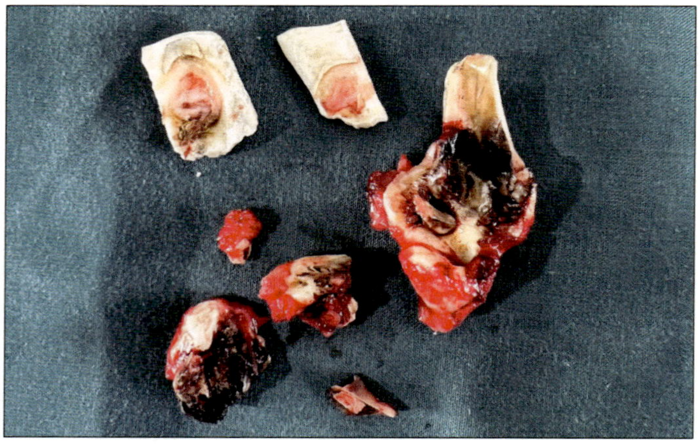

The tooth could only be extracted in in multiple pieces, due to the length of time elapsed since the disease process had begun. Image credit Dr Kirsten Jackson, Dental Vet.

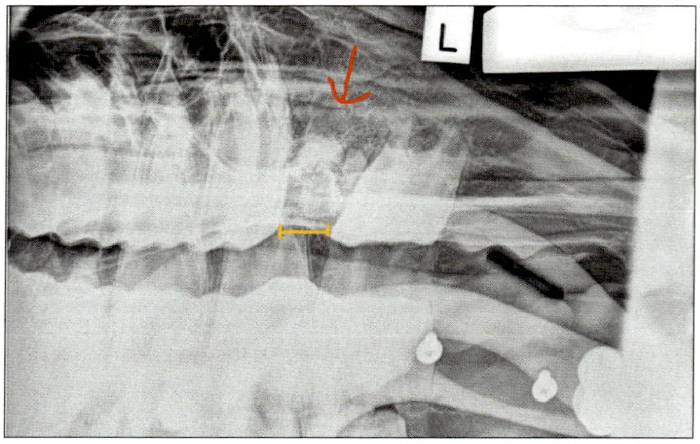

This radiograph shows the blunted roots (red arrow) and multiple fragments of the 207. Note the narrow width of the alveolar opening (orange line) into the mouth has become due to dental drift between the teeth adjacent to the 207. Image credit Dr Kirsten Jackson, Dental Vet.

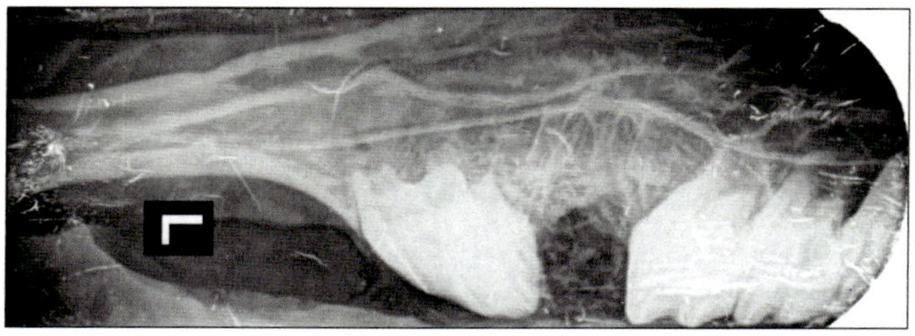

This intraoral postoperative radiograph shows not only that all dental fragments of 207 have been removed but also illustrates the severity of the dental drift of the 206 and 208 to close the gap where the fractured 207 previously resided. Image credit Dr Kirsten Jackson, Dental Vet.

Case Study #2

A FIVE-YEAR-old horse with a nearly two-year history of purulent discharge from a draining tract beneath a large, hard swelling on her ventral mandible due to an apical infection.

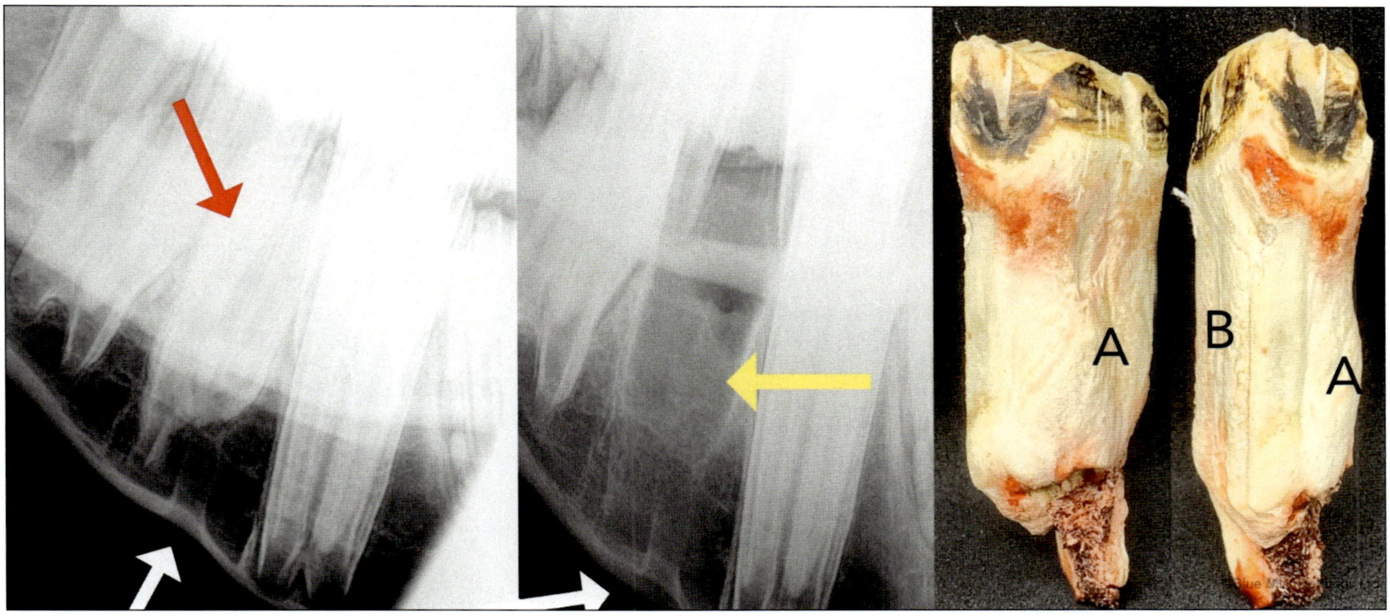

Five-year-old horse with a two-year history of recurrent purulent drainage from a large, hard swelling on her ventral mandible. The white arrows are pointing to the site of the draining tract through the bone of the ventral mandible. The red arrow is pointing to the affected tooth, which was extracted. The surface of the crown at (B) illustrates normal contour of the crown of the tooth, with none of the bulging caused by the apical infection at (A). Two years previously, it was nearly identical to the tooth on its right. The yellow area is pointing at the empty alveolus in the post-extraction radiographs (middle). Image credit Author.

Radiographs had been taken nearly two years previously, which illustrated a draining tract through the bone and signs of apical infection, but extraction had not taken place. Radiographs on my first visit showed the previously straight roots (like those shown at B) had bulged outward (see A) and the ***apex*** of the infected tooth had blunted and degenerated, with cementoma formation. The change in contour of the apex was an impediment to extraction and made it extremely difficult, as the apical half of the tooth was significantly larger than the alveolus, but with patience and persistence, it was extracted whole. Post-extraction radiographs are essential to ensure all tooth material and cementomas have been completely removed.

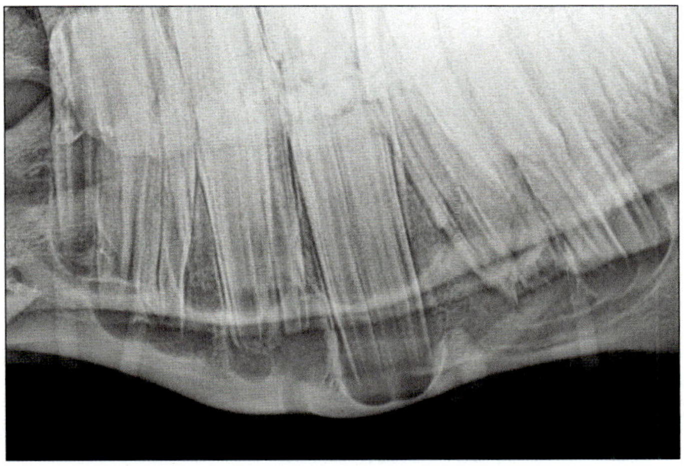

Radiographs taken two years previously showed a draining tract through the mandible, but none of the bulging reserve crown seen in the Pre-surgical radiograph (red arrow) in the figure Mandibular Draining Tract CT Extraction, above.

Tetanus cover (tetanus prophylaxis)

Extraction surgery opens the ***mucosa***, alveolar bone, and deeper structures to infection and the possibility of soil-sourced infection with *Clostridium tetani*, the bacterium which causes tetanus. Tetanus is a disease which affects most mammals, but horses and humans are particularly susceptible. The bacterium can enter the body from the soil through a wound (usually a puncture or other closed-over wound), where it multiplies in the absence of air and produces the toxin responsible for the clinical signs of this disease. A few weeks after infection, a horse begins to have increasingly severe muscle tremors and spasms, induced by sudden movement or noise. As the disease progresses, muscles begin to spasm all over the body, so severe they can break bones and the jaw can lock up, so they cannot eat. It progresses until it affects blood circulation and breathing. Approximately 80% of affected horses die. Horses which recover will usually do so in two to six weeks. However, it can usually be prevented by vaccination and regular boostering. Boostering a properly vaccinated equid for tetanus with a tetanus toxoid is essential. If a horse is *un*vaccinated or it has been more than around five years since last vaccinated, vaccinating for tetanus and at the same time administering a tetanus antitoxin may be indicated, but consult with your veterinarian, who will know the local requirements for this vaccine interval. See the next section for details about tetanus vaccination.

Tell Me More About Tetanus?

TETANUS TOXOID IS, in essence, tetanus toxin which has been modified to stimulate an immune response but not cause toxicity or disease. All going well, the horse responds to the vaccine by making its own antibodies to the toxoid. Therefore, coverage, or protection from tetanus depends upon the equid's immune system to find the toxoid and then react to it by making antibodies to try to destroy the toxoid. Unfortunately, this doesn't happen immediately. It takes about two weeks to get a protective level of antibodies, or coverage, for your horse. When your equid is revaccinated (given a "booster") in approximately a month or so, the antibody-making response will be kicked up higher and take most of a year or more to decline. This is the "initial series" you may have heard of. Your vet will advise on current recommendations for the number of boosters and time intervals required to maximize your horse's cover for your area and specific vaccine. Ask your veterinarian how often they recommend revaccination in future.

If my horse isn't vaccinated at extraction time, what do we do?

He can get his first tetanus, but tetanus coverage will only be available *after* the first two weeks has elapsed if he only gets a tetanus toxoid. That's when your vet may or may not recommend tetanus antitoxin. Tetanus antitoxin comprises pre-formed antibodies which are extracted and purified. It should only be used in emergency cases when a horse is not vaccinated and an injury occurs. Properly performed ***odontoplasty*** is not an emergency. So, the take-home lesson here for first-time vaccinates is to please have your horses vaccinated at least one month before planned odontoplasty, or extraction or other surgery, and have them boostered when your vet is there for the dentistry, then keep them current. If you keep your horses vaccinated for tetanus, then they'll never need a tetanus antitoxin. Just remember (not dentistry for a moment) the small puncture wounds your horses sustain in the mud of winter may never be noticed, and if your horse is covered, so much the better! Talk with your vet

Don't All Wolf Teeth Need Extraction?

REMEMBER THAT ALL extractions must be treated the same with respect to pain relief and method, regardless of their class, including wolf teeth. See Chapter 15, Veterinary Specific Procedures: Extraction Considerations.

AS DISCUSSED EARLIER in Chapter 8, Secondary forms of Dental Disease: Wolf Teeth, not all wolf teeth need extraction, but some absolutely do. Bitted riding with any of the following conditions can cause pain and behavioral problems if the wolf teeth are allowed to remain in place.

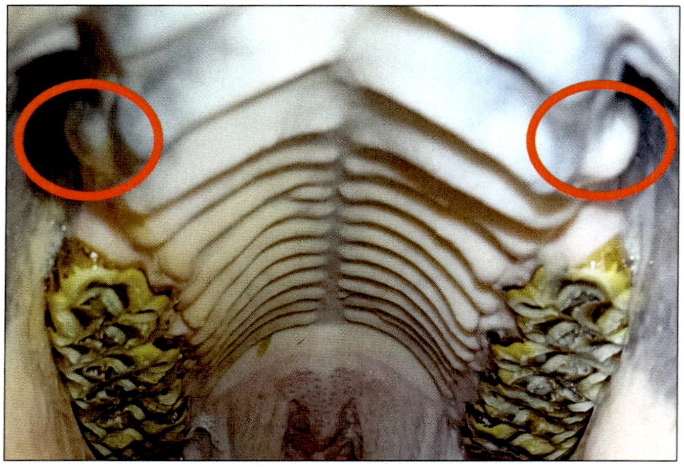

This horse is unlucky enough to have two unerupted maxillary wolf teeth. Image credit Dr Elke Pollaris.

loose or Mobile Wolf Teeth

Fractured or mobile (loose) wolf teeth likely cause pain whenever the horse moves its mouth or tongue... which is most of the time. These teeth should be extracted.

Wolf teeth which are separated from the first cheek tooth

These will be unstable and likely to fracture or become mobile, both of which are painful and need addressing.

Unerupted, or blind, wolf teeth

When a bit hits them, it will cause pain and possibly behavioral issues. They are often missed on an oral examination. If these are mandibular, the situation becomes even worse. I have seen these unerupted

Wolf Teeth Requiring Extraction

Condition	Explanation
Fractured	Broken wolf teeth may have painful pulp exposure
Filed to gumline	Tooth likely has a painful pulp exposure
Mobile	Loose tooth painful, especially when hit by bit
Distant from '06	No support from adjacent tooth, liable to fracture
Unerupted	Tooth is under the gingiva, painful when hit by bit
Mandibular	Mandibular wolf teeth will be painfully hit by bit

Wolf teeth requiring extraction, and the reasons for it. Image credit Author.

mandibular wolf teeth in two half-brothers. Each horse had the same unerupted wolf tooth, which had its occlusal (or what should be the occlusal) surface directed mesially and ***buccally***.

Mandibular wolf teeth

First, because they are likely to be damaged by concussion from a bit, and second, because they are so often missed. They may also be unerupted, which makes them doubly hard to find. They may be ***palpated*** and seen on radiographs. Mandibular wolf teeth are rare, but they do occur. Because they cause so much grief to horses which have them, it is important to always palpate the bars of both the maxilla and the mandible during the initial examination.

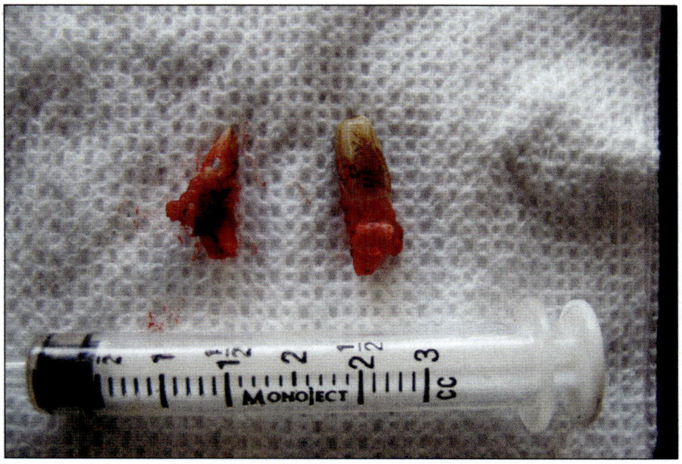

Two mandibular wolf teeth extracted from a thoroughbred. They had been fractured prior to extraction and portions were absent. Image credit Author.

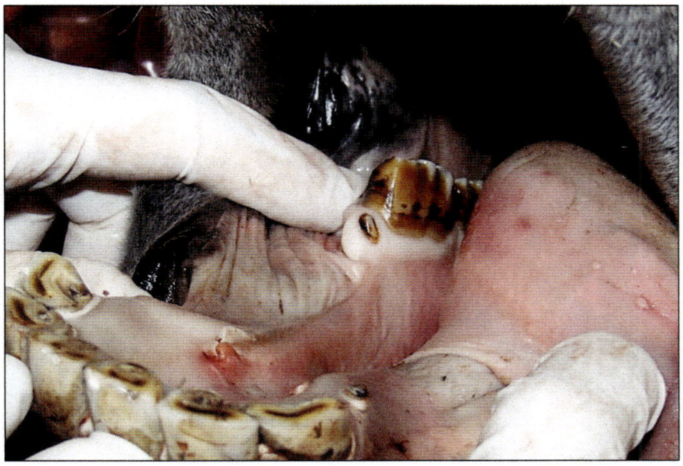

This mandibular wolf tooth in a cadaver appears to have been rasped down in the past. A dangerous procedure, which likely caused pulpitis and perhaps tooth death. Image credit Author.

Which wolf teeth may sometimes be left in place?

It is up to the discretion of the practitioner to determine if they think a wolf tooth will or will not be a problem, but here are some guidelines to help you understand the rationale behind these decisions. These may be left in place: wolf teeth which are not mobile nor fractured and reside flush against the first cheek tooth, especially if they are tucked in toward the palate. These will likely never contact a bit. Large, molarized, intact (non-fractured), non-mobile wolf teeth which are flush with the first cheek tooth are usually good candidates to stay in place as well. That being said, I once bought a horse which had been handled extremely roughly. He had large molarized wolf teeth. One had been loosened and one had broken clean off. It took some time to get him to respond quietly to a bit after properly extracting these teeth.

Filing off or breaking off wolf teeth... or any tooth, for that matter...

It is neglect and abuse to file or rasp the wolf teeth, or any teeth) into the pulps, much less down to the gumline instead of extracting them. No matter how small a tooth, it will still have live pulps. Filing them will cause pulp exposure, pain, likely pulpitis and tooth death, coupled with periodontal disease and draining tracts from possible osteomyelitis. This is never a good idea.

What Does Ongoing Post-Extraction Care Look Like?

YOUR VETERINARIAN WILL detail the immediate post-extraction care needed for your horse. Your horse will need dental care, including odontoplasty, at least every six months for the rest of its life due to a now-unopposed tooth or teeth. Equine incisors and cheek teeth must be opposed, or the elongation of the tooth or teeth opposite an extraction site will be unimpeded and result in abnormal mastication (chewing).

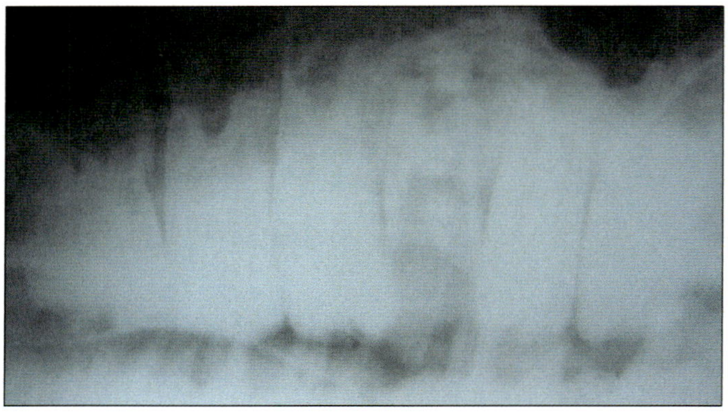

This horse had an incomplete extraction several years prior to my first examination. Despite the large proportion of tooth still in the alveolus, note the dental drift of the '08 and '10 into the space left by the extraction of the occlusal portion of the '09. Image credit Author.

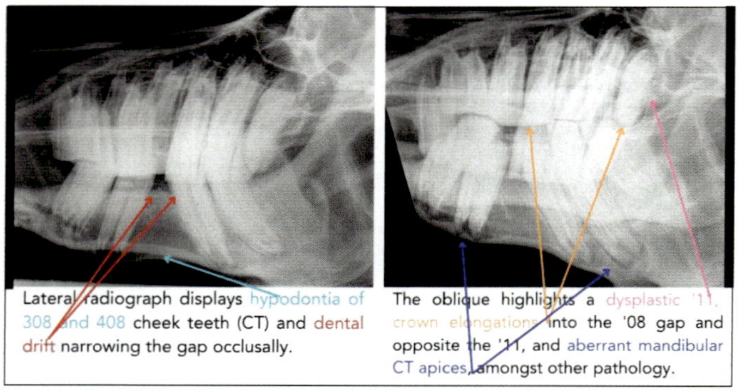

Note the dental drift in this miniature with hypodontia. Teeth will also drift post-extraction due to the angulation of the most mesial and distal cheek teeth trying to constantly press the arcade together like a brick wall. Image credit Author.

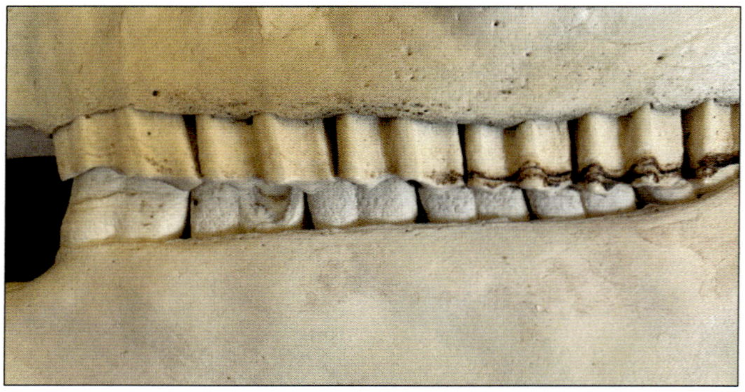

Note that even in a normal mouth, the teeth do not line up perfectly, i.e. the 208 is placed distally to the more mesial 308. This means crown elongation opposing an extracted tooth will affect all the teeth around it. And that is before considering dental drift, which will cause all teeth to be incorrectly opposed, with time. The six-monthly odontoplasty is essential to the care, comfort, and life of your horse post-extraction. Image credit Author.

Also, under normal circumstances, the outward angulation of the tooth roots forces the teeth in each cheek tooth arcade toward each other to form a solid unit like a brick wall. Once a tooth is removed from this arcade, however, the same forces from the tooth root angulation cause the teeth on either side of the extraction site to migrate towards the gap by dental drift. This will cause previously opposed teeth to not meet as they once did, further necessitating that six-monthly odontoplasty. Little may be done about this drifting, which will set off the rest of the teeth in the mouth in terms of occlusion.

In plain words, the teeth opposing the new gap will form ***crown elongations*** into the opposing jaw unless they are prevented from doing so. More than one tooth will be affected by this, as the tooth arcades normally do not line up the teeth perfectly adjacent to each other, i.e. the 208 does not fit directly over the 308, for example:

In severely neglected post-extraction or tooth loss patients, the unopposed teeth erupt until they erupt into the mucosa or even the bone of the mandible or maxilla from where the tooth was extracted. This is incredibly painful for the equid concerned. Unfortunately, it is not rare.

You can minimize the effects of extraction and dental drift by having odontoplasty performed on your horse every six months (unless your vet recommends more often) to prevent crown elongations from becoming a seriously painful problem to your horse.

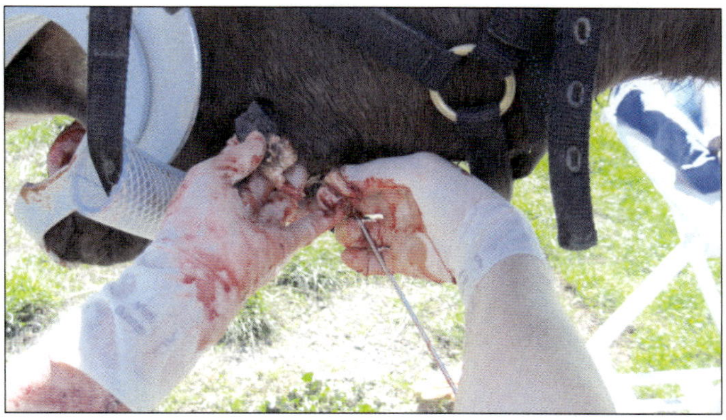

Post-operative care for this horse included oral saline flushes and cleaning and monitoring of the skin around the wound. Prior to extraction, she had a chronic mandibular draining tract from an apical abscess and fractured tooth root. She had a Steinmann Pin assisted repulsion of the broken root via the draining tract.

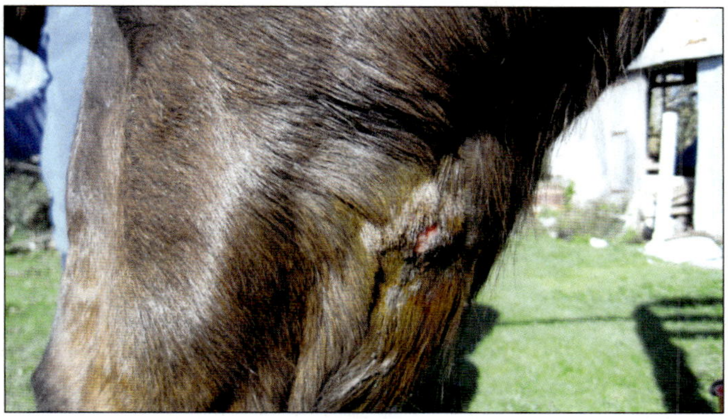

One week post-extraction of tooth and root fragment: little tissue reaction and cessation of discharge. Continuation of drainage could indicate a problem which your veterinarian should know about. Image credit this image and left, Author.

Special Challenges: Equid-Like Teeth in a 2000 kg Animal!

WHITE RHINOS AND other large ungulates pose many challenges for those desiring to perform dentistry on them. But with an awesome team like that of the Auckland Zoo in New Zealand, anything is possible. Pictured here is only a fraction of the support staff helping on the day. Veterinarians, vet technicians, zoo keepers, and the maintenance crew all help on the days the dental vet comes to town. This is only attempted with a crew of many vets and a huge support staff.

See the next page for Inkosi at the Auckland Zoo!

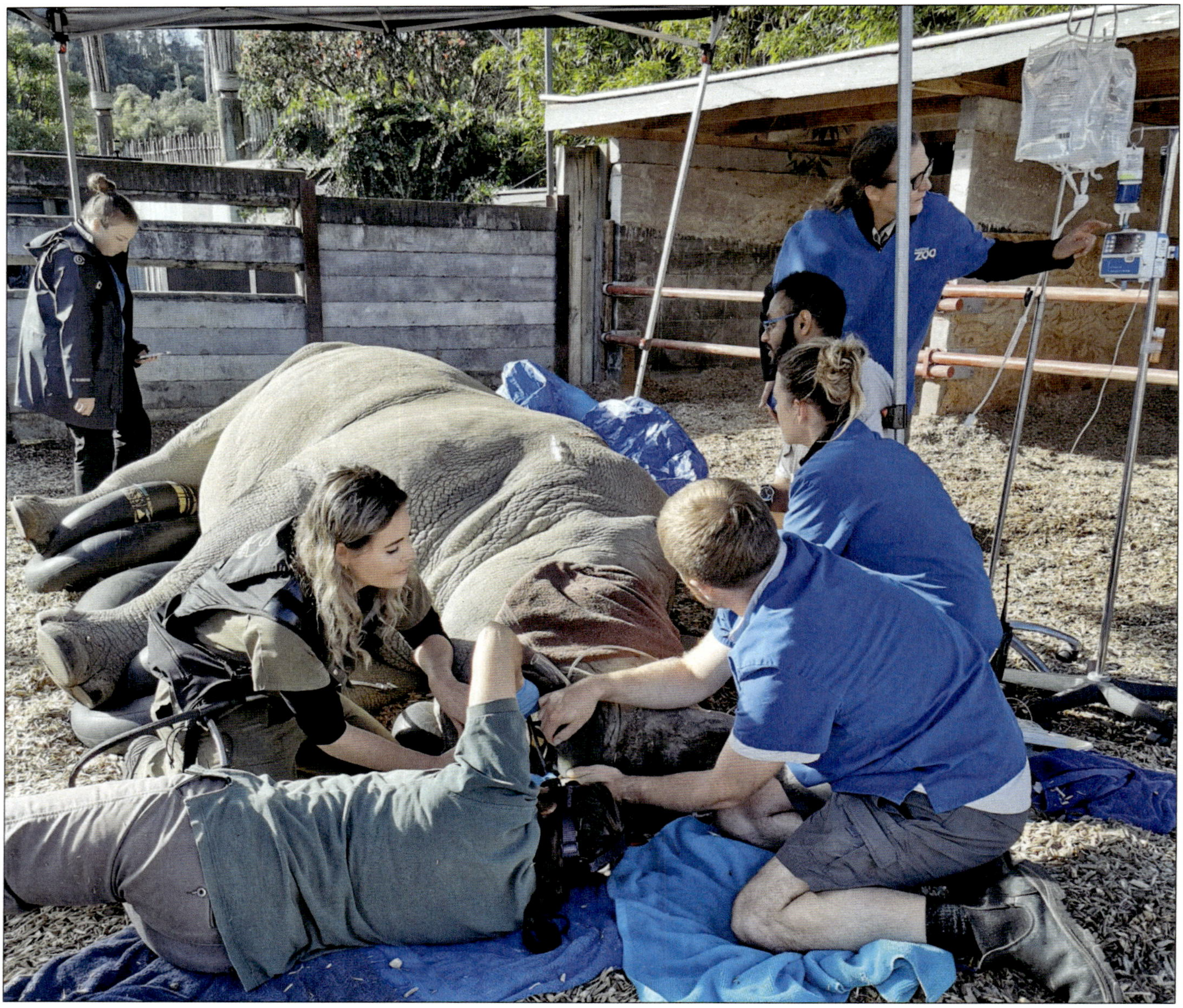

And sometimes one must lie down. Dr Elizabeth Thompson is lying on the ground, with her arm somewhere inside Inkosi's large mouth with a relatively small oral entrance. Inkosi is a nearly 2000 kg Southern white rhinoceros at Auckland Zoo in New Zealand, under a planned general anesthesia for dental care: odontoplasty!These animals receive the very best of preventative care. White rhinoceros teeth are similar to an equid, but four times larger and lack incisors and canines. The sheer size and mass of an adult white rhino make even the simplest procedures challenging on many levels, but the importance of dental care is well-recognized and prioritized by the zoo staff who care for these majestic animals. Image credit Amy Ross, used with permission of Auckland Zoo.

CHAPTER SIXTEEN

WHAT ARE ADVANCED DENTAL TECHNIQUES TO HELP MY HORSE?

EQUID ***VETERINARY*** DENTISTRY has evolved steadily over the past thirty years and many new techniques have been created and evolved in this time to the improvement of equine ***oral*** health. It's exciting to be a part of this. You can be, too!

What is Restorative Therapy in Equids?

RESTORATION (LIKE A filling in our own teeth) is an option in some cases for your horse. There are many dental specialist veterinarians performing these procedures now. See Chapter 6, Developmental and Acquired Conditions: Infundibular and Peripheral Caries. The purpose of applying restorations is to prevent or reduce the risk of ***pulp exposure*** or to protect a tooth.

Pulp exposure may occur or be in danger of occurring when a tooth is placed at risk by:

- disease such as ***infundibular caries***
- injuries such as tooth fracture
- tooth malformation
- endodontic therapy

To stop the progression of ***pathology***, equine dental veterinarians may utilize restoration, or "filling" with similar dental restoration materials to those used in human dentistry. Because equine teeth differ from those of humans in their composition and structure, extensive training in this technique is essential.

The goal of restoration is to stop progression of disease and create a functional tooth, or if the goal of a functional tooth is not achievable, at least stopping the progression of disease. Restoration involves thorough evacuation of any diseased ***tissue***, timely and correct application of the various layers of restoratives, and careful monitoring.

Factors which make this difficult include:

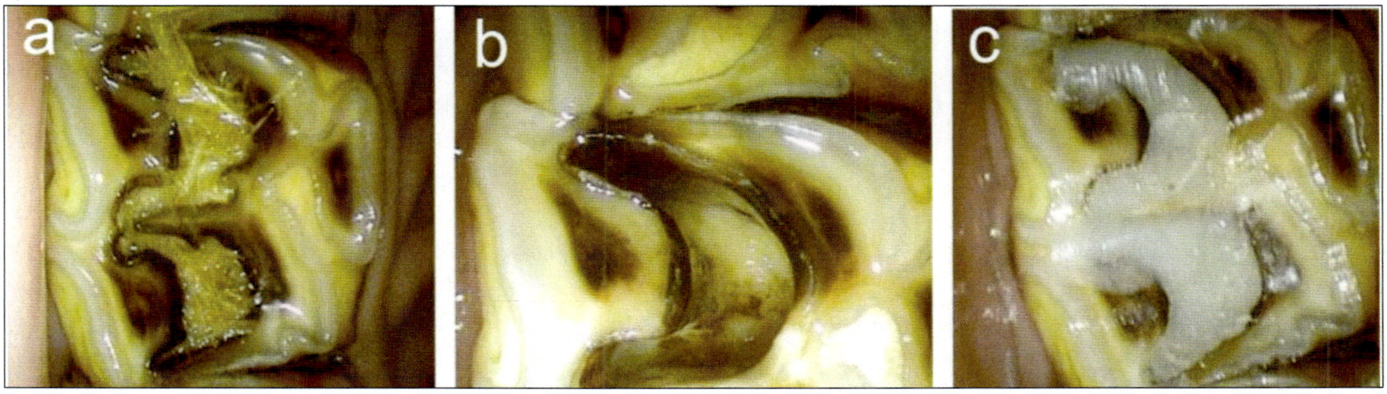

Stages of restoration of infundibular caries in equine cheek tooth 109; (a) grade 4 infundibular caries with food impaction in both mesial and distal infundibula; (b) fully prepared cavity prior to restoration, note cleanliness of apical region and visualization of enamel apex; (c) after restoration with dual-cured flowable resin composite. Image credit Dr Pearce C. (2020). Image originally published in Pearce C. Recent developments in equine dentistry. New Zealand Veterinary Journal 68, 178-86, 2020. ©NZVA

- the shape of the horse's mouth and placement of the teeth, necessitating working via mirror or oroscope at right angles to your field of vision.
- with the more distal teeth, working at a distance of a foot or more from the front of the mouth.
- grinding forces on the teeth from the opposing arcade may prevent retention of restoratives.
- working in a standing, sedated but not perfectly still patient.
- the degree of decay already present in the tooth when the horse is presented may not allow saving of the tooth by restoration.

And the list goes on!
But at least there are now choices.

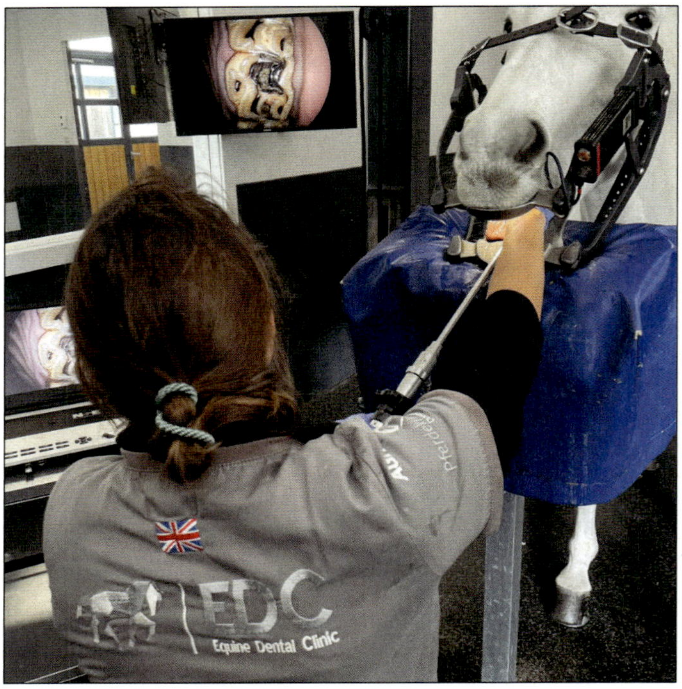

Restorative and endodontic therapy can help prevent a tooth affected by severe caries from fracturing apart. Dr Nicole du Toit of EDC (Equine Dental Clinic) is using an oroscope to view this horse's teeth in preparation for restorative therapy. Image credit Dr Nicole du Toit.

How is it Different From Endodontic Therapy?

What is endodontic therapy?

A tooth which has sustained damage to its pulp is extremely painful to the horse. The resultant pulpitis is the source of the pain. To relieve this pain, a dead tooth must be extracted or treated by a specialist veterinary dentist, if the specialist deems the patient an appropriate candidate for pulp canal or other endodontic therapy.

Endodontic therapy is treatment of a tooth which has sustained damage to the pulp, as an alternative to extraction. It consists of removal of damaged or dead pulp and ***dentin*** and replacement with the appropriate filling material. Vital pulpotomy is the endodontic technique used when a tooth is still alive, and a partial or total pulpectomy is used when the pulp and part of the tooth nourished by the pulp are dead.

Why perform endodontic therapy on horses?

Endodontic therapy is performed to:

- save the life of a tooth (vital pulpotomy) or
- enable a horse to retain a dead tooth without pain (partial or total pulpectomy), also called pulp canal therapy (like "root canal therapy", but in horses), and
- preserve the function of the tooth for as long as possible.
- keep a horse with pulpitis or a nonvital pulp exposure from having to stop its training or work schedule (while pain free!) for the time required to recover from an extraction.

The alternative to pulpotomy or pulpectomy is extraction. Successful endodontic therapy can prevent the problems previously discussed with the physical loss of a tooth, namely that the unopposed teeth will continue to erupt into the space created, and that ***dental drift*** will cause a shift of the rest of an arcade over time. Both problems cause serious difficulties for the horse, especially if it doesn't receive six-monthly quality dental care. See Chapter 15, Veterinary Specific Procedures: Ongoing Post-Extraction Care.

By using endodontic therapy, a tooth with a pulp exposure may survive, or an internally dead tooth (the parts of the tooth which were supported by the now-dead pulp) may remain in place. Due to the still-live ***periodontal tissues*** around it, this devitalized but filled tooth will continue to erupt, giving the opposing teeth something to grind against, as well as preventing the dental drift which would occur if the tooth were extracted. Unfortunately, a dead tooth is more brittle than a live one and is prone to eventual fracture.

Endodontic therapy sounds simple, but unfortunately, it is anything *but* simple. With appropriate training and instrumentation, *incisor* endodontic therapy is relatively straightforward. ***Cheek teeth***, however, are a different story altogether. Cheek tooth endodontics are extremely difficult by virtue of cheek tooth anatomy. There is very little room to work, and that room is often more than a foot inside the small entrance created by the horse's mouth... and one must work at 90 degrees to the mouth with the aid of endoscopic cameras. Challenging indeed.

Some veterinarians perform pulpotomy, or pulp canal therapy with only radiographs and oroscopic examination, but a prominent equine veterinary dental specialist recently said that a CT or MRI is recommended for every cheek tooth case being considered for pulpectomy. Or said another way, successful cheek tooth endodontic therapy may be improved by utilizing better visualization than can be achieved with radiographs and endoscopy alone, although some specialists are satisfied with their radiographs and oroscopy.

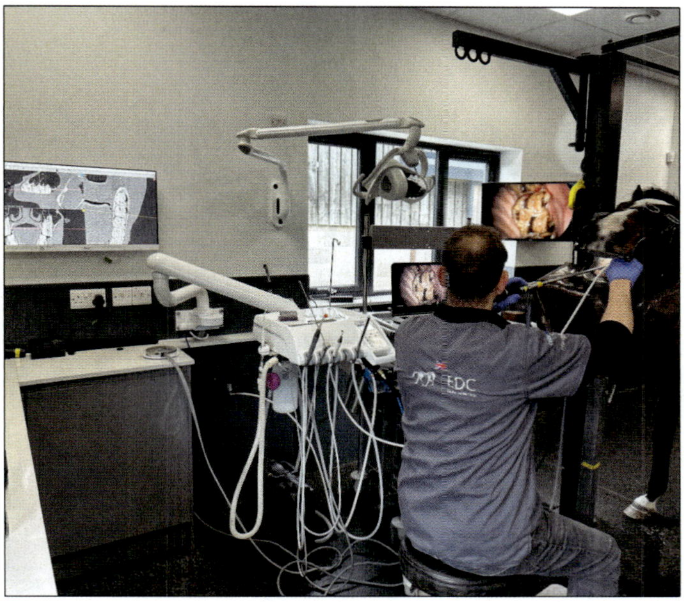

Access to the back of a horse's mouth for these involved procedures is challenging, even with the best of training, facilities, and equipment! Dr Chris Pearce of EDC shows how he works with oroscopic visualization plus previously taken CT images on the screen to the left. Image credit Dr Chris Pearce.

What is a Vital Pulpotomy, and is it Helpful?

VITAL PULPOTOMY IS our endodontic therapy answer to treatment of a recently injured, still vital (live) tooth which has sustained ***pulpar exposure***. It is the simpler of our options, but it is only available as an effective treatment within the first two to three days after injury.

Vital pulpotomy may be indicated in several cases:

- ***Iatrogenic*** pulp exposure from dental operator or surgeon
- Accidental pulp exposure, such as by dental fracture

Repair of pulp exposure

A vital pulpotomy is commonly used by a trained, experienced dental veterinarian to treat pulp exposure on teeth which have 1- sustained a fracture which has opened a pulp, but when the rest of the tooth is still alive and well, or 2- sustained an iatrogenic pulp exposure by a dental operator.

Fractured teeth are extremely painful to the horse if the fracture line enters or is near the pulp. The most common dental injury I see are fractured ***incisors*** sustained when one horse kicks another in the face, or when a horse runs into something more solid than they are. If we are aware a pulp exposure has occurred, we can help the horse by performing a vital pulpotomy.

The purpose of a vital pulpotomy is to provide protection from pulpitis for the pulp elements while formation of a ***dentinal bridge*** hopefully occurs inside the pulp chamber. Vital pulpotomy is performed under sedation with ***analgesia*** by your dental veterinarian. It is a procedure whereby a tooth with a pulp exposure has the pulp chamber evacuated past the area of exposure down to live, clean tissue, and the chamber is treated with various substances appropriate to equine teeth to encourage formation of a dentinal bridge. A tooth restoration is placed over the pulpotomy to provide more protection. See Chapter 10, Head Trauma and Dental Pathology: Accidental Pulp Exposure.

A dentinal bridge is a barrier created by the pulp laying down a layer of reparative (tertiary) dentin between the exposed pulp and the rest of the pulp. This is an attempt to seal off the rest of the pulp from the area of injury to prevent infection and death of the pulp, and thus save the tooth. If you see blood coming from what might be a fractured tooth, ring your dental vet right away! If a vital pulpotomy and restoration of that tooth (like a filling at your dentist) can be performed, you have a good chance of saving the tooth. Since the blood supply to a tooth is better in young horses due to the excellent blood supply in their wide-open apices, you have a better chance of saving the tooth than you would in a geriatric, but it's worth a try!

Partial or Total Pulpectomy (Like Human Root Canal)

PARTIAL OR TOTAL pulpectomy, the endodontic therapy which in humans is referred to as "root canal therapy", would best be described as a "pulp canal therapy" in horses, due to the differences in pulpar anatomy between people

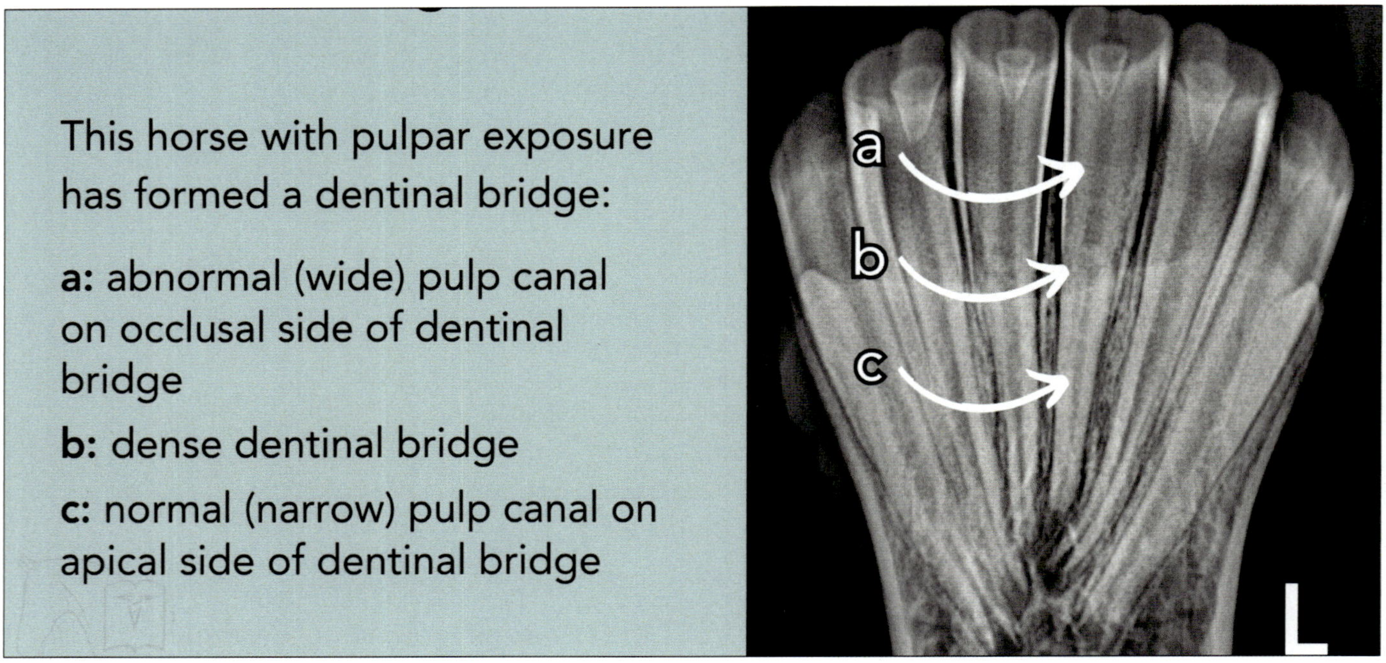

This horse had a pulpar exposure of his 301. Note the overly wide pulp at a) on the occlusal side of the radiodense dentinal bridge at b), which has formed to protect the normal pulp chamber at c), which is apical to the dentinal bridge. Image credit Dr Marieke van den Enden.

and horses. This has been used on incisors for a long time in equine veterinary dentistry with excellent results. The results in cheek teeth are more challenging and require significant investment in training, equipment, and materials to be effective. While endodontic therapy can keep that tooth in place as a space-occupier and help prevent the problems of drift and overgrowths, the internally dead tooth will be more brittle than a live tooth, and thus more liable to fracture in the future.

Endodontic treatment of incisors

Incisors have relatively wide and straight pulp canals, especially when compared to the cheek teeth. Endodontic therapy of incisors is currently being performed successfully by equine dental veterinarians and is a useful therapy to retain the use of an incisor without pain to the horse. If the endodontic therapy fails, the tooth must be extracted.

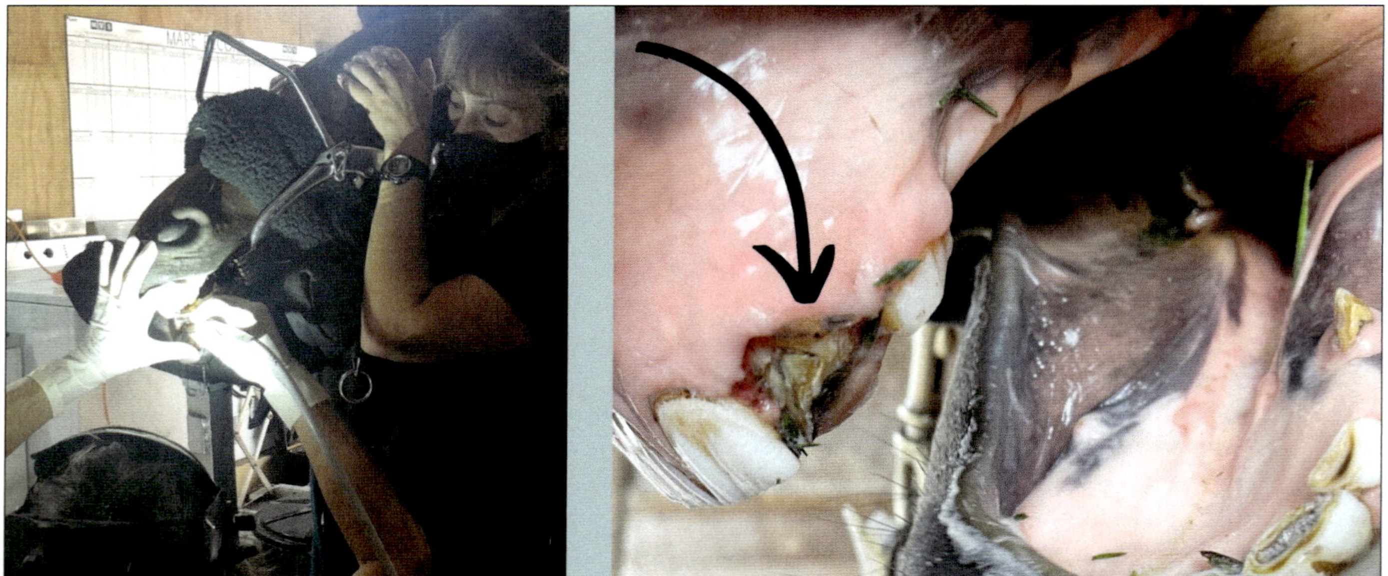

Fractured 202 and endodontic therapy on a young horse to save the tooth. Images credit Dr Stephanie Brooks.

Endodontic treatment of cheek teeth

The pulpar anatomy of equine cheek teeth make partial or total pulpectomies quite difficult. Equid cheek teeth have between five and seven pulp canals extending from a central pulp chamber toward the occlusal surface of the tooth. Fortunately or unfortunately, the number of pulp horns do not equal the number of tooth apices or roots, so not only do the canals interconnect... *randomly*, but the communications between them change over time. Both factors make it challenging to ensure your vet has effectively cleaned and completely filled the involved pulp or pulps. Without this thorough treatment, the pulp canal therapy might as well not have been done. CT is extremely helpful to fully visualize exactly where the pulps reside and whether complete cleaning and obturation (filling) of the pulp canals has been effective.

How successful is cheek tooth pulpectomy?

You as an owner must be prepared, if you wish to have pulpectomy endodontic therapy performed on your horse's cheek tooth, that this procedure will require multiple rechecks and likely repeat procedures, and they are not always successful. Failure is a possibility, at which time the tooth may require extraction. Textbooks and scientific literature claim success rates to be between 60 and 90%.

Orthodontics for Equids? Really?

MOST OF YOU will be familiar with the idea of orthodontics in humans: headgears, braces, and the like, to correct malocclusion. See Chapter 6, Developmental and Acquired Conditions: Malocclusions. In horses, it's a lot trickier. The narrow age ranges within which orthodontics must be utilized to have any chance of success make it even more challenging. Orthodontics may be used in foals with congenital malocclusions such as overbite, underbite, or wry nose, and may also be needed after mandibular or maxillary fractures. The type of orthodontics needed depends upon the degree and type of malocclusion as well as the age of the equid.

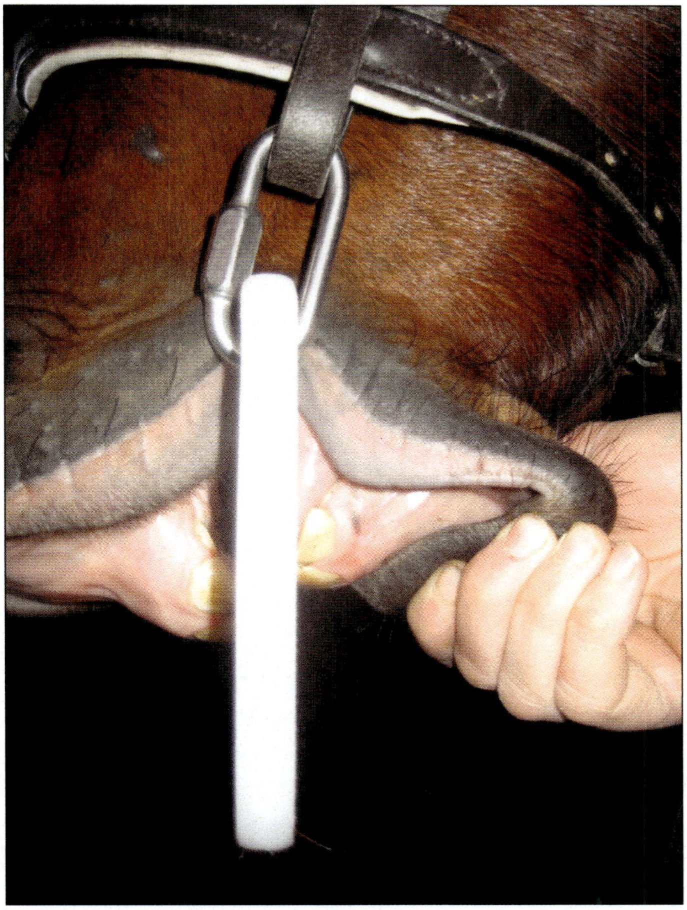

A bit plate may encourage correct occlusion in a young horse with overbite or overjet in a limited number of cases when used early enough. The below functional orthodontic appliance may have been more effective. Image credit Author.

For those who wore a headgear, like me, you'll remember how uncomfortable it was, and how you were meant to wear it for a certain number of hours per day. Try telling that to a foal who wants to nurse from its mother. There are functional orthodontic devices such as this bit plate, below, which may work on selected cases if worn by a young foal for a certain numbers of hours per day, but the "owner compliance" regarding keeping a device on a young, nursing foal will be limited by the owner's time and their willingness to make it work, the foal's compliance, and the mare's as well. Devices such as this must be used in extremely young foals to have the desired effect.

One of the most important concepts to understand concerning non-surgical orthodontic manipulation of the symmetrical equid malocclusions is that non-surgical correction must be attempted at a very young age. For this reason, the first neonatal foal check should include evaluation of the foal's bite. It is simple to do and can save everyone, including the foal, a world of heartache and pain.

Because of the issue of compliance, most foals whose malocclusion is amenable to use of a functional device will probably do best with a *fixed* functional orthodontic device. These may be applied by a dental specialist veterinarian and treated at the same time with ***odontoplasty***.

If a malocclusion is not amenable to the use of a functional orthodontic device, orthognathic surgery, or surgical orthodontics may be utilized to reposition portions of the ***mandible***, maxilla, or the entire jaw to correct function and esthetics (how it looks). These surgeries are used to correct the bite and misaligned jaws caused by trauma (e.g. fractures), unbalanced growth of the mandible vs. the maxilla, or misalignment of jaws, muzzle, and teeth (e.g. wry nose). Most of these surgical procedures can be performed a little later in life after skeletal growth begins to slow. These are extremely tricky surgeries which are best left to teams of veterinarians with advanced training in surgery, dentistry, ***anesthesia***, and imaging.

These corrections do not always work, but without them, the foal is doomed to a lifetime of pain.

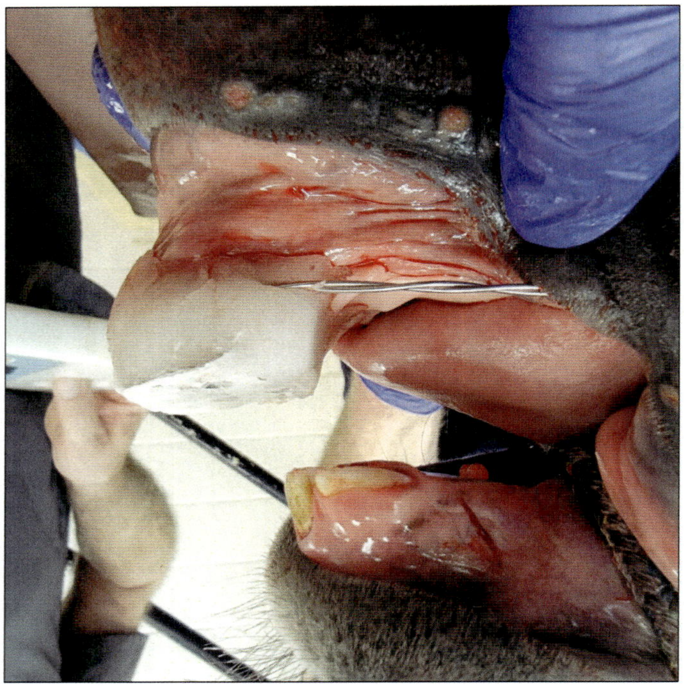

Functional orthodontic appliances are surgically fitted to a foal for treatment of MAL 2, or overbite or overjet. Yes, the person is upside down. So is the foal. Images credit to Cathie Heald Greenwell.

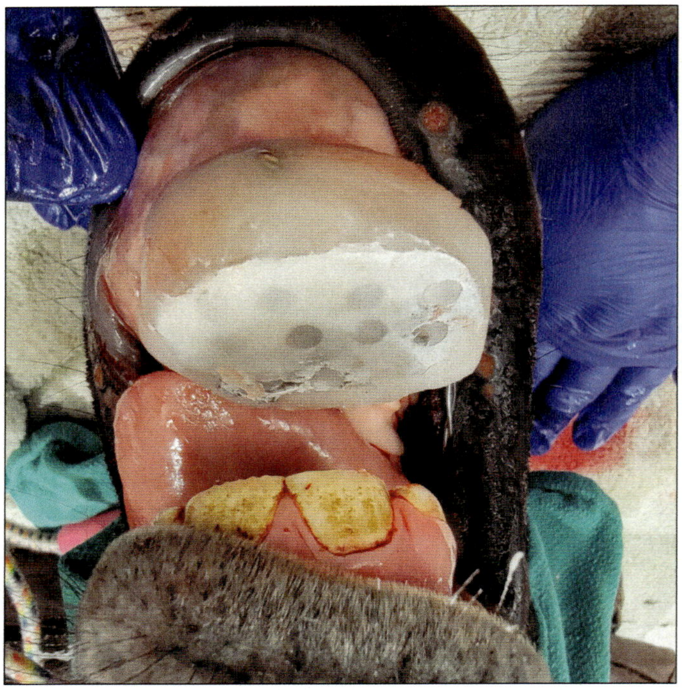

Front view of functional orthodontic appliances are surgically fitted to a foal for treatment of MAL 2, or overbite or overjet. Images credit Cathie Heald Greenwell.

So, what happens if I don't get my horse's severe incisor malocclusions corrected?

Malocclusions where the incisors do not meet will eventually cause severe problems and pain for your horse if not addressed. In a similar manner to how the cheek teeth apices are oriented mesially and distally to force the cheek teeth arcades into a solid, single unit, the muscles of the head are oriented to pull the incisors and cheek teeth against the opposing incisor arcade to achieve the huge forces required to bite hard feedstuffs. In other words, the muscles of the mandible and maxilla are designed to close the mouth in chewing, so these muscles are the strongest. The contact between the incisors serve to hold the maxilla and mandible in the correct places, but what if those incisors do not meet, as with an overbite or an underbite?

- These muscles pull hard against each other, causing the rostral portion of the mandible where the mandibular incisors are seated, to curl upward toward the palate, while the bone of the rostral maxilla curls downwards toward the mandible. They keep curling towards each other until they make contact and begin cutting into the soft tissues and bone of the opposing part of the mouth, if left long enough.
- The unopposed mandibular and the maxillary incisors are not grinding each against each other, and so crown elongation, or "overgrowth" occurs, and they get longer and longer, which compounds the problem just mentioned.
- The unopposed incisor pulps are likely very close to the occlusal surface, so if one performs odontoplasty on these teeth, pulp exposure would be highly likely when attempting more than the most minimal reduction.
- The cheek teeth may also be affected by this mandibular/maxillary misalignment, which allows mesial and distal hooks to form. These may worsen the incisor malocclusion.

So, you see it's not a mere matter of a "little malocclusion" here if correction is not attempted. The secondary changes from this malocclusion have severe implications as a foal grows. If correction is unable to be performed on these severely affected patients for whatever reason, euthanasia must be considered for humane reasons.

How Do Minimally Invasive Extraction Techniques Work?

SOME RELATIVELY NEW procedures have evolved which allow your dental veterinarians to intraorally extract difficult-to-extract teeth which once would have required extraction via trephination and repulsion or buccotomy. See Chapter 15, Veterinary Specific Procedures. These are helpful for teeth with:

- crown fracture so extensive there is nothing available to grip from inside the mouth (clinical crown absent).
- malformations of apices or crown.
- obstructed tooth eruption pathways.
- unstable teeth due to severe infundibular or endodontic decay.

What are some of these minimally invasive techniques?

These minimally invasive techniques include the MTE, or minimally invasive transbuccal extraction procedure, intraoral sectioning of the tooth, partial coronectomy, and Steinmann pin repulsion.

Minimally Invasive Transbuccal Extraction Procedure

This procedure is used after standard intraoral extraction techniques have been attempted and failed, and is useful for the above extraction challenges. A "lateral buccotomy" is a technique where a surgeon makes a flap on the side of the face over the affected tooth, but critical structures traverse this path, so it has largely been replaced by the minimally invasive transbuccal extraction (MTE) procedure. MTE is a minimally invasive version of a buccotomy which may be performed in the standing, sedated horse. This also takes significant advanced training and equipment to be used effectively. After proper pre-extraction sedation, perineural anesthesia, radiography, and intraoral extraction attempts (which include elevating the tooth from its alveolus before progressing to MTE), etc., MTE involves entering the oral cavity through only a tiny (5 mm) incision in the cheek and utilizing specially designed set of trochars, cannulas, and long instruments, and continuing with intraoral extraction of teeth where access was previously limited. MTE makes it possible to elevate and separate the tooth further, then drill and tap into the offending tooth, finishing with insertion of a screw with which the tooth may be extracted into the mouth.

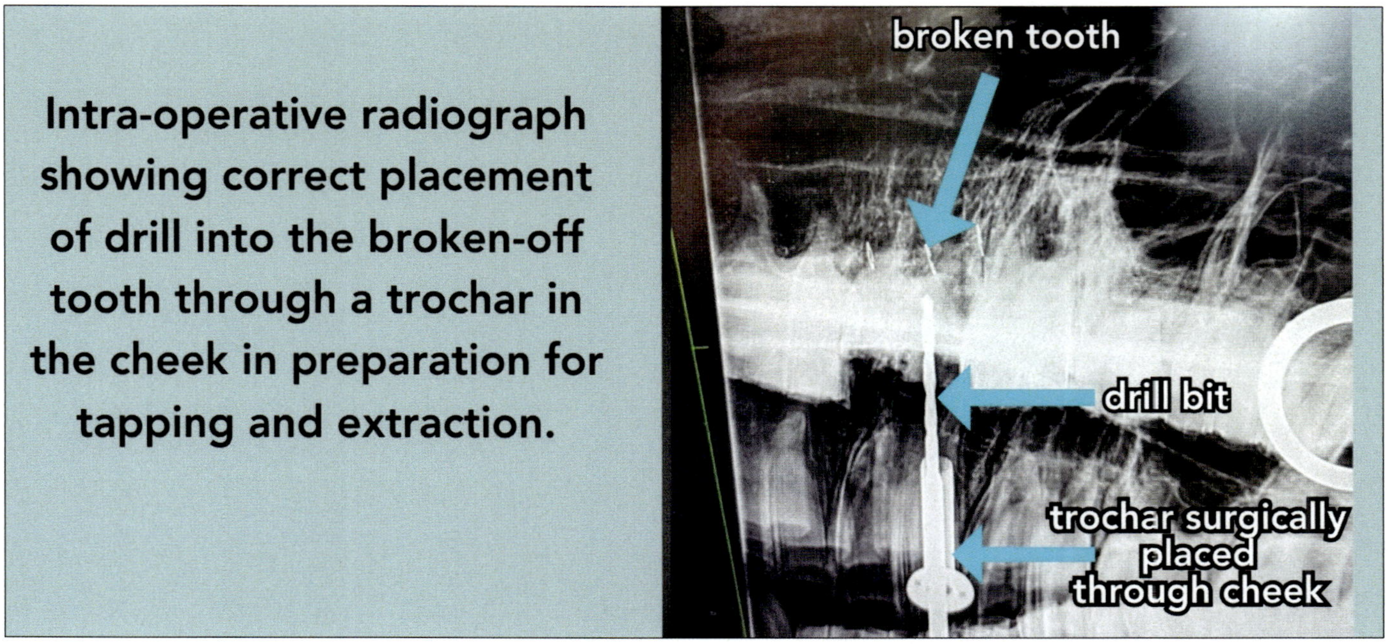

Minimally Invasive Transbuccal Extraction has been a welcome addition, allowing standing extraction of teeth which would have previously required general anesthesia and repulsion. Image credit Dr Olivia James.

This has made a world of difference to many horses, which in the past would have been subjected to general anesthesia plus trephination and repulsion. In the occasional case, a vet may have to resort to trephination and repulsion, but these are now thankfully few, with the advent of minimally invasive procedures.

Partial Coronectomy to Aid Intraoral Extraction of Teeth

Portions of crown may be sectioned off to allow more room between the tooth and the adjacent teeth to ease blocked extractions.

Intraoral Tooth Sectioning

The tooth may be cut longitudinally into half or into thirds, especially useful in teeth with diverging (spreading) apices or roots.

Minimally Invasive Steinmann Pin Repulsion Technique

While repulsion, per se, is an extremely destructive procedure, repulsion via a 2-3 mm Steinmann pin, can be an excellent way of helping a tooth exit an ***alveolus*** after other intraoral methods have failed, especially when a draining tract is present. After standard intraoral extraction procedures, this technique may be used to gently tap the tooth out of the alveolus.

These advanced extraction techniques require intensive veterinary dental training and extensive practice to master, in addition to specialized dental surgical equipment, so don't expect your general equine veterinarian to perform them, unless they have had the interest and instruction. They will certainly be able to refer you to a specialty practice to let you take advantage of these highly effective, new modalities for your horse.

CHAPTER SEVENTEEN

WHAT ABOUT MY BROODMARES?

BROODMARES, ALTHOUGH NOT ridden, still develop sharp points and every one of the dental problems listed throughout this book, such as cheek and tongue ***lacerations***, ***malocclusions***, ***periodontal disease***, sinus infections, ***EOTRH***, and loose teeth. Though she may never have a bit in her mouth, the pain from these pathologies can make her life miserable.

But They Don't Ever Have Bits in Their Mouths!

BROODMARES, ALTHOUGH NOT ridden, still develop sharp points and every one of the dental problems listed throughout this book, such as cheek and tongue lacerations, malocclusions, periodontal disease, sinus infections, EOTRH, and loose teeth. Though she may never have a bit in her mouth, the pain from these pathologies can make her life miserable.

As she ages, these conditions worsen and will cause her untold pain.

See:

Chapter 4, Examination of the Mouth
Chapter 5, About Dental Conditions
Chapter 6, Developmental and Acquired Conditions
Chapter 7, EOTRH
Chapter 8, Secondary Forms of Dental Disease
Chapter 9, Iatrogenic Disease
Chapter 10, Head Trauma and Dental Pathology
Chapter 11, Sinus Disease
Chapter 12, Special Equids: Geriatrics and Miniatures
Chapter 14, Odontoplasty vs. "Floating"...
Chapter 15, Veterinary Specific Procedures
Chapter 16, Advanced Techniques to Help Your Horse

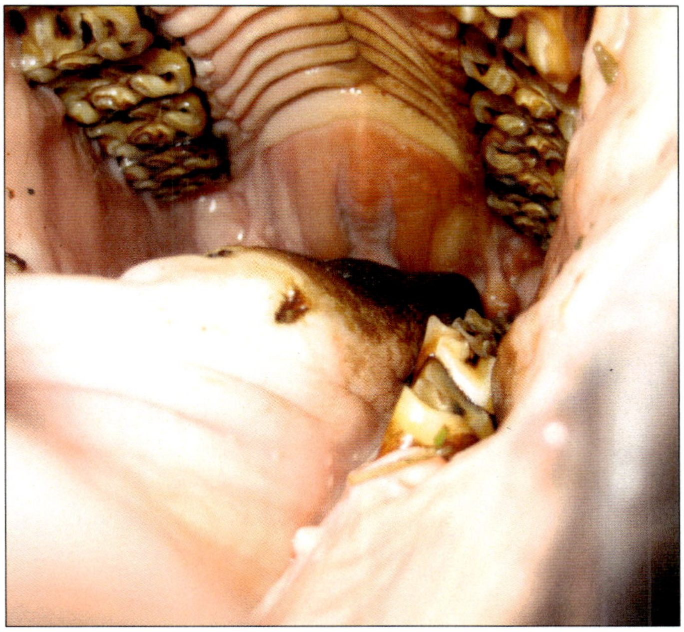

Sharp enamel points *on* ***lingual*** *mandibular* ***arcades*** *causing tongue lacerations. Image credit Dr Oliver Liyou.*

Does She Have Thorough Dental Examinations Yearly?

YOUR MARE MAY live with many other horses, but not be checked regularly, as often happens with broodmare bands. Has she taken a kick to the face and lives in quiet misery with a fractured tooth? We often don't notice the pain in these horses.

See:

Chapter 1, How do I Know My Horse has Dental Disease?
Chapter 10: Head Trauma and Dental Pathology.

"Well, She has Been Returning to Heat, and Last Year She Aborted her Foal…"

HAVE YOU EVER considered *this*? The bacteria entering the bloodstream from the periodontal disease she may have in her mouth won't help the expensive foal she carries. Studies on ***periodontal disease*** in both women and in dogs (different studies!) indicate periodontal disease may increase the likelihood of low birth weights, pre-term labor and late miscarriage, kidney disease, liver disease, vaginal disease, and cardiovascular disease. Studies in women also indicate that periodontal therapy may significantly reduce the rate of premature low birth weights. It behooves you to ensure your mare is receiving good dental care, including proper examination and odontoplasty at least yearly to ensure she is a fit as possible to be a mother to your next foal. More research on equids is needed in this area.

See:
Chapter 6, Developmental and Acquired Conditions
Chapter 7, EOTRH
Chapter 8, Secondary Forms of Dental Disease
Chapter 9, Iatrogenic Disease
Chapter 10, Head Trauma and Dental Pathology
Chapter 11, Sinus Disease

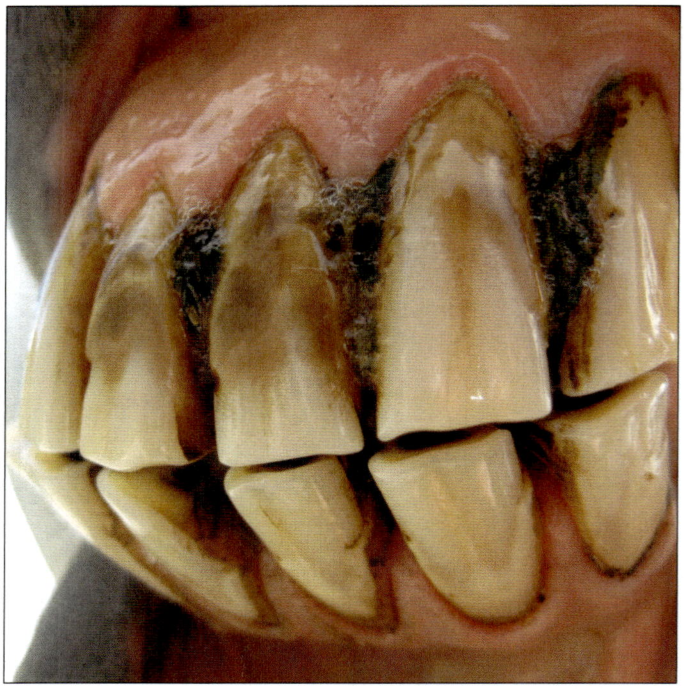

Broodmare with extremely painful periodontal disease, part of her EOTRH syndrome. Her teeth "had been ***floated****", but she hadn't had a dental examination in years, if ever. Image credit Author.*

Some of the Progeny of My Mares Seem to Have Poor Dentition. Why Might This Be?

TOOTH CREATION STARTS in the developing fetus inside the uterus of the mare. To give you an idea of when, it has been shown that the calcification of the deciduous cheek teeth, one of the later stages of tooth development, occurs by four months of gestation, and the calcification of the first permanent tooth buds begin at around ten months of gestation. That pretty much covers the whole of gestation and early foal life for development of all the teeth. Considering this timetable, recognize that the nutrition of the mare (a function of her dental health) may have implications in fetal tooth development.

See:
Chapter Three, Anatomy of the Mouth

Dentistry provided to broodmares has historically been perfunctory or non-existent, but there is no reason for this to occur. Thorough dental examination has often been bypassed as it was deemed unimportant, but broodmare owners should consider this much more seriously.

CHAPTER EIGHTEEN

HOW DOES FEEDING HEIGHT AFFECT OCCLUSION?

EVER THOUGHT ABOUT the level you place your horse's feed bucket, relative to the horse?

Why Should I Worry About Feeding Height?

IN THE WILD, and in a free-grazing situation with our domestic horses, horses spend at least sixteen hours per day grazing with their muzzles on the ground. Their anatomy has evolved with this eating style, and amongst other things, the inability to regularly eat with their head lowered may contribute to malocclusions. Conversely, allowing horses to eat with their muzzles down by the ground can contribute to better oral health and help improve some malocclusions.

When a horse lowers its head to eat, graze, or work and nothing (like a tight halter or cavesson) restricts its ***mandible*** from dropping toward the ground, moving ***rostrally*** with respect to the ***maxilla***, the occlusion between the upper and lower teeth is improved. However, as we saw in Chapter 4, Examination of the Mouth, when we discussed evaluation of the horse for for ***mesiodistal*** (sometimes known as ***rostro-caudal***) movement, we noted that when the muzzle is lifted, the mandible shifts ***caudally***, or backward. If a horse is fed up high and must continually eat with his head and muzzle raised, the mandible doesn't spend enough time moved rostrally (forward), and instead, remains mostly caudally (backwards). This may contribute to the development of distal ***hooks*** on the ***mandibular*** (lower) '11s and rostral hooks on the maxillary (upper) '06s. If these hooks develop, they restrict the rostral movement of the mandible and create discomfort and/or pain for the horse.

Odontoplasty, including a thorough examination and appropriate treatment to minimize these hooks and other malocclusions, plus routinely feeding the horse at ground level can assist in prevention of further hooks of this type.

Something to think about when you hang up that hay net or put their hay up into a high feeder... we won't even start talking about getting bits of hay in their eyes...

CHAPTER NINETEEN

HOW CAN YOU HELP YOUR VET HELP YOUR HORSE?

HERE ARE SOME more things you can do to make life easier for yourself and your veterinarian.

Can You Give Me a List of Things to Help My Vet?

SURE! Here you go!

1. Provide a safe place to work. This should be free of dangerous items a horse could back into or fall over. These same dangerous items could trip you up as well! Ideally, out of the weather.
2. Prepare your horse for examination and treatment by another person while taking safety precautions for yourself. It may take some persistence and effort, but it will be worth it in the long run. If the pre-sedation examination does not upset them, sedation will be much more effective. As always, take care when handling a horse, as per the Disclaimers! Helmets are always good around horses to protect your head!
    - 2.1. Ensure they can be quietly caught.
    - 2.2. Make sure they can be touched around the head, neck, chest, back, and rump without a fuss.
    - 2.3. They may be used to being bridled, but it is also a good idea for them to be accustomed to having their lips opened while standing quietly.
3. Provide access to clean water and power, preferably with an RCD, if their equipment requires it.
4. Pay on time, whatever your agreement. Better yet, pay on the day—many dental practitioners are solo vets who have little spare time and even less spare energy to chase debts so they can continue to pay their own bills.
5. Remember the differences between a basic tooth float and a thorough dental examination and odontoplasty. Consider the Eight Levels of Dentistry. A First Level through Fifth Level float requires little knowledge and minimal equipment. Its goals are simply rasping sharp points and overgrowths, if their instruments allow, and if the horse cooperates. Unfortunately, the information obtainable at this level about your horse's oral health and potentially needed treatments is severely limited. The Sixth Level exam is the first thorough exam which will allow odontoplasty to be performed.
6. Understand the costs of quality equine dental instrumentation and training. If you think saddles, bridles, feed, and dentistry are expensive, try purchasing dentistry instruments. If properly cared for, equine dental instruments will last a long time, but the initial outlay and ongoing required essential additions can be hefty. As a practitioner continues to add to their skill set to enable them to treat your horse's more involved dental cases, the required investment in equipment, training and time adds up.
7. Recognize that attaining expertise in equine dentistry requires huge investments of time and money. Merely the courses and journals one must assimilate to keep up with each month's new information do not come cheaply. Prices for conferences and wet labs (hands-on courses) in advanced techniques are steep, and attendance often requires overseas travel. Time away from practice also costs money.

8. Remember that health insurance for your horse, including dental coverage and surgical coverage, could literally save your horse's life when things get critical and expensive. This insurance is highly recommended for any horse.

All of these points help your veterinarian offer your equids the best possible care!

CHAPTER TWENTY

NOW IT'S UP TO YOU: HOW CAN YOU HELP YOUR HORSE? NTKs WHEN IT'S DENTISTRY DAY FOR YOUR EQUIDS!

IT TRULY IS up to you. I've written this book for you to learn all I could teach you of those dental ideas and solutions which are important to help you help your horse. Here are some "need-to-knows" (NTKs) for when someone is coming to perform dentistry on your horse.

How Do I Keep My Horse Safe?

I HAVE WRITTEN this book to give you the tools to understand enough about your horse's mouth in health and disease that you can make informed decisions and do your "due diligence", or check the qualifications and abilities of those you wish to use for your horse's dentistry. Only in this way can you offer your horse the level of dentistry you desire.

Not all dental training, certificated or not, is equal. Even if someone calls themself a "dentist", it doesn't mean they are the best choice for your horse, no matter now nice they are to your horse, and no matter how fancy their equipment. Many schools of dentistry create their own certification, and therefore they are not answerable to anyone but themselves. The dental education of non-***veterinary*** lay dental operators varies wildly, anything from "learning from a mate" to a formal program with examination. Most certifications, other than the BAEDT and the IGFP, are self-administered by their own training institute. These are not regulated by outside consumer bodies, may not be insured, and don't usually have a requirement for yearly continuing education.

Dental veterinarians have passed a five year (UK, NZ, Australia, etc.), six year (CA), or an eight year (USA) course in veterinary medicine, including anesthesiology, cardiology, critical care, endocrinology, ethics, neurology, physiology, radiography, surgery, etc., which enables them to properly care for the entirety of your horse, *including* their mouth, and have also obtained postgraduate training in equine dentistry. They are well-suited to take the best care of your whole horse, including its teeth. They are regulated by outside consumer bodies (veterinary boards administered by the government), are usually insured, and must usually complete continuing education on a yearly basis to stay up to date on current therapies and procedures, as well as to keep their veterinary registration or license current.

When someone is on-farm to perform dentistry on your horse, if they seem overzealous in their dentistry work, do not hesitate to stop them and discuss the situation. If they don't want to discuss it, or you are still in doubt, stop them and get a second opinion. Many veterinarians particularly trained in equine dentistry are happy to assist! The ***floating*** part of the odontoplasty should take less than one hour.

After floating or proper odontoplasty, regardless of any so-called "realignment", your patient should recover from sedation or treatment promptly, looking for food and be happy to eat after the proper time (about an hour) dictated by your veterinarian has elapsed.

After routine dentistry, horses should never:

- salivate excessively or drool
- have pink or red ***occlusal*** (chewing) surfaces*
- decline to eat or have a decreased appetite
- have swellings in the mouth
- gnaw on their knees or fences
- suddenly become reluctant to be bridled or haltered
- suddenly become reluctant to work
- be in any form of serious discomfort
- suddenly have any odd behavior changes

Especially importantly: the occlusal surfaces themselves should never be pink or red after treatment. This is a serious situation. If any tooth surfaces are exuding liquid of these colors or** are **these colors, this indicates the odontoblast processes of the pulp or the pulp itself have been exposed and vital pulpotomy or "pulp capping" is essential to prevent tooth death and loss down the line.

What is the Minimum Instrumentation Needed for a Thorough Dental Examination and Odontoplasty?

TO PERFORM DENTISTRY to a thorough level, or a level at which one can truly rule out dental disease as the source of your horse's "problem", be it behavioral or otherwise, your dental practitioner needs at minimum the following equipment:

- safe, full-mouth speculum
- large dose syringe or flushing unit to flush the mouth with water
- strong intraoral light source
- intraoral mirror
- dental picks and probes
- dental ***floats*** or a power floating unit
- veterinarian to examine and sedate the horse if a veterinarian is not to perform the dentistry
- an oroscope (if possible)

I once thought I did a pretty good job of dentistry until I started learning more about it and began looking much deeper. Sedation allows a thorough examination to be performed every time, not just when the horse prefers. It is also recommended for the safety of the owner or handler as well as for that of the horse. Visualization of many small intraoral structures is next to impossible in the unsedated horse, and international standard of practice in veterinary equine dentistry dictates that these structures be evaluated. The use of X-rays by your veterinary dental practitioner enables diagnosis, treatment, and monitoring of more challenging conditions.

Red Flags: Which Instruments Can Seriously Damage My Horse?

Power instruments are not for the untrained or minimally trained!

Power dental instruments are replacing many hand floating instruments for the educated equine dental practitioner. Used judiciously in well-trained hands, they are a time- and effort-saving tool. They allow the operator to treat specific teeth in the mouth and leave the mouth of every horse the best they can possibly make it, while minimizing wear and tear on their own body. Proper use of instruments and water minimizes the potential for thermal (heat) damage to the tooth pulps. Power dental instruments should never be used by untrained floaters or practitioners untrained in their use, as damage can occur rapidly. Whether using power or hand instruments, your equine dental practitioner should understand and consider that the pulp chambers may reside as little as less than one to four millimeters beneath the surface of a crown elongation (tooth overgrowth). Removing more than this, whether by grinding or cutting, may expose pulp. If any pulp is exposed, indicated by a pink or red spot on the surface of the tooth, vital pulpotomy, (pulp-capping procedure) is needed, ideally within 24–36 hours, to prevent potential death of that tooth within the next one to five years. This is a "painful procedure" and is entering live ***tissue***. As such, this procedure should only be (and depending upon your location, may legally *only be*) performed by a veterinarian.

What are molar shears or molar cutters, and how are they dangerous?

While molar shears or cutters are not power instruments, they are probably even more dangerous for two main reasons:

First, their usage is not incremental, as is odontoplasty, and they do not allow the operator to evaluate the distance to live pulp, which increases the risk of ***pulpar exposure***. When you transversely (across) cut off a piece of tooth with this modified bolt cutter, you cannot see if pulp is in the way of your cut. These have historically been used for long crown ***eruptions***, or ***overgrowths*** on teeth which were not in apposition to another tooth. As mentioned previously, the position of the pulp in an "unopposed" tooth is extremely close to the occlusal surface and pulps can readily be exposed.

Second, teeth cut with molar cutters tend to crack on a longitudinal, or ***apex***-to-occlusal line, which will require extraction of a previously-live tooth (significance: still alive, painful, and stuck tightly in place), which will shortly die, causing excruciating pain to your horse before that happens, but will be difficult to remove in its entirety. Molar cutters are best used as bolt cutters for cutting steel, which is not alive.

The only exception to *not* cutting across a tooth is during extraction of a tooth: for a veterinarian to section a tooth in a transverse plane (cutting across the tooth) by a sectioning bur or molar cutters. This is only necessary when a cheek tooth is partially extracted but is too long and is blocked from fulling exiting the ***alveolus*** due to lack of available height in the mouth. This tends to occur in young horses (relatively long cheek teeth) with a small mouth.

Cut-off wheels? How can they hurt my horse?

The flat surface of a powered cut-off wheel may be safely used in a sedated horse by a veterinarian to carefully reduce tooth overgrowths by grinding with the *flat* of the blade, when coupled with water cooling and careful observation. This is *not* the same as using the edge of the cut-off wheel. When the sharp edge of a cut-off wheel is used to cut transversely across a tooth, cutting off a slice of ***crown elongation***, the operator may expose living pulp or some of the pulp's tiny extensions, both of which endanger the life of a tooth. Vital pulpotomy by a veterinarian is indicated if a pulp exposure or near-pulp exposure occurs. See Chapter 3, Anatomy of the Mouth and Chapter 9, Iatrogenic Disease.

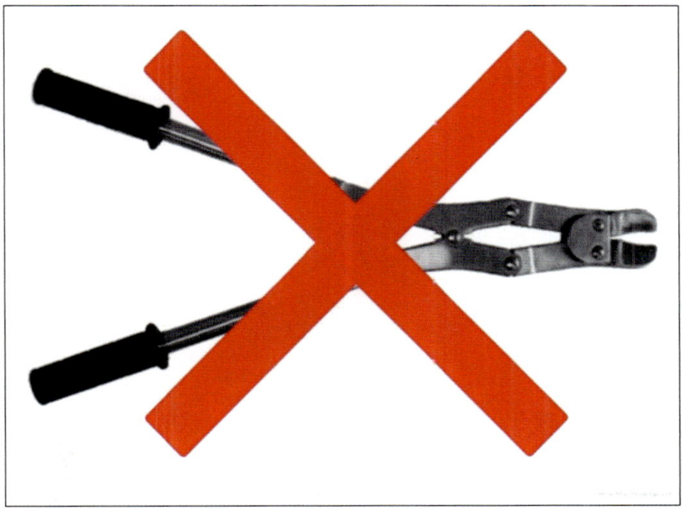

Molar cutters are best used as bolt cutters for cutting steel. Not for teeth, which are best left alive. Image credit Author.

How could one-sided or unilateral gags be seriously dangerous?

These go by the name of Bayer, Schouppe, spool, coil, Landmeisser, wedge, and the like. They have a bite piece which fits between the ***cheek teeth*** made of either:

- cylindrical spring steel or a solid metal cylinder (the "spool" types), or
- a wedge of metal, plastic, or rubber (the wedge types).

The only benefit from using either of these types of gag is slightly easier floating of the teeth because one side of the mouth held open to some degree. However, these gags are not recommended because at best, they do not

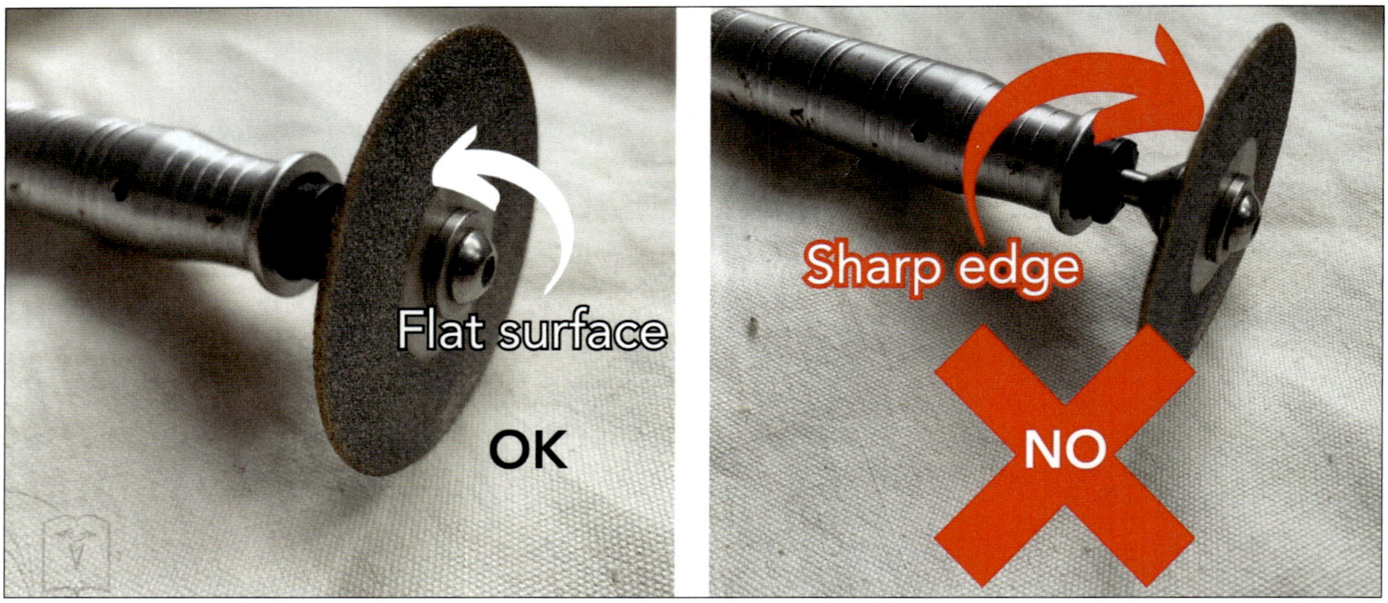

Using the sharp edge of a cut-off wheel to slice across a live tooth is contraindicated, as it is likely to lead to pulp exposure and tooth death. The flat side may be used carefully with intermittent water cooling and observation to watch for disappearance of dentinal staining to prevent pulp exposure, as with other power dental instruments. Image credit Author.

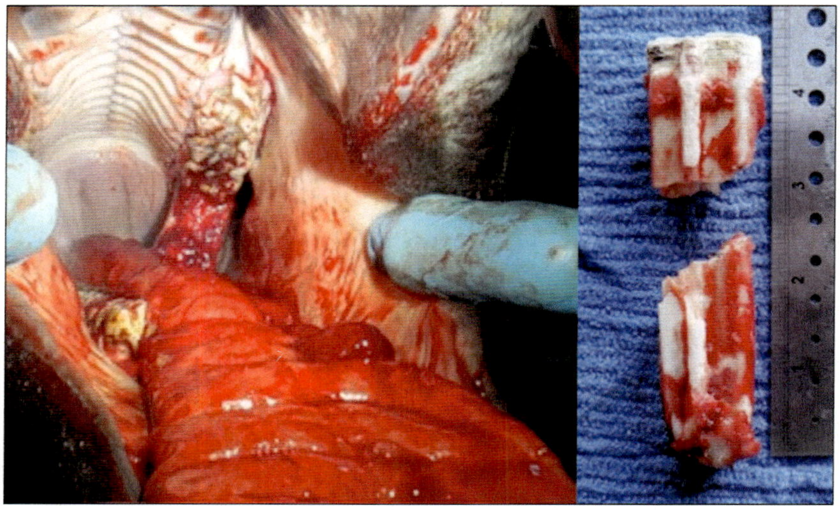

The Only Humane Use for Molar Cutters. This tooth was too long to come out into the mouth when it was being extracted intraorally and had to be cut. Molar cutters should ONLY be used on teeth which are in the process of being extracted by your veterinarian. Unmarked images credit Cathie Heald Greenwell, graphic credit Author.

significantly assist in examination or floating, and at worst, they frequently cause serious damage. The reasons for this are as follows:

- A horse masticates (chews) a lot with a unilateral (one-sided) gag in place. This makes it difficult to examine the teeth, which is the primary purpose of a dental examination, which should be performed before the teeth are filed.
- As the gag occupies mouth space on the side where it is placed, the tongue is pushed toward the other side where examination or floating is being attempted. This decreases visibility inside the mouth, already minimal at this level, and making floating more difficult.
- The temporomandibular or jaw joint, commonly known as the TMJ, may be damaged when a horse bites down hard on the unilateral gag, putting all strain on only one side at a time.
- If the gag slips from *between* the teeth to the *inside* of the arcade (to the palatal and lingual sides of the arcade), the palatine artery may be ruptured. It bleeds. A lot. For a long time.

- Most seriously, however, the danger of fracturing cheek teeth is very real. The cylindrical shape of the "spool" types causes the entire force of both sides of the strong masseter (chewing) muscles to be focused on a narrow line across two opposing teeth, which may lead to a fractured cheek tooth or teeth, with severe consequences. A fractured tooth needs to be extracted. A fractured tooth will cause your horse a lot of pain until the tooth is discovered and extracted. Make no mistake, cheek tooth extraction is a major surgery, especially because that recently-healthy tooth will be firmly stuck in place. And the worst thing? ***The fracture never had to happen in the first place.***

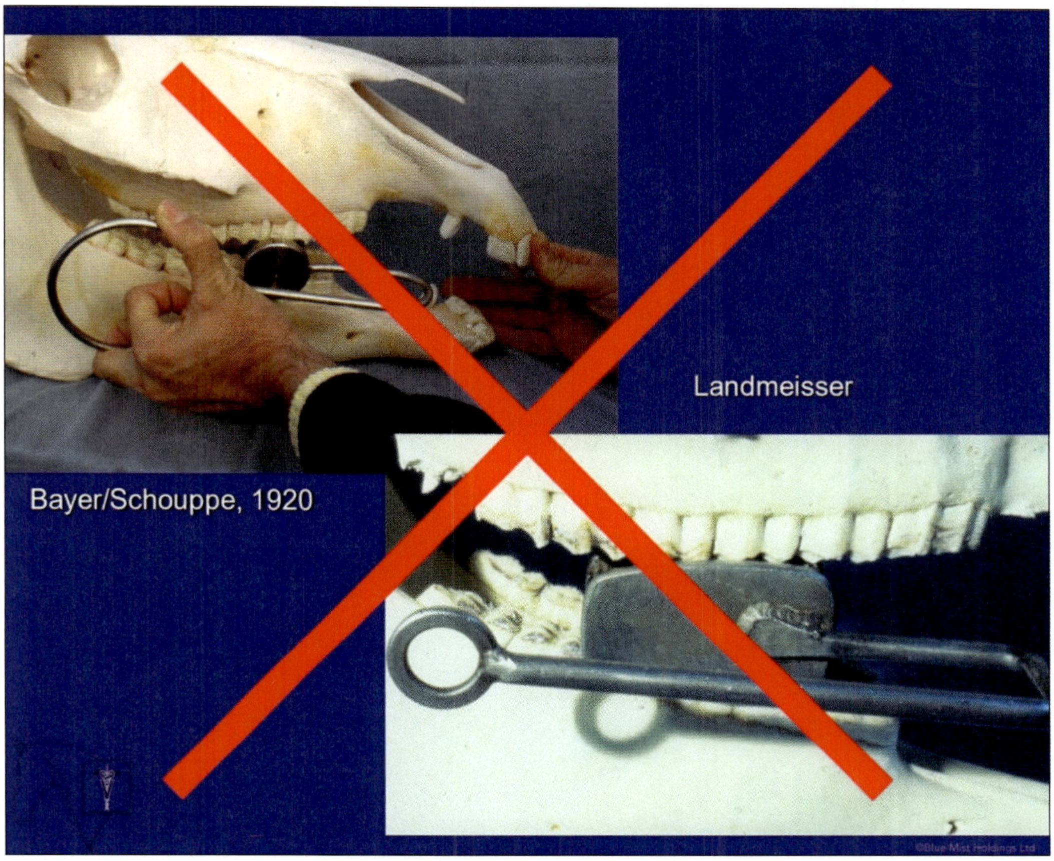

*The image shows two of the many NON-recommended gags which are sometimes used at The Second Level: Shown are the Bayer/Schouppe (1920) and the Landmeisser. These can seriously damage teeth and other **tissues**, including the fracture of cheek teeth. Image credit Dr Jack Easley, red cross graphic credit Author.*

What about a captive bolt percussion tooth cutter, that "chips" off the tooth? They're slick!

These captive bolt tooth cutters are *not* slick--they are dangerous to your horse. These are placed over a crown elongation and with a slam of the attached weight, cut off the elongation in one go, at whatever level they are placed (or slip to). By now you understand what can also happen. Not only will it remove the elongation, but it may also cause unintended tooth fracture and expose pulp, which will cause a pulpitis, and likely tooth death. It can be disastrous for the horse. If it has a weakened jaw, e.g. from underlying ***osteomyelitis***, this captive bolt percussion tooth cutter could fracture the skull. I think it's fair to say these are ***contraindicated*** *(unless used on a tooth to be extracted by a vet during its extraction, but there are much safer options.)*

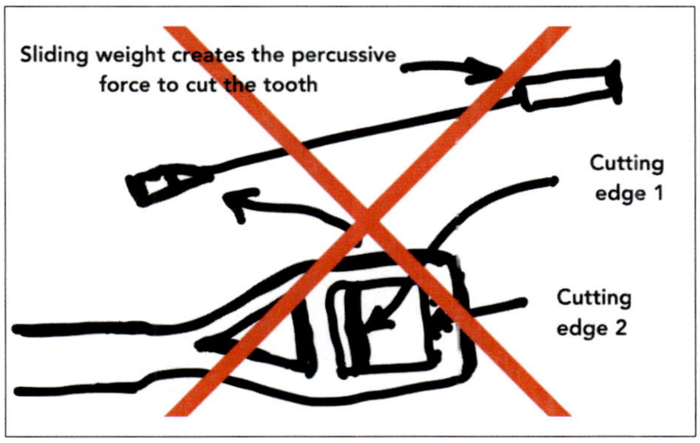

These captive bolt percussion tooth cutting tools (I won't grace them by calling them "instruments") are one of the most dangerous tools in a horse's mouth because they fracture tooth material indiscriminately as well as cause pulp exposures, or worse. Image credit Author.

How Frequently Does My Horse Need Dental Examination and Odontoplasty?

HOW FREQUENTLY ARE dental examination and treatment recommended? Keeping in everything we've discussed in this book, you'll now know this frequency depends on the horse's age and use: once to twice yearly for younger horses from birth to eight or nine years of age and at least annually after that. For optimal performance, some horses, especially those sensitive horses with pronounced cingulae, may require six-monthly odontoplasty to perform precision work. Once your horses have had a pain-free mouth for a little while, believe me, you will know if they want their teeth attended to in less than the standard year. They will probably make sure you know.

In Conclusion...

I'VE NOW GIVEN you all the information I think you'll need to make informed decisions about the dental care of your horse.

Do with it what you will. I hope this helps you feel more comfortable with helping your horse get the best care you can offer him or her.

Kind regards,

Elizabeth Thompson BA (Hons) DVM MANZCVS GradDipTeach

Waihi, NZ 31 May 2024

PART TWO: QUESTION & ANSWER

Disclaimer

THESE DISCLAIMERS ARE DESIGNED TO HELP EDUCATE my readers about the risks involved in equine dentistry and emphasize the importance of safety and professional supervision.

1- **Purpose and Accuracy of Information:** The author is giving her best, professional advice in this book because she wants her readers to be informed. While every effort has been made to ensure the accuracy and completeness of the information provided in this book, the author, publisher, and contributors make no warranties or representations regarding the accuracy, reliability, or completeness of the content. Best practices for equine dentistry change over time and the author is under no obligation to update the book.

2- **General Disclaimer and Professional Advice:** The information provided in this book is for educational purposes only. It is not intended to be a substitute for professional veterinary advice, diagnosis, or treatment. Readers should always consult with a qualified equine dental veterinarian for specific advice and guidance tailored to their individual horses' health and/or or medical conditions. This book is not intended to teach the reader to perform dental examinations or treatment, and unless the reader is a qualified equine dental veterinarian, EDT, or trained lay dental operator legally allowed to practice dentistry in the area in which they work, they should not attempt any dental procedures whatsoever on their horse(s).

3- **Safety Precautions:** The author, publisher, and any contributors to this book strongly advise readers to exercise caution and follow appropriate precautions and safety measures when handling horses, especially during sedation of the horse, dental examinations and treatment. Always prioritize safety and take necessary precautions, many of which are detailed in the book, to minimize the risk of injury to both the horse and handler, with the goal of preventing accidents or injuries. Helmets and stout boots are essential.

4- **Assumption of Risk:** Readers of this book acknowledge and understand the inherent risks associated with handling horses, including but not limited to the risk of injury from being kicked, bitten, struck by a forefoot, or being hit by the horse's head or speculum by engaging in or attempting to perform any dental procedures. The reader assumes all risks associated with the use of this information, including but not limited to handling horses and any involvement with equine sedation or equine dental procedures.

5- **No Veterinarian-Client-Patient Relationship.** Reading this book does not establish a veterinary-patient or veterinary-client relationship between the reader, their equids or other animals, and the author.

6- **Professional Supervision:** Equine dentistry, like any activity with horses, is inherently dangerous and should be performed only by trained professionals. Should a reader choose to obtain proper training and certification, even then, they are advised to never attempt procedures beyond their level of expertise.

7- **Informed Consent:** These disclaimers are designed to help educate my readers about the risks involved in equine dentistry and emphasize the importance of safety and professional supervision.

8- **External Links and References:** This book may contain links to external websites or references to third-party products or services. These links and references are provided for informational purposes only and do not constitute endorsement or recommendation. The author, publisher, and contributors are not responsible for the content or reliability of any external websites or products mentioned in this book.

9- **Emergency Preparedness:** Readers are encouraged to have a thorough understanding of emergency response protocols and access to veterinary and medical care in the event of an accident or injury during equine dentistry procedures. Prompt and appropriate medical attention is essential in mitigating the severity of injuries.

10- **Jurisdictional Variations:** Readers should be aware that laws and regulations regarding equine dentistry vary by jurisdiction. This includes regulations regarding who may legally perform dentistry in the reader's area. It is the reader's responsibility to familiarize themselves with, and comply with, applicable laws and regulations in their area, whether these are at the city, state, province, county, or country level. Readers with specific legal questions or concerns are advised to consult with their own legal counsel for guidance on applicable laws and regulations in their jurisdiction.

CHAPTER TWENTY-ONE

WHY ARE THERE DENTAL RECORDS IN THE FIRST PLACE?

"Saying floating is all a horse needs is like saying if you brush your teeth, you won't get cavities, periodontal disease, or cracked teeth."
–Jack Easley, DVM, MS, DBVP (EqPract), AVDC (Equine)

Q1:

I hadn't seen my dental practitioner recording any dental records, and he's never given me one. When I asked him about this, he said he doesn't keep records because if he forgot to write something down, he could get in trouble for not having performed that part of a dentistry. Can you explain this?

A:

Sorry, I cannot explain this. I wonder how he keeps track of the progress of the equids he is treating. Your ***veterinary*** dental practitioner will be keeping records, as records are important to monitor your horse's response to treatment, or in other words, to record how your horse's mouth is improving or deteriorating over time. Veterinarians are also required to do so by law. Conscientious non-veterinary EDTs and lay dental operators will keep records as well. Even if they don't provide the record to you, a professional vet or non-vet practitioner will keep records so they can offer your horse the best possible care.

With respect to the last part of your question, there is no regulation on whether non-veterinarians must keep records in much of the world, but I for one want to give your equid the best possible care, which requires monitoring response to treatment, so I keep extensive records. It takes time to do so, but your doctor or veterinarian would not be around long if they neglected something so basic as keeping patient records.

To see what there is in your horse or donkey's mouth to keep records on, and why it's important, see:

Author Preface, #5

Chapter 2, Eight Levels of Equine Dentistry

Chapter 2, Eight Levels of Equine Dentistry, Terminology

Chapter 3, Anatomy of the Mouth

Chapter 4, Examination of the Mouth.

CHAPTER TWENTY-TWO

ISN'T ALL DENTISTRY THE SAME?

"Many people don't understand that when you have an emergent, objectively established truth by the methods and tools of science, you do not have the luxury of standing in denial of it because it is true, whether or not you believe in it."
—Neil deGrasse Tyson

Q2:

My trainer thinks my horse is misbehaving because he has mouth pain, but I've had the "dentist" to him, and he says his mouth is fine. What can I tell my trainer to get him to understand?

A:

Your trainer might well be correct. To find out, I would recommend you start by reading:

Chapter 2, Eight Levels of Dentistry

If a thorough examination has not been done, I would recommend you have it done. A thorough examination includes flushing the mouth with plenty of water, so it is clean, and using a full-mouth speculum, a strong light, and a mirror or oroscope (an oral endoscope), with picks and probes, under sedation. Sadly, without all of this, and a Seventh Level examination, your operator could not have visualized (seen) the whole mouth well enough to tell if there is, or is not, anything wrong in your horse's mouth.

The minimum list of what your dental practitioner needs (and knows how to use) is:

- safe, full-mouth speculum
- large dose syringe or sprayer on a hose to carefully flush the mouth with water
- strong light source
- intraoral mirror
- dental picks and probes
- a thorough understanding of the job they're trying to do, and effective training
- a veterinarian to examine and sedate the horse, if a veterinarian is not to perform the dentistry

You, as the owner, are the person who can specify the level of dentistry your horse receives, as you are paying the bill. However, you cannot rule out mouth pain if your horse's mouth has not been fully examined, either. So, I hope you can find someone who can do a thorough job at this, so you can go back to your trainer and let them know if your horse truly does, or does not, have evidence of dental pain, and what has, or can, be done to alleviate it.

Further, you are the only person who can safeguard your horse's mouth, as you're the one hiring the dental practitioner. The only way you can do that is by learning everything you can about your horse's mouth, hence this book.

See also:

Chapter 3, Anatomy of the Mouth

Chapter 4, Examination of the Mouth

and the rest!

CHAPTER TWENTY-THREE

HOW CAN WE SAFELY SEDATE MY OLDER HORSE AND STILL GET THE JOB DONE?

"First, then, let there be no mistake about the age. If the horse has lost his mark [...] not only will the purchaser's hopes be blighted, but he may find himself saddled for ever with a sorry bargain."
—Xenophon, On Horsemanship, Gutenberg translation

Q3:

I have a 28-year-old Friesian which when sedated for a dental ***float*** is wobbly, while he is still alert. Is there a sedative used for senior horses that helps to alleviate this issue?

A:

A good and important question!

Tricky sedation for older, anxious, or painful horses

Effectively and safely sedating anxious, extremely painful, and/or older horses can be tricky. Anxiety in these horses, usually due to a combination of moderate to severe long-term ***oral*** pain plus the smarts which old horses tend to acquire, causes release of chemicals in their bloodstream which help them override the sedative drugs usually used. You may have seen these sedated horses seem alert, while they're ataxic (wobbly). There are several problems here:

- Geriatrics may have compromised (poor) ability to metabolize and eliminate (clear out) sedation drugs.
- Geriatrics may want to fight with us because of dental or generalized musculoskeletal pain. Administering intravenous pain relief prior to sedation may help here.
- Anxious horses' sympathetic (fight or flight fear) response may let them overpower the drugs.
- Repeatedly administering drugs when a horse "won't sedate" still means they are in their system, but not effective. However, when the anxiety or fear goes, the horse may "crash", or become extremely sedated and possibly go down. Not ideal for a geriatric.

These horses may become very sleepy and probably more ataxic (wobbly) when the vet stops working in their mouth.

I used to struggle with this, but a board-certified veterinary anesthesiologist gave me a new protocol. Those disastrous old-horse and anxious-horse sedations rarely occur now for me. I use this technique with most of the anxious horses in my practice.

Twenty minutes before your vet expects to begin work, your horse may be injected intramuscularly in their own paddock near to where the dentistry will be performed (but be sure other horses cannot push it around) with an ***anxiolytic*** (anti-anxiety) drug and a small dose of the standard sedation and pain relief drugs. I leave it alone where it comfortable, without stressing, it for the next 20 minutes. The anti-anxiety drug keeps the horse from working itself up and overriding the other drugs later.

After this time, the horse can be quietly led to the ***stocks*** or working place and standard sedation drugs administered at a low dose . Giving the anxiolytic after they have become wound-up hasn't been effective in my hands.

Horses sedated with this regimen appear quite awake, but they don't seem to care what you're doing, which differs vastly from sedation without the anxiolytic. It's important that everyone takes their time and does not stress the horse at all. This will give your vet the longest-lasting sedation time, with less anxiety and ***ataxia,*** to allow completion of their work.

It's important for everyone to take their time and not stress the horse at all.

I have found the horses given this sedation regimen appear awake but are rarely ataxic. However, they don't seem to care what you're doing, which usually very different from doing it without the anxiolytic.

See:

Chapter 12, Special Equids: Geriatrics and Minis

Chapter 15, Veterinary Specific Procedures: Tricky Sedation for Older, Anxious, or Painful...

CHAPTER TWENTY-FOUR

WHAT IS "QUIDDING" AND HOW IS IT RELATED TO MY HORSE'S TEETH?

"The basis of modern clinical therapy is diagnosis. This presupposes that disease can be accurately identified and then effectively eliminated by the application of appropriate therapy. It would seem, therefore, that information obtained in making a diagnosis is the foundation for successful treatment. Discipline must be exercised in collecting material for a meaningful diagnosis."
—Jack Easley, DVM, MS, DBVP (EqPract), AVDC (Equine)

Q4:

I have a miniature donkey that ***quids.*** He drops lumps of twisted up hay and stores food in the sides of his mouth. He's choked three times since starting this habit. I'm sure it's tooth related. But how, exactly?

A:

That sounds like ***quidding***, or dropping "quids" of wadded up hay or grass. Choke frequently occurs when a horse isn't chewing its food properly, resulting in large wads (quids) of long hay or grass stems that get stuck in the esophagus.

The underlying issue here, or the reason he's quidding, may be ***oral*** pain, which is causing him to chew insufficiently, and the feed just wads up instead of progressing. It sounds like he's also packing his cheeks with feed material. Correcting the reason for the pain usually corrects this problem.

The list of dental diseases which can cause problems like this includes, but isn't limited to:

- Retained deciduous teeth. You didn't mention this miniature donkey's age, but like all miniature breeds, they tend to retain their deciduous teeth and get impacted teeth because of lack of space in the mouth, so it's important they are checked every year by an equine dental veterinarian with postgraduate training in equine dentistry. They can get into some serious problems if they're not treated early. There is so little room in their head for their oversized teeth that we must provide them with special care. See:
  - Chapter 12, Special Equids: Geriatrics and Minis
- Crown elongations (including ***sharp enamel points*** and more) due to malocclusion, combined with lack of correct ***odontoplasty***, or tooth ***floating***, causing ***ulceration*** of the inside of the cheeks (***buccal mucosa***) cause pain and quidding. See:
  - Chapter 6, Developmental and Acquired Conditions, and Chapter 8, Secondary Forms of Dental Disease.
- ***Periodontal*** disease, which progresses quickly with the help of the bacteria and feed material packed into the food wads in the cheeks. See:

  - Chapter 5, About Dental Conditions
  - Chapter 6, Developmental and Acquired Conditions.

- Fractured or loose tooth or teeth. See:

  - See Chapter 6, Developmental and Acquired Conditions
  - See Chapter 8, Secondary Forms of Dental Disease, and Chapter 10, Head Trauma and Dental Pathology.

- Missing tooth or teeth with crown elongations of the teeth opposing the missing-teeth-gap. This restricts the normal lateral (sideways) jaw movement and may progress to the extent of the elongated tooth protruding into the soft ***tissue*** (or even the bony tissue) of the opposite jaw. See:

  - Chapter 6, Developmental and Acquired Conditions
  - Chapter 8, Secondary Forms of Dental Disease
  - Chapter 10, Head Trauma and Dental Pathology

- "***Dental drift***" of teeth after loss or extraction of a tooth and neglecting the six monthly-for-life requirement of "odontoplasty", or tooth floating. See:

  - Chapter 15, Veterinary Specific Procedures, Ongoing Post-Extraction Care.

- ***Pulp exposure*** and pain causing incorrect chewing of feed materials. See:

  - Chapter 6, Developmental and Acquired Conditions
  - Chapter 8, Secondary Forms of Dental Disease
  - Chapter 9, Iatrogenic Disease,
  - Chapter 10, Head Trauma and Dental Pathology.

- Foreign body in the back of the mouth or tongue (stick, piece of wire, etc.) preventing donkey from chewing correctly. See:

  - Chapter 10, Head Trauma and Dental Pathology, and Chapter 11, Sinus Disease.

- Supernumerary (extra) teeth, which are usually not opposed by teeth in the opposite jaw, leading to over growths (as above). See:

  - Chapter 3, Anatomy
  - Chapter 6, Developmental and Acquired Conditions
  - Chapter 8, Secondary Forms of Dental Disease,
  - Chapter 10, Head Trauma and Dental Pathology.

Be sure any pelleted ration which may require soaking, such as sugar beet, has been appropriately soaked to manufacturers specifications.

There are other conditions which may cause choke, which your veterinarian can rule out, including neurological dysfunction.

Truly, though, most of these conditions may be prevented by at least once-yearly veterinary dental examination and as-needed therapy. Unfortunately, when we breed equids, we have not been selecting for good tooth occlusion, or bite, so we need to take care of them.

CHAPTER TWENTY-FIVE

CAN MY HORSE'S DENTAL ISSUES AFFECT HER EYES?

Q5:

Can teeth affect a horse's eyes? I have an older mare who has a constant dripping from only her right eye. It makes the skin beneath it soggy and painful. She has no swelling or tenderness in her mouth, and she eats well on both forage and grain. Can any kind of dental issue (major or minor) cause an infection or blockage of the ***nasolacrimal duct***? And, if so, how does this happen?

A:

Yes, dental disease can affect a horse's eyes, but a much more common cause of unilateral (one-sided) constant discharge in the absence of eye pain or cloudiness is blockage of a nasolacrimal duct. This can occur from ***inflammation*** or an infection in the nasolacrimal duct from bacteria and contaminated material moving down the duct from that right eye itself.

Has your ***veterinarian*** examined her? Has her nasolacrimal duct been flushed? I would suggest you consult your veterinarian, who will probably examine the eye first, then check the nasolacrimal duct for patency (whether or not fluid can be flushed through it) with fluorescein dye, then treat as they see fit.

With regards to the dental question, has she had a thorough ***oral*** and head examination, including a tooth-by-tooth probing for ***pulp exposure***, especially the most ***distal cheek teeth***? Percussion of her ***sinuses***?

See:

Chapter 3, Anatomy of the Mouth

Chapter 10, Head Trauma and Dental Pathology

Chapter 11, Sinus Disease

CHAPTER TWENTY-SIX

WILL EXTRACTING MY OLD HORSE'S BROKEN TOOTH BE TOO HARD ON HIM?

Q6:

My 23-year-old horse has a fractured "molar" discovered at last dental examination and had been ***quidding*** his food. Initially, he had swelling, which disappeared with sulfa medication and has not returned. He has no problem with grass and his teeth are ***floated*** every year, but he has lost weight. I plan to feed a senior feed next winter. I wondered if extraction of the fractured tooth is an option or if would make matters worse? If he has no infection, wouldn't it be better to leave what remains to "hold" the neighboring teeth from caving in? Is it possible that the fractured tooth could grow faster to the height of the other teeth? His front teeth look funny. Some of them are very brown and they look awfully long. There is grass and feed packed in between his teeth, but he doesn't want me to touch them so I can't pull the grass out. His mouth smells. What can I do?

A:

It sounds like you have your work cut out for you! It would be a good idea to get your dental ***veterinarian*** to examine and X-ray your horse's teeth to determine the exact problems your horse has in his mouth. Only then will you have the full picture.

The pulp, or the live, painful part of the tooth may be only 2-6 millimeters beneath the surface or sides of a tooth, so there may be ***pulp exposure*** and pain from the fractured ***cheek tooth***. If the tooth fracture extends into live, painful, ***tissue***, there will be infection and pain. That's probably why he's eating small bites and quidding.

If he has a fractured tooth, it should probably be extracted as soon as possible, unless it's just a tiny chip off the outside (***buccal, lingual*** or ***palatal*** chip) which hasn't caused pulp exposure. The fractured tooth will probably not erupt faster, and it may already be dead, which is termed a non-vital pulp exposure. The fact he's an older horse means the pulp chamber is smaller and has a poorer blood supply than would a younger horse, and he is unlikely to be able to seal off the live portion of his tooth to keep it alive. The signs he's showing in his ***incisors*** may indicate he may also have ***EOTRH***, Equine Odontoclastic Tooth Resorption and Hypercementosis. Additionally, leaving the tooth in place if it is falling apart won't stop dental drift.

See:

Chapter 6, Developmental and Acquired Conditions

Chapter 7, EOTRH

Chapter 9, Iatrogenic Disease

Chapter 10, Head Trauma and Dental Pathology.

Sometimes it's hard to tell your horse is in pain

Regarding showing pain, this horse *is* showing signs of pain, we just need to learn how to listen to them: the quidding, the smaller bites, and the weight loss are all signs of discomfort in the mouth, or pain. There is some recent excellent research which has been published in the past few years about facial expressions and pain levels. It's described in Chapter 1. Sometimes it's hard to tell when they're in pain, but believe me, a fractured tooth will be causing him pain every time minutes of every day, especially when he chews (which is most of the day...). Please get your dental veterinarian to look at your horse as soon as possible.

See:

Chapter 1, How do I Know My Horse Has Dental Disease?

Chapter 2, Eight Levels of Dentistry

Chapter 4, Examination of the Mouth

Chapter 5, About Dental Conditions

Regarding the post-extraction requirements for horses and their owners, you are right to be cautious about tooth extraction and ongoing sequelae. As you mentioned, extraction of a tooth (or tooth loss) in a horse results in a gap in that ***arcade***. It also means that the opposing tooth will no longer have anything to grind against. That opposing tooth will continue to erupt and without regular ***odontoplasty***, it will become a ***crown elongation*** which causes severe problems to your horse as it erupts into the opposing jaw. Not a nice situation for the horse. If it's left too long, one cannot reduce (grind away) the full excess length without exposing the pulp, or live portion of the tooth, so please schedule your veterinarian for those six-monthly dental visits before they leave your place. The teeth will also undergo ***dental drift***, whereby the teeth will, in effect, attempt to close the gap to stabilize the arcade, which is designed to function as a unit. The six-monthly odontoplasty won't stop this drift, but it will keep the opposing teeth in check.

Also see:

Chapter 15, Veterinary Specific Procedures: Extraction Considerations

Chapter 15, Veterinary Specific Procedures: Ongoing Post-Extraction Care

Remember that while the ongoing requirement for six-monthly dental examination and treatment seems onerous, it is much better than the pain your horse will be experiencing from a fractured tooth and likely pulp exposure, and maybe EOTRH.

CHAPTER TWENTY-SEVEN

WHAT WAS ALL THAT DUST WHEN MY HORSE'S TEETH WERE FLOATED?

Q7:

When my horse was having his teeth ***floated*** with a power instrument the other day, there were great clouds of dust coming from the horse's mouth. What is this, and is it important?

A:

The dust you were seeing the other day was most likely ground tooth dust combined with saliva containing bacteria and other microorganisms.

I hope the practitioner gave you a mask if he or she was making dust, and that either they were using a water-cooled instrument with constant water irrigation (as your own human dentist would) or rinsing the mouth frequently with cool water. Not only will water-cooling prevent the clouds of dust from entering the practitioner's and your lungs (not to mention your horse's), but just as importantly, it will cool the heat generated by the fast-moving disc against the tooth. Keeping the teeth cool is essential for your horse's tooth health. These are important for several reasons:

1 - Tooth dust is similar in structure to asbestos, which is dangerous to inhale.

2 - The dust will also contain aerosolized microorganisms (bacteria, viruses, fungi, etc) which could cause infections in those inhaling it.

3 - Friction from power grinding discs creates heat. If there are "great clouds of dust", it is likely water cooling is not being provided to your horse. Without cooling the teeth with water regularly, the heat can create "thermal (heat) damage", which can injure the live part of the tooth, called the pulp, or its tiny processes near the occlusal surface. If the teeth are heated without rapid cooling, a pulpitis may develop. If the tooth cannot overcome the pulpitis created by the heat, the tooth will die.

See:

Chapter 3, Anatomy of the Mouth

Chapter 9, Iatrogenic Disease

Chapter 14, Odontoplasty

CHAPTER TWENTY-EIGHT

DOES MY HORSE NEED HIS WOLF TEETH OUT?

Q8:

I have a 3-year-old Friesian filly that I will be starting next summer. I have been given (and read) conflicting opinions as to whether to have her ***wolf teeth*** removed. If they need to be removed, when would be the best time to have it done? I have one horse that never had his removed and he has never had issues with the bit. I would like to avoid an unnecessary procedure if possible. I plan to ride her with a bit, but for pleasure riding only, not intense dressage or the like.

A:

This question is frequently asked. Unfortunately, the answer to your question depends upon the size and location of the wolf teeth, and whether they are in a position that could endanger them if a bit is pulled back hard against them. Often when this happens (even during pleasure riding, as unexpected things will happen) a wolf tooth (***premolar*** one/ ***Triadan*** 105, 205, 305, or 405) is contacted and damaged. Your horse is three years old, so whatever wolf tooth development will occur has likely already occurred or should have by six to eighteen months of age.

A wolf tooth can break, exposing pulp and resulting in ***inflammation*** and infection, or it may become loosened, or a combination of both. All of these will result in pain and if not noticed, and may contribute to training issues and attitude changes. If any of these wolf tooth injuries occur, the tooth should be removed in its entirety.

Regarding the relatively rare ***mandibular*** wolf tooth, whether they have erupted through the ***gingiva*** (tooth visible) or not yet unerupted (tooth still hidden beneath the gums, but erupted out of the bone), I always remove them. Mandibular wolf teeth are often situated further ***mesial*** to the ***cheek teeth*** than ***maxillary*** wolf teeth are, and they can be a huge problem in a bitted horse. Unerupted mandibular wolf teeth may be lying flat on top of the bone or directed ***mesially*** (forward) and ***buccally*** (outward toward the cheek). As you might imagine, the tender gingiva overlying these teeth is traumatized whenever the bit hits them, and this would cause no end of grief for your horse. Your ***veterinarian*** or EDT should always ***palpate*** the ***bars of the mouth*** between the ***incisors*** and the cheek teeth with their fingers to ensure no mandibular or maxillary wolf teeth are present under the ***mucosa***, and to check the bars for any signs of pain. Unerupted mandibular and maxillary wolf teeth are often invisible to the eye but are easy palpable with the fingers.

See:

Chapter 3, Anatomy of the Mouth

Chapter 15, Veterinary Specific Procedures

Chapter 15, Veterinary Specific Procedure: Do all Wolf Teeth Need Extraction? (a specific section of Chapter 15)

CHAPTER TWENTY-NINE

MY HORSE HAS A PROBLEM WITH HIS MOUTH, AND I JUST BOUGHT HIM!

Q9:

I just bought a horse, Doc, and I had a prepurchase done, but they didn't look in its mouth. Can you please come look at his mouth? He seems to shake his head a lot and doesn't want to be bridled.

A:

I show up, perform my standard ***veterinary*** physical exam (note ***mentation***, listen to its heart, trachea, lungs, abdomen, etc.), sedate the horse, open its mouth, and take a peek...

And find one of the ***cheek teeth*** is fractured down the middle, amongst other ***pathology*** including ***sharp enamel points*** and many ***buccal*** (cheek) ulcers.

What happens next? What was your agreement? This is not, I repeat ***not***, a cheap or simple fix, either for you or the horse. Whether or not the seller knew a fracture was present, it has likely now become your (painful and expensive) problem. The extent of the damage will need to be assessed by a dental veterinarian, who will benefit by any information you can get from the previous owner or trainer, such as any injuries they know to have occurred, when they occurred, and barring that, if there was any time the horse started showing any abnormalities in its eating, work, demeanor, etc.

Comprehensive horse health insurance, including dental surgery coverage, is recommended before you take a new horse home. Health insurance for your horse, including dental coverage and surgical coverage, is highly recommended for any horse.

See:

Chapter 3, Anatomy of the Mouth

Chapter 4, Examination of the Mouth: Special Dental Exams

Chapter 6, Developmental and Acquired Conditions

Chapter 10, Head Trauma and Dental Pathology

Chapter 15, Veterinary Specific Procedures: Extraction Considerations

Chapter 6, Developmental and Acquired Conditions

CHAPTER THIRTY

IS MY DENTAL OPERATOR KNOWLEDGEABLE? HOW DO I TELL?

Q10:

How can I tell if my dental practitioner knows what they're doing?

A:

When you understand the information in this book, you should be able to tell. Unfortunately, without learning this information, you're pretty much left to your own devices. This was my primary reason for writing this book. Most places in the world do not require any training, certification, continuing education, or competency assessed by a regulatory body to perform dentistry upon your horse. Usually, only registered, practicing ***veterinarians*** are required to have these. In some locations (some states in the USA, provinces in CA and and other places), equine dentistry is regarded as the practice of veterinary medicine and therefore limited to veterinarians. Whether it is *enforced* is an issue, so check with your country, state or province regulatory boards to find out. Veterinarians who have had postgraduate training in equine dentistry, EDTs (by the definition put forth in the Author Preface) along with dental veterinarians and their well-trained equine dental technicians who work directly with them, can offer your horse the best modern equine dentistry has to offer.

See:

Author Preface, #5

Chapter 2, Eight Levels of Equine Dentistry

Chapter 2, Eight Levels of Equine Dentistry: What Does the Title of the Person...

CHAPTER THIRTY-ONE

IS MY HORSE TOO OLD FOR DENTISTRY?

Q31:

"The last ***vet*** who saw my horse said it was too old to have dentistry" or "the last vet who saw my horse said it was too old to be sedated".

A:

This is rarely, if ever, the case.

There are special anesthetic techniques which help support the aging body systems of a horse, including ***anxiolytic*** drugs (drugs which decrease anxiety), which let your vet use lower dosages of short-acting drugs for sedation. The use of strong ***stocks*** (stationary or portable) can also help by providing a supportive wall for them to lean against.

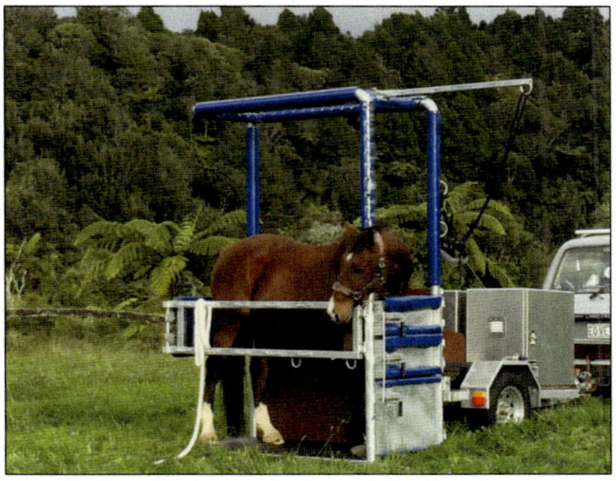

Equi-Still Portable Equine Stocks offer your horse support while examination and treatment are performed. Image credit Author.

The ***pathology*** in the mouth of older horses requires care. Aged horses with severe dental pathology are unfortunately more common than they should be. They end up with severe ***crown elongations (overgrowths)***, sometimes growing into the opposing ***maxilla*** or ***mandible***. By the time they slow down or stop eating, the pathology will be indeed severe and will take multiple visits to safely reduce these elongations without exposing pulps.

See:

Chapter 12. Special Equids: Geriatrics and Minis.

CHAPTER THIRTY-TWO

DO VETS KNOW ANYTHING ABOUT EQUINE DENTISTRY?

Q32:

"But they don't teach ***vets*** very much about dentistry in veterinary school, do they?"

A:

This may or may not be true, depending upon where your veterinarian went to veterinary school, but there is more to "dentistry" than simply placing a ***float*** into a mouth and rubbing back and forth. There are other structures and organ systems in the body than just the teeth, and they are interconnected. The myriad of subjects taught in veterinary school which pertain to the ***oral*** cavity (mouth), the supporting bones of the head, the musculature, the nerves, arteries, veins, the rest of the anatomy, the ***pathologic*** conditions, the pharmacology, the immunology, the diseases, etc., the list goes on. For the most part, equine or mixed practitioners with postgraduate training in equine veterinary dentistry can offer you the very best modern equine dentistry has to offer.

See:

Author Preface

Chapter 2, Eight Levels of Dentistry: What Vets Do...

Chapter 15, Veterinary Specific Procedures

Chapter 16, Advanced Techniques Available

CHAPTER THIRTY-THREE

I HEARD MY DONKEY/MINI/PONY/? DOESN'T NEED DENTISTRY!

Q33:

"Donkeys don't need dentistry."

"Ponies don't need dentistry."

"Minis don't need dentistry."

"My grandfather's horses never needed dentistry."

A:

Ever heard these comments?

Just because it wasn't done, doesn't mean it *shouldn't* have been done. Medicine has changed and times have changed.

Donkeys, ponies, and miniature horses (*especially* miniature horses) *do* need dentistry. In the wild, natural selection would "select for" horses with good teeth, meaning that equids with poor teeth didn't flourish when times were lean, and were slower than their other herd mates... resulting in their being killed by predators and not remaining in the gene pool to reproduce. The other result of this is that those horses with good teeth survived to breed and create more horses with "good teeth". For thousands of years, fortunately or unfortunately, we have bred horses for things like speed, pulling ability, or performance of one type or another. Unfortunately, in more recent times, we rarely focused on the things we couldn't see... their teeth. With our feeding horses and protecting them, without natural selection to weed out the horses with poor dentition (teeth), we need to do dentistry, because we have created painful situations for our horses by our lack of consideration for the genetics of their dentition. While we were selecting for these performance traits we desired, we even bred horses of different skull types together: cold bloods and hot bloods to get a "warmblood", which may have even worse mouths.

For a start, see:

Chapter 12, Special Equids: Geriatrics and Miniatures

Then read on to these pages!

Chapter 1, How do I Know My Horse Has Dental Disease?

Chapter 2, The Eight Levels of Equine Dentistry

Chapter 3, Anatomy of the Mouth

Chapter 4, Examination of the Mouth

Chapter 5, About Dental Conditions

Chapter 6, Developmental and Acquired Conditions

Chapter 7, EOTRH

Chapter 8, Secondary Forms of Dental Disease

Chapter 9, Iatrogenic Disease

Chapter 10, Head Trauma and Dental Pathology

Chapter 11, Sinus Disease

Chapter 12, Special Equids: Geriatrics and Miniatures

CHAPTER THIRTY-FOUR

WHAT IS THE DRIFTY THING HORSE TEETH DO AFTER EXTRACTIONS?

Q14:

My horse had an extraction in the back of his mouth and the guy who extracted it told me to have dentistry done in six months because of some kind of drift thing. I'm wondering why I need to do this. Can you please explain it?

A:

Your ***vet*** was probably talking about two ***occlusal*** problems called "***dental drift***" and ***crown elongation*** ("***overgrowth***") of teeth following an extraction. Equine ***cheek teeth*** and ***incisors*** must be opposed (the ***mandibular*** teeth meeting the opposing ***maxillary*** teeth), or the tooth or teeth opposite an extraction site will be unimpeded and overgrow, resulting in elongations of the remaining teeth. These overgrowths, unless the horse has regular ***odontoplasty***, (usually 6 monthly), can erupt until they are digging into the opposing jawbone. You could imagine what that would feel like when they are grazing sixteen hours per day. To make it even more complicated, the teeth on either side of an extraction site will migrate towards the gap, a phenomenon called dental drift, due to the direction of the tooth roots, moving the teeth towards each other. Little may be done about this drifting itself, which will cause misalignment with the rest of the teeth in the ***arcade*** as well, but the effects can be minimized by regular odontoplasty. Crown elongations will thus begin in other teeth as well, so those six-monthly dental examinations and odontoplasty are essential. If they are left longer and one tries to reduce the length of the overgrown teeth flush with the rest of the teeth, ***pulp exposures*** may result. The six-monthly frequency of odontoplasty helps prevent this.

See:

Chapter 5, About Dental Conditions: Some Diseases Caused Indirectly From Poor Dentition

Chapter 6, Developmental and Acquired Conditions: Malocclusions

Chapter 15, Veterinary Specific Procedures: Extraction Considerations

Chapter 15, Veterinary Specific Procedures: Ongoing Post-Extraction Care

CHAPTER THIRTY-FIVE

BROODMARES AREN'T RIDDEN, SO THEY DON'T NEED DENTISTRY, DO THEY?

Q35:

My broodmares never have a bit in their mouths, so I've never had their teeth ***floated***, but my son says they need it. I don't believe it. Why would they?

A:

Broodmares are just as prone to ***crown elongation*** (***overgrowths***) as any other domestic horse, which causes ***sharp enamel points*** that can lacerate the ***buccal*** (cheek) walls as well as the tongue, causing constant misery. They also get other malocclusions, ***periodontal*** disease, ***EOTRH***, tooth loss in extreme cases, and any of the other painful conditions experienced by their ridden counterparts.

She may live with many other horses but not be checked regularly, as often happens with broodmare bands. Has she taken a kick to the face and lives in quiet misery with a fractured tooth? We often don't notice the pain in these horses.

See:

Chapter 1, How do I Know My Horse has Dental Disease?

Chapter 10: Head Trauma and Dental Pathology.

In addition, what about those expensive foals they're carrying? The ***periodontal*** disease may put those foals at risk. Details of this specifically in Chapter 17, What About My Broodmares?.

Also see:

Chapter 2, Eight Levels of Dentistry

Chapter 4, Examination of the Mouth

Chapter 14, Odontoplasty

Chapter 17, What About My Broodmares? (again...)

Tooth creation starts in the developing fetus inside the uterus of the mare. To give you an idea of when, it has been shown that the calcification of the deciduous cheek teeth, one of the later stages of tooth development, occurs by four months of gestation, and the calcification of the first permanent tooth buds begin at around ten months of gestation. That pretty much covers the whole of gestation and early foal life for development of all the teeth. Considering this timetable, recognize that the nutrition of the mare may have implications in fetal tooth (and other) development.

Also see:

Chapter 3, Anatomy of the Mouth

CHAPTER THIRTY-SIX

CAN I LEAVE MY HORSE'S WOLF TEETH IN?

Q36:

I hear you can leave some ***wolf teeth*** in. Is that true?

A:

Sometimes they don't cause a problem and can remain in the mouth. If they sit right up against the first ***cheek tooth*** and are tucked inside, toward the palate, they may never cause a problem to a bitted horse. If they are solid, molarized teeth against the first cheek tooth and you have good hands for riding, they also may not require removal, unless you fall off with the reins in your hand. Often when behavioral problems arise, people tend to point to the wolf teeth.

The following wolf teeth really need to be extracted:

- Fractured or mobile (loose) wolf teeth likely cause pain whenever the horse moves its mouth or tongue... which is most of the time. These teeth should be extracted.
- If wolf teeth are not adjacent to the first cheek tooth, they are at high risk, and this is one of the indications for extraction.
- Unerupted, or "blind", wolf teeth
- Mandibular wolf teeth

See Chapter 8, Secondary Forms of Dental Disease: Wolf Teeth

See Chapter 15, Veterinary Specific Procedures: Wolf Teeth Extraction

See Chapter 15, Veterinary Specific Procedures: Do All Wolf Teeth Need Extraction?

APPENDICES

RECIPE: NON-SUGARY HORSE (AND DOG!) TREATS!

All my fiction books have recipes.
So, I didn't see why this one shouldn't– just because it's a veterinary book!

My horses and dogs love these bikkies (or cookies, to those of you in the States and Canada!).

Many commercial horse treats contain high levels of sugar and molasses, both of which are seriously bad for equid teeth. I don't cringe when they take these goodies from my hand, because while they contain a little sugar from the carrot and apple (in the applesauce), this recipe doesn't include molasses or other *concentrated* sugars. If you're a child, make sure to get your mum's permission and help first!

Preheat oven: to 350 deg F (200 deg C)

Mix well in a large bowl or bucket:

- 3c oats (human-type steel cut is good)
- 3c grated carrot (either finely grated or chopped fine in food processor)
- 3c applesauce (unsweetened)
- 3c flour

Prepare cookie sheets by either greasing with oil, covering with parchment or baking paper, or using silicon tray covers.

Roll out dough on a floured board and cut out like cookies, or simply drop by tablespoonfuls onto a tray as you would for drop cookies, whichever you prefer.

Bake until set, around 15 minutes.

Store in an airtight jar or cookie tin in the fridge. If storing in the tack room, remember that the mice and rats would like them too, so a metal container might be a good idea!

Bon appétit!

About the Author

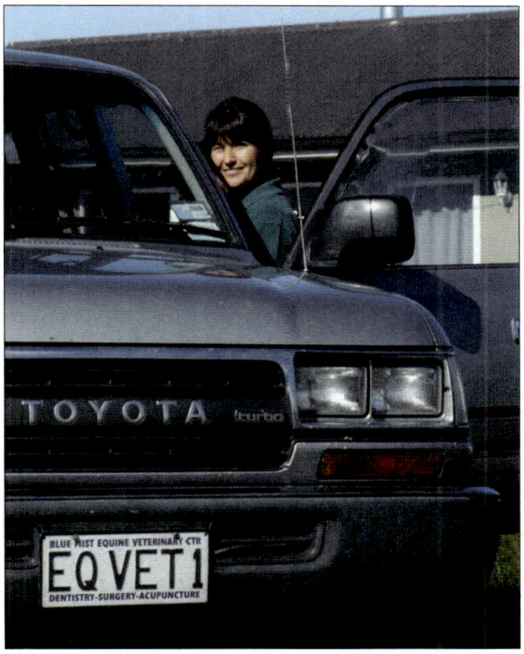

DR ELIZABETH (LIZZI) Thompson grew up riding wild in the Santa Cruz Mountain redwoods, became an equine veterinarian at UC Davis School of Veterinary Medicine and practiced in the Gold and Pony Express Country of California before emigrating to New Zealand. She has two wonderful boys, a grandson, and an awesome partner in that sea of green. When she's not writing, she's swinging a rapier or shooting a bow in medieval garb, riding or driving a carriage, playing in the garden or with her Dexters on her hobby farm, singing, cooking, or looking into a horse's mouth in her equine veterinary dental practice.

Qualifications and Honors:

Lizzi graduated from UC Santa Cruz in 1984 with a BA in Biology (Honors), from UC Davis School of Veterinary Medicine in 1988 with a Doctorate of Veterinary Medicine, and from University of Waikato (NZ) in 2012 with a Graduate Diploma in Teaching (Secondary Biology and Chemistry).

She achieved her Membership in the Australia New Zealand College of Veterinary Scientists (ANZCVS) in 2007 in Equine Dentistry.

She is the 2023-25 President of the Dentistry Chapter of the ANZCVS and sits on the NZEVA Equine Dental Subcommittee.

Awards:

Dr Thompson is multiply published and awarded in special interest magazines and veterinary periodicals. Lizzi's veterinary professional writing awards include the Jonathan Hope Award for the Best Practitioner Publication (NZ) for both 2010 and 2023.

Under her writing pseudonym Lizzi Tremayne, with her debut first-in-series historical fiction novel *A Long Trail Rolling*, she was Winner True West Magazine Best Western Romance 2016, Winner RWNZ Pacific Hearts 2014 for the best unpublished manuscript, Winner RWNZ Koru Award 2015 for Best First Book, Koru Award 2015 for 3rd Place Best Long Novel, and Finalist 2015 Best Indie Book Award.

Bibliography and Further Reading

MESSAGE FROM THE AUTHOR:
The information presented throughout this book has been sourced from the excellent writings below and translated into a horse owner's language. The author is indebted to every one of these authors and researchers, leaders in this field, and claims only the mistakes, which are hers alone. Her most profound thanks to them all.

Abusallamah, A. (2014). *Histology of Dentin*. Retrieved from www.Slideshare.Net/DrAbusallamah/Histology-of-Dentin.

Ask, K., Rhodin, M., Rashid-Engström, M., Hernlund, E., & Andersen, P. H. (2024). Changes in the equine facial repertoire during different orthopedic pain intensities. *Scientific Reports*, *14*(1). https://doi.org/10.1038/S41598-023-50383-Y

Auer, J., & Stick, J. (1999). *Equine Surgery 2nd ed* (2nd ed.). WB Saunders Co.

Baker, G., & Easley, J. (2005). *Equine Dentistry* (3rd ed.). Elsevier Saunders.

Barakzai, S. Z., Finnegan, C., & Boden, L. A. (2009). Effect of 'tongue tie' use on racing performance of Thoroughbreds in the United Kingdom. *Equine Veterinary Journal*, *41*(8), 812–816. https://doi.org/10.2746/042516409X434134

Barton, A. K., Troppenz, A., Klaus, D., Lindenberg, I., Merle, R., & Gehlen, H. (2023). Tongue ties do not widen the upper airways in racehorses. *Equine Veterinary Journal*, *55*(4), 642–648. https://doi.org/10.1111/evj.13867

Barton, A., Lindenberg, I., Einspanier, A., Merle, R., & Gehlen, H. (2022). Evaluation of the effect of tongue ties on stress parameters, behaviour and heart-rate variability in racehorses. *Animal Welfare*, *31*(2), 231–241. https://doi.org/10.7120/09627286.31.2.007

Bettiol, N., & Dixon, P. M. (2011). An anatomical study to evaluate the risk of pulpar exposure during mechanical widening of equine cheek teeth diastemata and 'bit seating.' *Equine Veterinary Journal*, *43*(2), 163–169. https://doi.org/10.1111/j.2042-3306.2010.00138.x

Björnsdóttir, S., Frey, R., Kristjansson, T., & Lundström, T. (2014). Bit-related lesions in Icelandic competition horses. *Acta Veterinaria Scandinavica*, *56*(1), 40. https://doi.org/10.1186/s13028-014-0040-8

Borkent, D., & Dixon, P. M. (2017). Equine peripheral and infundibular dental caries: A review and proposals for their investigation. *Equine Veterinary Education*, *29*(11), 621–628. https://doi.org/10.1111/eve.12497

Borkent, D., Reardon, R. J. M., McLachlan, G., Smith, S., & Dixon, P. M. (2017). An epidemiological survey on the prevalence of equine peripheral dental caries in the United Kingdom and possible risk factors for its development. *Equine Veterinary Journal*, *49*(4), 480–485. https://doi.org/10.1111/evj.12610

Carmalt, J. L. (2003). Understanding the equine diastema. *Equine Veterinary Education*, *15*(1), 34–35. https://doi.org/10.1111/j.2042-3292.2003.tb00210.x

Carslake, H. (2009). Suture exostosis causing obstruction of the nasolacrimal duct in three horses. *New Zealand Veterinary Journal*, *57*(4), 229–234. https://doi.org/10.1080/00480169.2009.36907

Cohen, S., & Burns, R. (2002). *Pathways of the Pulp* (S. Cohen & R. Burns, Eds.). Mosby.

Cox, A., Dixon, P., & Smith, S. (2012). Histopathological lesions associated with equine periodontal disease. *The Veterinary Journal*, *194*(3), 386–391. https://doi.org/10.1016/j.tvjl.2012.04.026

Dacre, I. (2005). Equine dental pathology. In G. Baker & J. Easley (Eds.), *Equine Dentistry* (2nd ed., pp. 91–109). Elsevier.

Dixon, P. (2006). Cheek Teeth Diastemata and Impactions. *AAEP Focus on Dentistry*, 68–82.

Dixon, P. M. (2014). A review of swellings of the frontal region of the equine head. *Equine Veterinary Education*, *26*(7), 365–371. https://doi.org/10.1111/eve.12187

Dixon, P. M. (2020). Treatment of equine oro-nasal and oro-maxillary fistulae. *Equine Veterinary Education*, *32*(9), 471–478. https://doi.org/10.1111/eve.13127

Dixon PM. (2011). Dental anatomy. *Proceedings of the American Association of Equine Practitioners: Focus on Dentistry*, 8–24.

du TOIT, N., BURDEN, F. A., & DIXON, P. M. (2009). Clinical dental examinations of 357 donkeys in the UK. Part 1: Prevalence of dental disorders. *Equine Veterinary Journal*, *41*(4), 390–394. https://doi.org/10.2746/042516409X368912

du Toit, N., & Rucker, B. (2013). The gold standard of dental care: the geriatric horse. In *Veterinary Clinics of North America: Equine Practice* (Vol. 29, pp. 521–527).

Dunlop, C. (2007). Personal communication re: sedation older horses. In *Personal Communication*.

Earley, E., & Rawlinson, J. (2013). A new understanding of oral and dental disorders of the equine incisor and canine teeth. In *Veterinary Clinics of North America: Equine Practice* (Vol. 29, pp. 273–300).

Earley, E. T., & Reiswig, J. D. (2020). Equine Dental Floating (Crown Odontoplasty). *Veterinary Clinics of North America: Equine Practice*, *36*(3), 501–526. https://doi.org/10.1016/j.cveq.2020.08.011

Easley, J. (2006). Equine Dental Developmental Abnormalities. *Proceedings of the American Association of Equine Practitioners: Focus on Dentistry. Indianapolis.*

Easley, J., Dixon, P., & du Toit, N. (2022). *Equine Dentistry and Maxillofacial Surgery* (J. Easley, P. Dixon, & N. du Toit, Eds.; 1st ed.). Cambridge Scholars Publishing.

Englisch, L. M., Rott, P., Lüpke, M., Seifert, H., & Staszyk, C. (2018). Anatomy of equine incisors: Pulp horns and subocclusal dentine thickness. *Equine Veterinary Journal*, *50*(6), 854–860. https://doi.org/10.1111/evj.12841

Ferguson MWJ. (1991). Colyer's Variations and Diseases of the Teeth of Animals. *Journal of Anatomy*, *176*, 219–220.

Greet, T. (2005). The management of oral trauma. In G. Baker & J. Easley (Eds.), *Equine Dentistry* (2nd ed., pp. 79–86). Elsevier.

Hall, M. (2014, May 1). Wounds to the skull, sinuses, incisive injuries. *Equine Wound Healing Workshop*.

Henry, T. J., Puchalski, S. M., Arzi, B., Kass, P. H., & Verstraete, F. J. M. (2017). Radiographic evaluation in clinical practice of the types and stage of incisor tooth resorption and hypercementosis in horses. *Equine Veterinary Journal*, *49*(4), 486–492. https://doi.org/10.1111/evj.12650

Heun, F., Schwieder, A., Hansmann, F., Bienert-Zeit, A., & Hellige, M. (2022). Dentigerous cysts with exostosis of the temporal bone in horses – A new variant diagnosed by computed tomography. *Equine Veterinary Education*, *34*(5). https://doi.org/10.1111/eve.13577

Jackson, K., & Kelty, E. (2023). Recent advances in the treatment and prevention of equine peripheral caries. *Journal of the American Veterinary Medical Association*, 1–8. https://doi.org/10.2460/javma.23.01.0036

Jackson, K., Kelty, E., & Tennant, M. (2018). Equine peripheral dental caries: An epidemiological survey assessing prevalence and possible risk factors in Western Australian horses. *Equine Veterinary Journal*, *50*(1), 79–84. https://doi.org/10.1111/evj.12718

Jackson, K., Kelty, E., & Tennant, M. (2021). A new equine peripheral caries grading system: Are the caries likely active or inactive? *Equine Veterinary Journal*, *53*(4), 780–786. https://doi.org/10.1111/evj.13359

Jackson, K., McConnell, E., Kelty, E., & Tennant, M. (2021). Traumatic injury to the parotid salivary gland or duct and the subsequent development of ipsilateral severe peripheral dental caries in two horses. *Equine Veterinary Education*, *33*(2). https://doi.org/10.1111/eve.13197

Jackson, K., Weber, L. M., & Tennant, M. (2016). A Retrospective Study of the Effectiveness of Four Different Treatments of Periodontal Disease in Equine Cheek Teeth. *Journal of Veterinary Dentistry*, *33*(2), 83–89. https://doi.org/10.1177/0898756416661624

Klugh, D. (2010). *Principles of Equine Dentistry* (1st ed.). CRC Press. https://doi.org/10.1201/b15198

Knox PM, Crabill, M., & Honnas, C. (2005). Mandibular and maxillary fracture osteosynthesis. In G. Baker & J. Easley (Eds.), *Equine Dentistry* (2nd ed., pp. 313–324). Elsevier.

Laukkanen, T., Karma, L., Virtala, A. M., Mykkänen, A., Pehkonen, J., Rossi, H., Tuomola, K., & Raekallio, M. (2023). Behavioral Signs Associated With Equine Cheek Tooth Findings. *Journal of Equine Veterinary Science*, *121*. https://doi.org/10.1016/j.jevs.2022.104198

Latimer-Marsh, L., Hazel, S., Santos, L., McGreevy, P., & Frankiin, S. H. (2017, November). The effect of tongue-tie application on stress responses in resting horses. *13th International Conference of International Society for Equitation Science.*

Limone, L. (2020). Update on Equine Odontoclastic Tooth Resorption and Hypercementosis. In *Veterinary Clinics of North America: Equine Practice* (Vols. 36, 3, pp. 671–689).

Liyou, O. (2009). Equine oral examinations and their effects on the reported incidence of pathology. *Proceedings of the Australian College of Veterinary Scientists Science Week, Annual Conference.*

López, N. J., Smith, P. C., & Gutierrez, J. (2002). Periodontal Therapy May Reduce the Risk of Preterm Low Birth Weight in Women With Periodontal Disease: A randomized Controlled Trial. *Journal of Periodontology*, *73*(8), 911–924. https://doi.org/10.1902/jop.2002.73.8.911

Lorello, O., Foster, D., Levine DG, & et. al. (2016). Clinical treatment and prognosis of equine odontoclastic tooth resorption and hypercementosis. *Equine Veterinary Journal*, *48*, 188–194.

Marcantonio Coneglian, M., Duarte Borges, T., Weber, S. H., Godoi Bertagnon, H., & Michelotto, P. V. (2020). Use of the horse grimace scale to identify and quantify pain due to dental disorders in horses. *Applied Animal Behaviour Science*, *225*, 104970. https://doi.org/10.1016/J.APPLANIM.2020.104970

Merillat, L. (1906). *Veterinary surgery. Volume 1: Animal dentistry and diseases of the mouth* (Vol. 1). Alexander Eger. https://archive.org/details/veterinarysurger00meri/page/n13/mode/2up

Mohammadi, Z., & Abbott, P. (2009). The properties and applications of chlorhexidine in endodontics. *International Endodontic Journal*, *42*(4), 288–302.

Moore, N., Schroeder, W., & Staszyk, C. (2016). Equine odontoclastic tooth resorption and hypercementosis affecting all cheek teeth in two horses: clinical and histopathological findings. *Equine Veterinary Education*, *28*.

Nickel, R., Schummer, A., & Sack, W. (1979). *The Viscera of the Domestic Mammals* (2nd ed.). Verlag, Paul, Parey.

Offenbacher, S., Katz, V., Fertik, G., Collins, J., Boyd, D., Maynor, G., McKaig, R., & Beck, J. (1996). Periodontal Infection as a Possible Risk Factor for Preterm Low Birth Weight. *Journal of Periodontology*, *67*(10S), 1103–1113. https://doi.org/10.1902/jop.1996.67.10s.1103

Pascoe, J. (1991). Complications of dental surgery. *Proceedings of the Annual Convention of the American Association of Equine Practitioners*, 141–150.

Pearce, C. (2020). Recent developments in equine dentistry. *New Zealand Veterinary Journal*, *68*(3), 178–186. https://doi.org/10.1080/00480169.2020.1722971

Pollaris, E., & et. al. (2019). Bit-Induced Lesions in the Equine Mouth: Prevalence and Association with the Bit. *28th European Veterinary Dental Forum, Book of Proceedings*, 126–127.

Popesco, P. (1977). *Atlas of Topographical Anatomy of the Domestic Animals* (2nd ed., Vol. 1). WB Saunders.

Thompson EA. (2014). Diastemata in the equine. *VetScript*, *27*(8).

Roßgardt, J., Heilen, L. B., Büttner, K., Dern-Wieloch, J., Vogelsberg, J., & Staszyk, C. (2022). The Equine Dental Pulp: Histomorphometric Analysis of the Equine Dental Pulp in Incisors and Cheek Teeth. *Veterinary Sciences*, *9*(6), 261. https://doi.org/10.3390/vetsci9060261

Smedley RC, Earley ET, Galloway SS, Baratt RM, & Rawlinson JE. (2015). Equine Odontoclastic Tooth Resorption and Hypercementosis: Histopathologic Features. *Veterinary Pathology*, *52*(5), 903–909.

Staszyk, C., Bienert, A., Kreutzer, R., & et. al. (2008). Equine odontoclastic tooth resorption and hypercementosis. *Veterinary Journal*, *178*, 372–379.

Staszyk, C., Wulff, W., Jacob, H., & Gasse, H. (2006). The periodontal ligament of equine cheek teeth: the architecture of its collagen fiber apparatus. *Journal of Veterinary Dentistry*, *23*, 143–147.

Thompson EA. (2008). Considerations in the decision for tooth extraction in the horse. *Proceedings of the Annual Seminar of the Equine Branch of the New Zealand Veterinary Association Annual Conference*, 83.

Thompson EA. (2009a). Equine Dentistry - Part 2: Origins of dental pathology, preventative techniques and equipment, equine veterinary dental education. *VetScript*, *22*(5).

Thompson EA. (2009b). Equine Dentistry - Part 3: Comparison of cheek tooth extraction techniques. *VetScript*, *22*(6), 14–20.

Thompson EA. (2009c). Equine dentistry: Part 1: The veterinarian's role, clinical signs, how dental problems emerge. *VetScript*, *22*(4), 7–10.

Thompson EA. (2010). Apical infection and extraction in a Warmblood cross mare. *VetScript, 23*(10), 24–28.

Thompson EA. (2012). Pitching at the right level. *VetScript, 25*(3), 8–10.

Thompson EA. (2014). Diastemata in the equine. *VetScript, 27*(8).

Thompson EA. (2015). Dental considerations in equine head trauma. *VetScript, 28*(1), 20–24.

Thompson EA. (2021). Tips and tricks for effective dental radiology. *Equine Veterinary Practitioner, 46*(1), 19–23.

Thompson EA. (2022). EOTRH syndrome: what do we know about this enigmatic condition? *Equine Veterinary Practitioner, 47*(2), 27–32.

Timothy, A. O. O. (2014). Do dental abnormalities predispose horses to colic? *Journal of Veterinary Medicine and Animal Health, 6*(7), 192–197. https://doi.org/10.5897/JVMAH2014.0290

Tinsley, T., Fogle, C., Means, E., & Robertston, J. (2023). The prevalence and risk factors of dental disease found in 100 miniature horses. *Frontiers in Veterinary Science, 10*. https://doi.org/10.3389/fvets.2023.1239809

Tremaine H. (2020). Update on the management of equine periodontal disease. *BEVA - Annual Congress*. https://www.ivis.org/library/beva/beva-annual-congress-birmingham-2018/update-on-management-of-equine-periodontal-disease

Tuomola, K., Mäki-Kihniä, N., Valros, A., Mykkänen, A., & Kujala-Wirth, M. (2021). Bit-Related Lesions in Event Horses After a Cross-Country Test. *Frontiers in Veterinary Science, 8*. https://doi.org/10.3389/fvets.2021.651160

Tuomola, K., Mäki-Kihniä, N., Valros, A., Mykkänen, A., & Kujala-Wirth, M. (2021). Risk factors for bit-related lesions in Finnish trotting horses. *Equine Veterinary Journal, 53*(6), 1132–1140. https://doi.org/10.1111/evj.13401

Verwilghen, D., Easley, J., Zwick, T., Uhlhorn, M., Grulke, S., Simhofer, H., Townsend, N., Liyou, O., Bodeus, F., Zani, D., Vlaminck, L., Pearce, C., Staszyk, C., & Bienert-Zeit, A. (2022). Equine Suture Exostosis: A Review of Cases from a Multicenter Retrospective Study. *Veterinary Sciences, 9*(7), 365. https://doi.org/10.3390/vetsci9070365

Weller, D., Franklin, S., White, P., Shea, G., Fenner, K., Wilson, B., Wilkins, C., & McGreevy, P. (2021). The Reported Use of Tongue-Ties and Nosebands in Thoroughbred and Standardbred Horse Racing—A Pilot Study. *Animals, 11*(3), 622. https://doi.org/10.3390/ani11030622

Wilson, G. (2004). Module 10. In *Equine Dentistry, course notes*. Postgraduate Foundation in Veterinary Science, University of Sydney, Australia.

Wilson GJ. (2000). *Equine Dentistry: A manual for equine veterinarians and equine dentists* (1st ed.). The Post Graduate Foundation in Veterinary Science of the University of Sydney.

Wilson, G.J. & Walsh, L. (2005). Temperature changes in dental pulp associated with use of power grinding equipment on equine teeth. *Australian Veterinary Journal, 83*(1–2), 75–77. https://doi.org/10.1111/j.1751-0813.2005.tb12201.x

IMAGE, EDITORIAL, AND GRAPHICS CREDITS

The author is exceedingly grateful to the following veterinarians, technicians, patient owners, photographers, and friends who have provided images and editorial assistance for this book. I couldn't have done it without you. My humblest thanks to you all.

Cover:

On the cover: Sue Paterson's mare "Connie", always obliging, shows off her teeth.

Photo: Joan E. Gilchrist.

Cover Layout and Design in Canva by Blue Mist Holdings Ltd., [Elizabeth Thompson, BA(Hons) DVM MANZCVS (EqDent) GradDipTeach(SecSci)] DBA Blue Mist Equine Veterinary Centre and Equi-Still Portable Equine Stocks and Dental Instrumentation, Waihi, NZ

Interior:

Amy Ardern, BS DVM MANZCVS(Equine Dentistry), Taranaki, NZ

Glenn Beeman, BSc DVM MANZCVS(Equine Dentistry), Mountainview Equine Ltd., Ashburton, NZ

Ingrid Bill, DVM, Ontario, CA

Holly Blue, BVSc, Blue Blood Equine and Worm-Ed, Auckland, NZ

Stephanie Brooks, BVBio/BVSc DVM, Matamata, NZ

Cathie Heald Greenwell, Equine Veterinary Practice, LLC, Shelbyville, KY 40065, USA

Professor Padraic M Dixon, MVB PhD FRCVS DiplomaEVDC(Equine) RCVS Specialist in Equine Surgery(Soft Tissue) European Specialist in Equine Dentistry, 9 Durham Rd, Edinburgh, EH15 1NU, Scotland, UK

Jack Easley, DVM MS DABVP(Equine Practice) AVDC(Equine), Equine Veterinary Practice, LLC, Shelbyville, KY, USA

Nicole du Toit, BVSc MSc CertEP PhD DipEVDC(Equine) MRCVS European and American Specialist in Equine Dentistry, Equine Dental Clinic LTD, Glebe Farm, Wimborne St Giles, BH21 5NR, Dorset, UK

Ashleigh Fisher, BVSc MANZCVS(Equine Dentistry), NZ

Joan E. Gilchrist, Auckland, NZ

Maxwell Hall, BVSc(Hons) MANZCVS(Equine Surgery) DipECVS, AUS

James Hewitt, MEng(Cantab.), UK

Barbara Hunter, DVM DACVS-LA, Matamata, NZ

Kirsten Jackson, BSc BVMS(Hons) PhD MANZCVS(Equine Dentistry), Dental Vet Pty Ltd, Forrestdale, Western Australia, AUS

Olivia James, BVSC(Hons) MANZCS(Equine Dentistry) CMAVA DICEVO DAVDC(Eq), Australian Veterinary Equine Dentistry, AUS

Oliver Liyou, BVSc MANZCVS(Equine Dentistry), https://portasafestocks.com Vanessa Marsh, BSc MHSc(Occ Health) DipMgt Cert Teach, NZ

Vanessa Marsh, BSc MHSc(Occ Health) DipMgt Cert Teach, NZ

Greg Miller-Hard, Pahoia Point, NZ

Matthew Mole, Waihi, NZ

Georgina O'Neill, BVBio/BVSc. Darling Downs Vets, QLD, AUS

New Zealand Veterinary Association, permission to use images originally published in Pearce C. *Recent developments in equine dentistry*. New Zealand Veterinary Journal 68, 178-86, 2020. ©NZVA

Laurinda Oliver, BSc BVSc MS DACVS(LA), NZ

Christopher Pearce, BVSc CertEM(IntMed) CertES(Soft Tissue) DipEVDC(Equine) BAEDT MRCVS EBVS European Veterinary Specialist in Equine Dentistry RCVS Recognized Specialist in Equine Dentistry, Equine Dental Clinic LTD, Glebe Farm, Wimborne St Giles, BH21 5NR, Dorset, UK

Elke Pollaris, MSc PhD DipEVDC(Equine), Equine Clinic De Morette, Edingsesteenweg 237, 1730 Asse, Belgium

Katrina Price, Thames, NZ

Amy Ross, DipVN CertAM-CWA RVN, Auckland NZ

Ruth V. Sobek, DVM, Palos Verdes, CA, USA

Manfred Stoll, DVM FNCED Diplomate EVDC(Equine) Eq Praktischer Tierarzt Zusatzbezeichnung/WBE Zahnheilkund Pferd Bleidenstedter Weg 7, D-65329 Hohenstein, DE

Elizabeth Thompson, BA(Hons) DVM MANZCVS(EqDent) GradDipTeach(SecSci), Blue Mist Holdings Ltd , DBA Blue Mist Equine Veterinary Centre and Equi-Still Portable Equine Stocks & Dental Instrumentation, Waihi, NZ. https://equistillstocks.com

Elliot J. Thompson, BSc(CompSci) BSc(Neuroscience), NZ

Tracy Tinsley, DVM, Elite Equine Mobile Dentistry, Holly Springs, NC, USA

Marieke van den Enden, DVM MANZCVS(Equine Dentistry), The Dental Vet, Cust, NZ

Professor Dr Denis Verwilghen, DVM MSc PhD DES DiplECVS Dipl EVDCeq MRCVS, Goulburn Valley Equine Hospital, Congupna, VIC, AUS

Prof Jenny Weston, BPhil BVSc PGDipEdAdmin PhD, Academic Lead of Veterinary Science, Dean of Veterinary Education, Massey University School of Veterinary Science, Palmerston North, NZ

Software Credit:

Interior Graphics created in Canva. Interior Layout and Design created in Scrivener, Vellum, Affinity Publisher, and Affinity Designer by Blue Mist Holdings Ltd., [Elizabeth Thompson, BA(Hons) DVM MANZCVS(EqDent) GradDipTeach (SecSci)] DBA Blue Mist Publishing, Blue Mist Equine Veterinary Centre, and Equi-Still Portable Equine Stocks and Dental Instrumentation, Waihi, NZ

THANK YOU

I hope you enjoyed the book! If so, could you please...

1 - Leave a short review on your favorite online retailer,
Bookbub, Goodreads and your favorite social media.
I'd be grateful for your help in spreading the word to help more horses!

2 - Join the *Equine Vet Today VIP List* by using the QR code or going to:
https: //bit.ly/EqVetToday

Sign up for the Equine Vet Today VIP list!

3 - Join *Lizzi Tremayne's Fiction Author VIP List* by using the QR code or going to:
https: //bit.ly/44oYeOR

Sign up for the Lizzi Tremayne VIP list!

As an independent (Indie) author and publisher, I'd sure appreciate it!
Thanks again! See you at the online course!

With kindest regards,
Dr Elizabeth (Lizzi) Thompson

ALSO BY LIZZI

Elizabeth Thompson also writes fiction as Lizzi Tremayne!

***The Long Trails* Series**

A Long Trail Rolling (Book One)

The Hills of Gold Unchanging (Book Two)

A Sea of Green Unfolding (Book Three)

The Long Trails Box Set

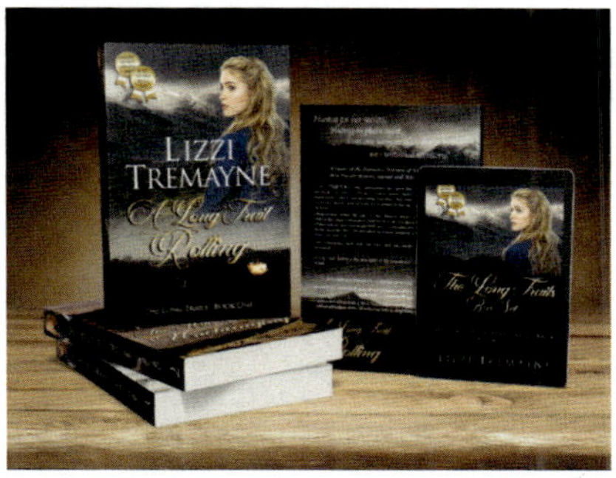

The *Once Upon a Vet School* Series

~Vet School 24/7~

Fifty Miles at a Breath

Lena Takes a Foal

~Practice Time~

Greener Pastures Calling

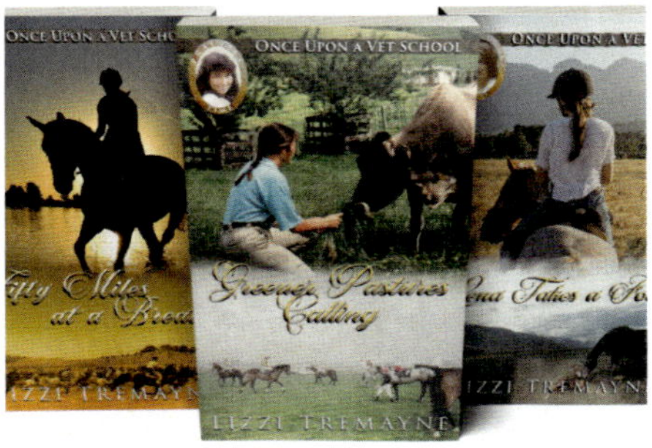

Multi-Series Samplers

Lizzi Tremayne First Chapter Sampler

There are many books and courses coming up!

You can sign up right here to be kept updated about upcoming Releases in the Equine Vet Today or Lizzi Tremayne's fiction stories!

Join the the ***Equine Vet Today VIP List*** with the QR Code or at: https: //bit.ly/EqVetToday

Join ***Lizzi Tremayne's Fiction Author VIP List*** with the QR Code or at: https: //bit.ly/44oYeOR

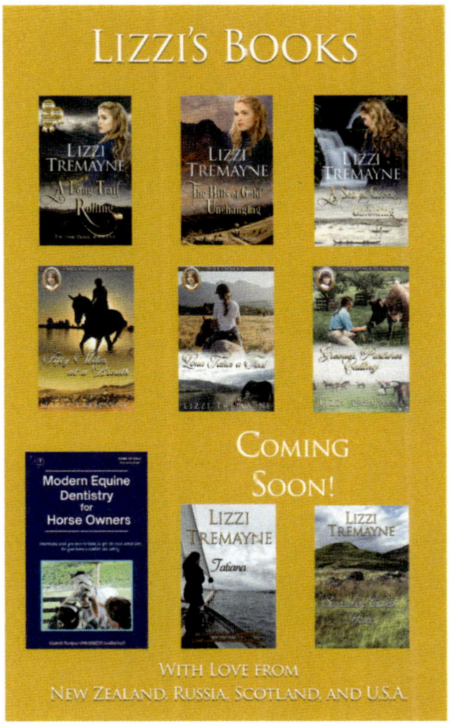

GLOSSARY

abrasion: Tooth wear produced by interaction between teeth and other materials such as feed or grit picked up while eating.

acute: A condition in its early, or immediate stages; depending upon the condition, this may be a period from minutes to months.

alveolus: The bony socket of the mandible or maxilla into which a tooth is anchored.

analgesia: A pain-free state without loss of consciousness. E.g. pain relief from use of anti-inflammatories.

anesthesia: A state achieved when there is a decreased sensations of touch, pain, temperature, and reflexes, with or without loss of consciousness.

anxiolytic: Anti-anxiety.

apical/ apex/ apices: The part of a tooth or tissue which is toward the apex or root, the opposite end from the occlusal surface.

apical infection: Infection or inflammation of the pulp. This is also called pulpitis, apical infection, tooth root infection, apical abscessation or peri-apical infection.

arcade: A tightly packed row of cheek teeth in the equid mouth. There are four arcades in each mouth: numbered (Modified Triadan System) 100, 200, 300, 400, for the horse's top right, top left, bottom left, and bottom right, respectively. As you look into the mouth, the 100 arcade is on *your* top left, and progresses to the 200 and on, clockwise.

ataxia: Wobbliness.

attrition: Wear (e.g. of a tooth) through tooth-to-tooth contact.

bars of the mouth: The bony portion of the mandible and maxilla between the canines and the premolars. Covered with thin, sensitive mucosa.

brachygnathism: Also known as parrot mouth, overbite, and overjet, brachygnathism is a congenital deformity in which the upper incisors are further rostral than the lower incisors. This must be checked with the head in a neutral position. Opposite of prognathism. "Brachy": short, "gnath": jaw, or mandible.

buccal: Adjacent to the cheek, i.e. the portion of a tooth closest to the cheek.

calculus (tartar): Accumulation of mineralized (calcified) plaque on the exposed portion of the teeth. Commonly seen on equine canines and in gingival areas affected by periodontal disease.

canines: The teeth between the incisors and the premolars. Evolved as fighting teeth, they are usually present in males and sometimes in mares.

caries (pl. caries): Two kinds of caries exist: **peripheral caries** and **infundibular caries**. They are like our cavities, which are also called caries. Caries affects first the soft cementum, then the dentin (harder than cementum but softer than enamel), and last, the enamel.

—**peripheral caries:** The degradation or erosion of the cementum covering the enamel of the outside of the tooth.

—**infundibular caries:** The degradation of the cementum lining the infundibulum of the teeth. Sugars in the diet and acidic feeds have been shown to be significant in caries formation.

caudal: Toward the tail of the horse. As opposed to rostral, or toward the "rostrum", or nose. Used on the parts of the horse outside the mouth. If referring to the inside of the mouth, "distal" is the correct term.

cementum/cement: A bone-like, relatively flexible, calcified tooth layer. Together with the dentin, they support the more brittle enamel from cracking under stresses of mastication (chewing). There are two types:

—***infundibular cementum:*** Lines and fills the infundibulum, and

—***peripheral cementum:*** Covers the periphery of all teeth and makes up a substantial part of the equine crown.

cheek teeth: The large, rectangular teeth in the distal part of the mouth. Six cheek teeth packed tightly together in each quadrant function as a single grinding unit.

chronic: A condition which has continued past the acute stage; depending upon the condition, this may be anywhere from weeks to months, and continuing indefinitely.

cingulum (pl. cingulae): Vertical enamel ridges on the buccal side of the maxillary cheek teeth. If these ridges are pronounced, with attrition their occlusal edges may turn into sharp enamel points which can create painful cheek ulceration.

continuous eruption: When a tooth continues to *grow* and erupt into the mouth throughout life, such as seen in rat and rabbit incisors. Differs from ***prolonged eruption***, as seen in equids.

contraindicated: Not advised, e.g. rasping teeth until pulp horns are exposed is *contraindicated.*

crown: The part of a tooth which contains enamel. It is in the far side of the tooth from the apex, or root tip, (which has no enamel). This may be:

—**reserve crown:** The unerupted portion of crown which is still inside the alveolus or socket.

—**clinical crown:** The erupted portion of crown which is visible in the mouth.

crown elongation: In general, elongation of a tooth, in a hypsodont, by continued eruption ("overgrowth"). Used here as excessive eruption of the tooth crown past the level of the adjacent teeth.

cup: Viewed on the occlusal surface of an incisor, it is the remnant of the infundibulum, and is filled with air or feed.

cupped: A stage of tooth wear where the crown is exposed past the infundibulum, but there is still exposed crown above the gingiva.

deciduous teeth: The baby teeth which will be exfoliated and (usually) replaced by the permanent teeth.

dental drift: In an equid, the drifting of the teeth adjacent to the site of an extraction towards each other, in effect attempting to close the gap. Unfortunately, this creates more malocclusion issues. Because of the absent tooth and dental drift, a horse requires examination and odontoplasty approximately every six months for its whole life to prevent severe malocclusions.

dental star: Viewed on the occlusal surface of an incisor, it is the remnant of the retreating pulp, and is filled with secondary dentine.

dentigerous cyst: A congenital malformation resulting in the development of cystic lesions within the temporal region (base of the ear), usually containing dental structures.

dentin/dentine: A mineralized, but relatively soft, ivory-like component of teeth which, along with the cementum, supports the more brittle enamel. Dentin gradually fills the pulp chamber with secondary dentine as the tooth ages.

dentinal tubule: Linear, parallel, microscopic tubules (like straws) in the dentin in which the odontoblast processes reside. They run in an apical to occlusal surface direction. See Bibliography for *Abusallamah, A. (2014)* for awesome electron microscopy images of dentinal tubules and odontoblast processes. Shows graphically why we shouldn't over-float or overheat teeth.

diastema (pl. diastemata): Two kinds of diastemata exist:

—physiologic diastema: The *physiologic* (normal) diastema is that *toothless* portion of the mandible or maxilla between the incisors (or canines) and the cheek teeth (or wolf teeth), also called the "bars of the mouth". The bit fits within this normal gap between teeth. This term is going out of use, allowing the word diastema to be reserved for a...

—pathologic diastema: A *pathologic* diastema is an abnormally wide gap between two teeth of the usually solid arcade of incisors or cheek teeth. It may or may not have food pocketing, filled with decaying feed material. Pockets, if present, may extend far toward the root or apex of the tooth. This is a serious disease of the ***periodontium,*** making a *pathologic diastema* part of periodontal disease. Diastemata may be classified as an open or a valve diastema.

dietary abrasive forces: Forces generated by rough foodstuffs grinding against the teeth in chewing. These forces result in increased abrasion of the occlusal surfaces of the teeth.

distal: Away from the midline, especially inside the mouth. The distal surface of a tooth is that surface furthest from the midline, which is the interdental space where the '01 and '01 meet. If looking at the outside of the head or horse, one uses "caudal".

edentate: Having no teeth.

enamel: The hardest calcified dental tissue in the body. It is extremely strong and wear resistant, but unfortunately it is brittle, so it needs support from the softer dentine to keep from fragmenting. It covers dentine in the crown of the teeth.

ensilaged feeds: Feeds such as hay treated to increase the forage value by inoculating them with microorganisms and fermenting them anaerobically (wrapping bales to keep the air away) which partially breaks down the feed and releases additional nutrients to the animals consuming the ensilaged feed. The low pH of the resultant feed *may* increase the likelihood of caries (peripheral and infundibular) and other dental disease, but this has not been fully proven.

EOTRH: *Equine odontoclastic tooth resorption and hypercementosis*, an extremely painful disease of horses around or over 15 years, where the internal portions of the teeth undergo variable levels of resorption (demineralization) and/or proliferation of the cementum (hypercementosis) around the surface of the teeth. Accompanied by severe periodontal disease, and often, tooth death. Radiographs are required for diagnosis and treatment at this point is extraction of affected teeth to relieve the pain. Extraction is curative, and horses usually do well once affected teeth are removed.

erosion: Dissolution of hard tissue (e.g. dissolution of cementum by acidic substances).

exfoliate: To shed or lose, as in a tooth.

expired: The wear stage past cupped, where the whole occlusal surface of the tooth is worn down to the level of the gingiva and the roots are still connected to each other by a thin crown.

expired with retained tooth root: The final stage of tooth wear where the tooth is worn to the gingiva, but the remains of the roots are no longer connected by the crown.

fistula (pl. fistulae): A tract, such as an open tract between a sinus and the mouth.

float (n.): An instrument used to file or rasp equid teeth.

float/floating (v.): Removal and shaping of a tooth crown to eliminate soft tissue trauma by reducing sharp enamel points and relieving malocclusions of the clinical crown. Compare to **odontoplasty**.

gingiva/l: The gums, or the epithelial tissue immediately surrounding the teeth and alveolar bone. It is a keratinized (and therefore toughened) oral membrane.

hard feed: Term for grain, in UK, NZ, and Australia, and possibly other places.

heterotopic or ectopic teeth: Inappropriate positioning of the erupting permanent teeth.

hooks: Overgrowths of teeth, usually on the end of a tooth row.

hypsodont: Long crowned teeth which erupt throughout the animal's life until the teeth expire.

iatrogenic: Caused by the operator, as in *iatrogenic pulpar exposure,* which is pulp exposure caused by removing too much tooth and exposing one or more tooth pulps.

idiopathic: Of unknown cause.

in occlusion: In contact with the tooth or teeth in the opposing arcade.

incisors: The teeth in the most rostral or mesial portion of the mouth. There are three in each quadrant, also called the central (most mesial), intermediate, and corner (most distal) incisors.

inflammation: The process which occurs in the body in response to injury, whereby the body releases chemicals into a specific area or generally into the body. This may be beneficial, such as when they are needed to fight infection, or detrimental, such as in cases of non-septic arthritis (in response to repeated injured, cascades of similar chemicals are released, which cause pain and break down tissues in the repeatedly injured area), or full-body, chronic inflammatory disease such as rheumatoid arthritis (where the immune system responds inappropriately and releases similar chemicals into the body, causing pain and tissue destruction).

infraorbital canal: A bony tube much like a hard, thick straw lined with soft tissue which begins at the base of the eye socket and opens onto the surface of the maxilla at the infraorbital foramen. A nerve and an artery run inside the canal.

infundibular caries: See caries, above.

interproximal space: The space between two adjacent teeth.

labial: Toward the lips.

lacerations: Cuts into a tissue, (e.g. into the gingival mucosa by sharp points).

lateral excursion to molar contact: The distance the centerline of the mandibular incisors needs to move to the side until they begin to separate, which is when the cheek teeth come into contact.

lingual: The portion of a tooth or tissue which is adjacent to the tongue.

mandible: The jawbone. It holds the mandibular teeth.

mark: Viewed on the occlusal surface of an incisor, it is the remnant of infundibulum, and is filled with cementum.

masticate/ mastication: Chewing and grinding feed by the horse's teeth to break it down into more easily digestible particles.

maxilla: The part of the skull which holds the maxillary, or upper teeth.

mentation: The horse's mental state: e.g. alert, bright, dull, anxious, or worried.

mesial: Toward the midline of the mouth, or the interproximal space between the '01 and '01, or the interdental space between the central incisors.

mesiodistal movement: The distal movement of the mandibular incisors with respect to the maxillary ones as the head is raised to a neutral position from a lowered position, or as head is continued to be raised. If there is little to no mesiodistal movement, there may likely be malocclusions preventing it. Sometimes known as rostro-caudal movement.

midline: In the oral cavity, the vertical line drawn along the interproximal space between the central ('01s) incisors.

molars: There should be three of these teeth in each cheek tooth arcade, or twelve molars total, consisting of only permanent teeth, with no corresponding deciduous precursors. They lie distal to the premolars and begin to erupt at around one year of age.

mucosa (oral): The epithelial tissue lining the inside of the mouth (the oral cavity) from the lip margins up to the area of the tonsils.

nasolacrimal duct: A soft tissue duct which carries tear fluid from the eye into the nasal cavity. The order of flow inside the nasolacrimal duct is from the eye through the: lacrimal puncta - bony lacrimal canal - lacrimal sulcus - nasolacrimal puncta - and out into your nose. The nasolacrimal duct carries the tears which make your nose run when you cry.

occlusal: The portion of a tooth which occludes or is in contact with the opposing tooth when chewing.

odontoplasty: The *informed* redefining, contouring, or rasping of the teeth. To achieve the "informed" portion of this definition requires a thorough oral examination be performed prior to rasping teeth, otherwise it is simply waving a rasp around in the darkness. The crown reduction which is performed *after* a thorough examination dictates which teeth should have their crowns shaped and reduced, and exactly how this should be done to relieve malocclusions of the clinical crown and reduce interference from other teeth. It is vital to only shape within the safe range of pulp- and odontoblast-free areas on the surfaces of the crown. Compare to **floating.**

oral: Pertaining to the oral cavity; in the mouth.

osteomyelitis: Infection of a bone or bones.

overgrowths: See ***crown elongation***.

palatal: The portion of a tooth or tissue adjacent to the palate.

palpate: To feel with the hand or fingers.

pathology: A disease or medical condition; the structural and functional deviations from the normal that constitute disease or characterize a particular disease.

periodontium: The tissues surrounding and supporting the tooth. These include the periodontal gingiva, periodontal ligament, alveolar bone, and subgingival cementum.

periapical abscessation: A pus-containing abscess around the apex (root end) of a tooth.

perineural anesthesia (nerve blocks): Temporary anesthesia created by injecting local anesthetics near a nerve which innervates (supplies sensation to) a surgical treatment, other treatment, or diagnostic area so the patient does not feel pain in the area supplied by that nerve. This minimizes sedation drugs required for the horse and makes the sedation and anesthetic period smoother for the patient.

periodontal: Around the tooth or pertaining to the soft tissues around the tooth.

periodontal ligament: The strong, collagenous fibers which anchor the cementum covering a tooth to the bony alveolus (socket). This holds a tooth in place.

peripheral caries: See ***caries,*** above.

permanent teeth: Teeth which should replace the deciduous teeth (incisors x01-x03, premolars—cheek teeth x06-x08) or be the first teeth to erupt into their place (molars—cheek teeth xx9-x11). They remain in place once they are erupted until they are completely worn or lost due to disease.

premolars: There should be three or four of these teeth in each arcade, or twelve to sixteen premolars total. The first premolar is called the ***wolf tooth***, (a ***vestigial*** tooth—an evolutionary remnant of a once-functional tooth), which may or may not have a premolar. It normally lies directly mesial to the second, larger, premolar. The second to fourth premolars each have a deciduous tooth and later, a permanent tooth. These are the first three of the cheek teeth.

prognathism: Also known as sow mouth, monkey mouth, or underbite. A congenital deformity in which the mandibular (lower) incisors are more rostral than the maxillary (upper) ones. Opposite of brachygnathism. "Pro": projecting, "gnath": jaw, or mandible.

prolonged eruption: Eruption whereby a tooth of a set length continues to erupt into the mouth through the life of the tooth until the tooth expires, or runs out, such as seen in equids. Differs from ***continuous eruption,*** as seen in rat and rabbit incisors.

pulp/ar exposure: Exposure of the pulp by damage to the overlying dentin, cementum, and enamel, or a combination of these. This may occur because of a tooth fracture or from over-attrition due to overly abrasive feeds (accidental pulp exposure) or due to over-grinding by a dental operator (iatrogenic pulp exposure) with hand or power floating instruments, excessive heat generation without water cooling, excessive pressure, chemical injury or by cutting teeth with a cut-off wheel or molar cutters. Pulp exposure may cause pulpitis and tooth death if the tooth is unable to fight the infection or damage to the tooth or teeth.

purulent: Containing or discharging pus, a clear to white to green exudate consisting of bacteria, white blood cells, and other body fluids; indicates infection.

putrefaction: Rotting of tissues, caused by bacterial and other microbial degradation of tissue.

quidding: Dropping lumps of chewed and spirally matted feed from the mouth.

rasping: Colloquial term for odontoplasty or "float".

rostral: Toward the rostrum, or nose. Used on the exterior of the horse (or outside of the mouth, anyway). If describing anatomy inside the mouth, mesial is the more correct term.

rostro-caudal movement: A term for mesiodistal movement. The caudal or distal movement of the mandibular incisors with respect to the maxillary ones as the head is raised to a neutral position from a lowered position, or as head is continued to be raised. If there is little to no rostro-caudal (mesiodistal) movement, there may likely be malocclusions preventing the movement.

sharp enamel points: Sharp points which develop primarily from enamel ridges left behind during mastication (chewing) due to the anisognathia between the upper and lower jaws of the horse. They tend to form on the buccal edges of the maxillary cheek teeth and the lingual edges of the mandibular teeth. Referred to as SEPs.

sinuses: Fine, bone lined structures inside the head lined with delicate soft tissue which clean and moisturize the air moving through them on its way from the nostrils toward the lungs. Several of the cheek teeth apices/roots reside inside them, causing problems for the sinuses when apical infections or abscesses are present.

stocks: A structure, usually made from robust wood or steel, designed to contain and support the horse (especially when sedated), making it easier and safer for everyone, including the horse. See example of Equi-Still Portable Equine Stocks at https://equistillstocks.com/equistill/.

subocclusal secondary dentine (SO2D): The secondary dentin/dentine which is laid down by the retreating pulp and lies between the live pulp and the occlusal surface of a tooth in a hypsodont tooth. The more occlusal portion of this SO2D stains brown in the presence of feed pigments and may be used as a "color coding" to help prevent pulp exposures during odontoplasty.

tartar (calculus): Accumulation of mineralized (calcified) plaque on the exposed portion of the teeth. Commonly seen on equine canines and in gingival areas affected by periodontal disease.

temporomandibular joint (TMJ): The jaw joint.

tooth bud: The immature precursor of a tooth in a dental follicle which will become a tooth when it matures. usually found in a young animal.

tooth eruption: A progressive protrusion of the tooth out of its alveolus (tooth socket).

tooth growth: Growth of the tooth from its apical, or root, end. *Incisors* grow slowly for approximately seventeen years. The *cheek teeth* only grow until two years after teeth are erupted into the mouth, then they ceases growth, and no longer lengthens. They only *appear* to lengthen over time, but that is due to *eruption*, and not actually growth, or lengthening of the tooth.**tissue:** Structure made up of cells or minerals May be *soft tissue* (e.g. muscles, organs, glands, layers of the gut from the mouth to the anus) or mineralized *hard tissue* (e.g. bone, teeth).

Triadan nomenclature: This book uses a Modified Triadan System for naming teeth. See Anatomy chapter for details.

ulceration: An oral ulcer, defect, or hole in the mucosa, (in this book, in the mouth) usually caused by a sharp enamel point cutting into and/or abrading away the gingiva. These are painful to the horse and may be exacerbated (made worse) by pressure over the side of the horse's cheek, as from a halter or bridle. Careful odontoplasty (floating), which minimizes the sharp points, allows them to heal, usually within a few days.

vestigial: A small, nonfunctional evolutionary remnant of a historically functional tooth.

vet: Abbreviation, here, for a veterinarian who is registered and licensed in their place of practice. Veterinarians have completed a full course in veterinary medicine at an accredited veterinary school and are licensed to practice in the country (and state, in the USA) in which they are practicing medicine and dentistry. They have a full working understanding of anatomy, physiology, anesthesiology, cardiology, critical care, endocrinology, microbiology, neurology, radiology and radiography, surgery, dental pathology, infection control, nutrition, health and safety, ethics, current legislation, etc., which enables them to properly care for the entirety of your horse. They are examined before being allowed to practice by government regulatory agencies and are subject to ongoing comprehensive regulation as to their continuing education and quality of practice, and they are usually insured. If you have a horse, you know that *things* happen. Your vet can best help him when those *things* happen. The teeth are live tissue and are not an isolated part of your horse. They have nerves plus a (very good!) blood supply, and they are attached to ligamentous tissue which anchors them to bone. All these tissues need the proper veterinary care, as does the rest of your horse. Sedation is not something to be taken lightly. In untrained hands, sedation drugs and the results of sedation in an animal that outweighs us by ten times, can be lethal—not only for your horse, but those around him, including you and yours.

wolf teeth: Small vestigial teeth usually found just mesial to the maxillary '06s and occasionally the mandibular '06s. They are usually tight against the '06s, but occasionally a space separates them. Wolf teeth do not function in mastication.